Nurses' Aids Series

PÆDIATRIC NURSING

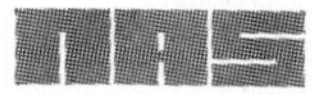

THE NURSES' AIDS SERIES

The Nurses' Aids Series, to which this book belongs, provides a series of up-to-date textbooks in the various fields of knowledge required by the modern nurse. The series covers the subjects included in the syllabus of the General parts of the Register, and, in addition, includes volumes on certain specialized subjects such as pre- and post-operative nursing, orthopædic nursing, ear, nose and throat nursing, and theatre technique.

Each volume is a complete textbook on its subject and is written, except in a few instances, by a Nurse Tutor at a leading hospital. The whole series aims at providing concisely, clearly and simply just that quantity of information which the nurse needs to possess, contained in compact and well-illustrated books at a price within the means of any nurse. If one can judge from the popularity of the series, this aim has been achieved, and the student nurse has at her disposal a set of convenient, up-to-date, comprehensive textbooks.

THE GENERAL EDITORS

NURSES' AIDS SERIES

PÆDIATRIC NURSING

M. A. DUNCOMBE

S.R.N.; R.S.C.N.; S.C.M.; Froebel Teacher's Certificate.

Matron, Queen Victoria Hospital, East Grinstead; President of the Association of British Pædiatric Nurses; Examiner to the General Nursing Council for England and Wales; formerly Lady Superintendent of Nurses, Evelina Children's Hospital; sometime Administrative Sister, the Hospital for Sick Children, Great Ormond Street, London.

with Foreword by

P. R. EVANS

M.D., M.Sc., F.R.C.P.

Children's Physician and Director of Department of Child Health, Guy's Hospital; Physician, the Hospital for Sick Children, Great Ormond Street, London.

SECOND EDITION

LONDON

BAILLIÈRE, TINDALL & CASSELL

1965

First published August, 1961
Reprinted July, 1962
Reprinted January, 1964
Second edition July, 1965
Reprinted February, 1967

7–8 HENRIETTA ST.
LONDON W.C.2

FOREWORD

In the early days of the treatment of tuberculous meningitis with streptomycin there was a five year old boy who was cured of meningitis but who seemed to be a human "write-off"—blind, deaf, spastic and mindless. It was the Ward Sister who persisted, got him to play with a string of little toys, and heard him say, fingering them in turn: "One—two—three—four . . ." So he *had* a mind, and he has since been educated.

That was a great perception; that was Sister Duncombe, now Matron, and still as distinguished in mind as in manner. She is not interested only in the very young, but has similar intuitive understanding of the puzzled student nurse—floating perhaps between the Scylla of barrier nursing and the Charybdis of leaving a crying infant to cry alone.

Such humanity and depth of feeling combined with breadth of knowledge might suggest impatience with practical details, but Miss Duncombe is meticulous in nursing and has the commonsense which is needed when a complex technical problem has to be pruned to essentials. She is just the person to write a thoroughly practical text-book (such as this one) on a sound basis of academic knowledge.

I am glad to welcome the new edition of *Pædiatric Nursing*. This book deserved to succeed and has done so. Now it has been carefully revised and is better than ever. It is a book for nurses, for nurses training in children's hospitals or departments, for nurses who mainly look after adults but have some children in their care, for sisters who teach nurses. There is another who is likely to want it too—the nurse who has left hospital for marriage and has a family of her own. All will find it reliable, interesting and delightfully illustrated.

May 1965 PHILIP EVANS

PREFACE

This volume of the Nurses' Aids Series was originally written for nurses training for the General Register, but its warm reception in children's hospitals and schools of nursing where nurses train for the special Sick Children's Register has shown that there was a great need for a textbook suitable for use by a much wider section of student nurses than was originally envisaged. The book has in fact established itself as a textbook for the basic three-year training, as well as for the integrated courses of four years' duration and the 13 or 15 month post-registration courses.

Practical details and practical advice have been included throughout the book for the reason that nurses used to handling adults may find certain aspects of sick children's nursing not only different but sometimes a little frightening. I hope therefore that the information the nurse will find in *Pædiatric Nursing* will make her care of sick children easier and more efficient and, by giving her a greater confidence, will enable her to develop a happy relationship with her young patients.

I have been most fortunate to have been able to enlist the help of Miss Beryl Gibbs in the preparation of this new edition. Miss Gibbs has had wide experience as a pædiatric ward sister and has for some years been Sister in charge of the Children's Ward at Orpington Hospital, where both medical and surgical conditions of children from birth to 15 years are treated. In addition Miss Gibbs has taken pædiatric outpatients' clinics and thus has had the opportunity of being in constant touch with all modern aspects of child care. Her experience coupled with her knowledge of the kind of teaching nurses need, and the difficulties they encounter when they start nursing sick children, have been of great assistance to me in revising the book and bringing it up to date.

The chapter on infant feeding has been re-written and simplified. Other sections have been re-arranged, such as the one on rheumatic and allied conditions, and a short chapter on communicable diseases has been added. I have included many new illustrations, and it has been possible this time to arrange for every illustration to appear beside its relevant text. As in the first edition, some diseases which nowadays are rarely seen in the British Isles have been included for the benefit of nurses working in the Commonwealth and other far-off English-speaking countries, in the hope of helping these nurses in the care of sick children under different conditions and with different facilities.

Many nurses in training are apprehensive of babies and sick children; others do not realize how much their treatment differs from that of adults. Proper understanding should dispel both fear and misconception. If this book helps nurses to enjoy their work in the children's ward and rouse their interest in this demanding but fascinating branch of nursing, I shall be amply rewarded for the time and work involved in its preparation.

Once again I owe a debt of gratitude to Dr. P. R. Evans for reading the new text, and this time also to Dr. Peter Swift for valuable advice given whenever approached by Miss Gibbs; to Miss Treadgold for her delightful drawings, to Mr. C. Engel, Mr. Boorer of *Nursing Times* and all who have assisted with the production or loan of the photographs for the illustrations. Several pædiatric tutors have made suggestions and helped in bringing the text up to date. Many others have through teaching, lectures and articles greatly influenced what I have written and helped me in many different ways. To all I am deeply grateful for assisting me to produce a textbook which should play its part in creating confident, competent and happy sick children's nurses.

May, 1965 M. A. DUNCOMBE

ACKNOWLEDGEMENTS FOR ILLUSTRATIONS

We gratefully acknowledge permission to reproduce illustrations as follows: to *Nursing Times* for Figs. 9, 12, 16, 17, 39, 40, 43, 49, 54, 55; to *Nursing Times* and *Guy's Hospital Gazette* for Figs. 36, 37; to William Heinemann Medical Books Ltd. for Fig. 48 (from *Child Health and Pædiatrics*); to *British Medical Journal* for Figs. 56, 57; to *Nursing Times* and Warwick Hospital Medical Illustration Department for Figs. 60, 61. Oxygenaire Ltd. kindly supplied the block for Fig. 10 and Armour Pharmaceutical Co. the photograph for Fig. 18.

CONTENTS

1*

1

THE HEALTHY CHILD

Introduction

The nursing of sick children is a far more complex and difficult task than many people would suspect. To deal successfully with them, some knowledge of children in health, their growth and their behaviour is necessary, for only then can deviations from the normal, such as are caused by sickness, stress and separation, be fully understood.

Many detailed studies of children have enabled pædiatricians and psychologists to work out average standards of mental and physical development at any given age. But no two children are alike, and norms and milestones must never be taken too literally. Each child is an individual with his own pace of development which is influenced by many factors such as his constitution, his surroundings, his family, his opportunities for experience, the physical and mental care he receives and the emotional security he is able to achieve.

The *average standards* are known as norms or milestones. They should be familiar to those who deal with children in health and sickness, but it is important to realize that variations of up to 10 or 15 per cent. below or above that standard may still be considered within normal limits. For that reason many pædiatricians now refer to developmental progress as a percentile of the average, rather than use rigid figures. Sometimes a line is drawn running diagonally across the weight chart, which is meant to indicate the "normal" gain of weight, but this is now frequently replaced by a shaded area covering from 30 to 45 per cent. below and above the average line. This allows for variations without causing alarm, and stresses the point that steady progress is of far greater importance than conformity with an arbitrary standard. For example, values which are not exceeded by 10 per cent. of all children are spoken of as 10 percentile. Values which are not exceeded by 90 per cent. of all children are spoken of as 90 percentile, and so on. Thus the range between the highest figure (90th percentile) and the lowest one (10th percentile) represents 80 per cent. of the measurements taken. If, for instance, a particular child has been measured (including weight, height, chest circumference, pelvic girth and head circumference) and the measurements are 25 per cent. below the accepted minimum, one would refer to this as 25th percentile. 25 per cent. of the children studied in order to obtain the average measurements would fall below that figure.

Antenatal Development

Development begins at the moment of conception and is most rapid before birth and during the first 18 months of life. The tiny, helpless creature we see at the time of birth is a perfect little being, capable of carrying on a life of his own, though only a few moments before he was completely dependent on his mother for all his vital processes and needs. He now has to breathe to obtain oxygen, to supply his own warmth and to obtain his own food by making the effort of sucking. His physical, mental and emotional growth, three completely interdependent factors, will be helped in greater or lesser measure by favourable surroundings, loving parents, a healthy and secure home and adequate educational and social services.

The Child at Birth

The average, new-born infant may be expected to weigh approximately 7½ pounds and to be 20 inches in length. The *head circumference* is approximately 13 inches, with a cranium which is disproportionately large compared with the face. The limbs seem short, in comparison with the body, and the head and abdomen large, in comparison with the thorax. *Subcutaneous fat* is sparse, the skin looks red and inelastic and the hair is as a rule merely a fine, down-like growth.

The *respirations* are rapid at 40 breaths per minute and are frequently irregular in rhythm and in depth. The *heat-regulating* centre is immature and variations in the body temperature may be sudden and considerable. The *pulse rate* is in the region of 120 to 140 beats per minute. The systolic blood pressure readings are between 60 and 80 and the diastolic between 50 and 60 millimetres of mercury. The *hæmoglobin* may be as high as 110 per cent. (16·3 grammes/100 millilitres).

The infant spends 20 to 22 hours asleep and rarely wakens except at feeding time. When awake, his *movements* are instinctive and reflex. The head turns towards the mother's breast in search of food. He can clasp his fist so tightly round an outstretched finger that he can be lifted up by it. If held in a "standing" position, he will make walking movements and he will kick and withdraw his leg if it is pricked or pinched. Breathing and sucking are also reflex actions. He has not yet gained control of his *eye movements* and squinting is a common and quite harmless feature. *Hearing* is present from birth and the infant will react to sudden or strong noises by reflex movements or by crying.

The First Year

During the first year development is astonishingly rapid and some progress can be noticed daily by those in close contact with the child. The *weight* increases by some 6 ounces a week in the first months of life, and the birth weight is usually doubled by the age of 5 months and trebled by the end of the first year.

The *head circumference* will have grown by 5 inches to 18 inches by the end of a year and it no longer seems disproportionately large in comparison with the body and face. The *respirations* are now regular and less rapid (approximately 24 respirations per minute when at rest). The *pulse rate* has dropped to 100 to 110 beats per minute and the *temperature* has become more stable.

The face and limbs are well covered with subcutaneous fat and there are dimples over the knuckles, elbows and knees. The *skin* is firm and elastic and no longer hangs in loose folds as in the newly born. The first set of *teeth* starts to come through at about 5 or 6 months and by the end of the first year the child is likely to have 8 or 10 teeth. The first down has been replaced by stronger *hair* and the soft *nails* are now fully developed and hard. The *eyes*, which in a majority of babies are blue at birth, are now a definite colour and the child is capable of focusing and of deliberate coordination.

While crying is not accompanied by tears in the first months, *lacrimation* has now become established. The infant masticates well by the age of one year and as a rule accepts solid food any time after he has reached the age of 4 to 5 months. During the latter half of the first year the child enjoys movement, and skills of many kinds are learned by constant experimenting. By 6 months many infants can *sit up* if supported, by 9 months they sit upright without difficulty and soon after that become expert in rolling from back to front and propelling themselves along by creeping, rolling or pushing themselves around on their seats. They pull themselves up with the help of the bars of the cot or a chair and begin to make ready for the *first steps*, which they are likely to achieve by the age of 12 to 16 months. When awake, the one-year-old "toddler" is incredibly active but he still requires between 12 and 16 hours of sleep a day. Some mothers manage to keep their children *dry and clean* in the day time by the age of one year, though relapses and regression occur during difficult times such as teething or periods of sickness or separation.

This rapid progress is not confined to physical growth. From the young infant who is wholly mother-centred, he has developed into a one-year-old filled with curiosity and anxious to make contacts with others, provided strangers allow him to make their acquaintance slowly and approach him quietly. As experience is lacking the one-year-old knows no fear and delights in a game with all sorts of animals and moving objects. He still needs cuddling and physical contact with a familiar person or object, and the majority of children at this age have a precious "cuddly", a teddy bear or a soft doll. Curiosity often makes him want to "look inside" and, unless he is given suitable toys which allow for taking apart and opening and closing, he is easily labelled destructive and rough.

The Second Year

Throughout the next year the young child remains greatly attached to his mother and seems lost and afraid if she is out of sight for long. He is both a possessive and a jealous little creature and it takes a mother's tact and love to achieve smooth acceptance if there is a new arrival in the family. Disturbances during that period are not merely due to jealousy but also to the fact that the child is still upset by changes in the daily routine and expects his food and daily activities to be as he has always been used to having them. "Tomorrow" is a term that has no meaning and promises involving time have to be linked to familiar happenings such as "after tea" or "when Daddy comes home".

Gradually he develops greater independence and as he loves to imitate others he makes the first attempts at dressing and feeding himself. These first attempts will be slow and messy, but this is an important stage in the child's development and those who deal with children have to learn to curb their impatience and accept delays or messy clothes. *Play* and other activities continue to be essential to his development, and media such as sand and water, climbing frames and bricks should be available for all children of this age. By the age of two the toddler is able to build a tower of 6 bricks and he can carry a cup of water for a short distance without spilling it. His gait is fairly steady by this time and he can run and turn corners without having an accident. A favourite play material is paper which he enjoys folding into small parcels, and he likes handling it as he turns the pages of a book.

His love for *stories* is confined to a small repertoire which he likes to hear over and over again and he gets very upset when a variant is introduced. Nursery rhymes are popular at this stage and the two-year-old is often able to repeat parts of them and even knows short ones by heart and delights in reciting them. Physically he has grown much taller, with bodily proportions nearer to those of the fully grown child. The first set of teeth is about complete (20 in all).

After this, progress appears less rapid and milestones are less well defined and less striking. An important period begins approximately at the age of 3 to 3½ years. For the first time the child shows signs of *independence* and emancipation. He is no longer wholly dependent on his mother and at this stage he develops and exhibits a will of his own. *Temper tantrums* in response to frustration are common and unless the child is wisely handled, this may prove an exasperating period for the family. Much trouble may be caused by restricting the child in his activities during the early years of development. Every child needs a suitable place where he can play unrestrictedly and be untidy and where disorder, sand brought in from the garden, or water splashed all over the floor while bathing the dolly, cause neither damage nor an indignant outcry from mother or nurse. Children's *clothes* should be serviceable rather than fussy and should be easily mended and washed when torn and soiled. Rompers and dungarees are most suitable for girls as well as for boys as they give adequate protection from cold and dirt, are hard wearing and easily laundered. Furthermore the bib and braces help to keep knickers, cardigans and socks in place. Shoes should allow ample room for the toes and should have a small heel. Sandals are suitable both for indoor and for outdoor wear unless there is some orthopædic contra-indication.

The *toys* should be strong and suitable for the child's age. The desire to experiment is a natural drive and toys which allow for taking apart and "looking in" will encourage this urge and permit a certain measure of destructiveness which is natural in children. Such toys include ordinary boxes and tins, building bricks, strong wooden engines and trucks, soft animals and glove puppets. Sand and water and equipment which allows the child to imitate adult activities such as "cooking", "washing day", "going shopping" and "playing at doctor" and dressing up, are particularly popular and can occupy children for many hours while teaching them a variety of skills. Whatever toys or play material are given to the child, care must be taken to select ones that are safe. The colours should be fast and of a vegetable type, corners should be rounded and there must not be any sharp edges or nails on which the child could harm himself. If the toy can be taken apart, no part should be small enough for the child to swallow or inhale it or to push it up his nostrils or into his ears.

All children need to learn independence step by step. *Accidents* are miraculously uncommon when children are left to their own devices and it is essential that adults should be capable of watching them instead of stepping in and forbidding adventure with endless warnings to be careful. Constant nagging or cries of "don't do this" or "do that" cause children to become indifferent to them and eventually produce disobedience. Some parents expect standards of achievement and behaviour far beyond the child's developmental stage, and discouragement and indifference are bound to follow such an attitude.

Emotional Development

Children need love, sympathy and sincerity. Criticism should be of a helpful rather than a squashing character and at no time should parents mock their children's friends or their achievements, or the child may be discouraged from making friends and bringing them home. The ability to make friends and easy relationships is essential in a happy life and it should be fostered from the earliest days. The secure child is the one who is outgoing and capable of making friends; he is able to occupy himself and shows no fear of any natural situation such as being in the dark or being left alone for short periods of time. He is sure of his parents' love, and though most children go through a phase in which they imagine that their parents do not love them and want to get rid of them, these phases are of short duration and rarely have any serious significance.

Some children are "too good", as if wanting to please their parents, of whose love they are not sufficiently certain. Alternatively, they may be clinging or always wanting to attract attention, for the same reason. Manifestations of such *insecurity* may take a variety of forms, such as naughtiness, food fads, fits of temper tantrums or jealousy, and may even contribute to starting attacks of asthma. Parents can be helped to understand the significance of such behaviour and many will be able to deal with them wisely and successfully simply by giving the child a little extra time and showing more than the usual interest in him and in his activities.

Punishment, if given, should be severe enough to hurt, but should always be adjusted to the gravity of the offence and to the individual child's tolerance for punishment. It should neither be delayed nor allowed to continue for a long period and should be logically related to the offence committed. Once given, it should be forgotten. Children in hospital need rarely be punished and hitting children is strictly forbidden. Any disciplinary action should be taken only with the full permission and advice of an experienced ward sister, who frequently can cope with the situation in some far more satisfactory way than punishing the child.

Occasionally parents are worried about their children's interest in their bodies. This interest is entirely natural and need not be discouraged. Questions about the differences in the bodies of boys and girls should be answered simply and without embarrassment. The same applies to questions about sex. To children these questions are not very different from any others they may ask and it is usually only the embarrassment and the "hush-hush" attitude of the adult which suggests that there is something special or secret about them. The child who asks the question should have an immediate and straightforward reply. He is unlikely to absorb more than he can understand, and a child who really wants to obtain information will gain it elsewhere if satisfaction cannot be obtained at home.

Masturbation and body rocking, which gives pleasurable sensations of a similar kind, cause parents much anxiety. Frequently neither is of serious significance. The best way to deal with them is to keep the child well occupied and to make sure that he has sufficient activity during the day to ensure sound sleep at night. Tight knickers or pants should be avoided. Occasionally, however, masturbation may grow into a real problem and, when it is coupled with other signs of disturbance, a pædiatrician or child psychiatrist should be consulted.

Food fads and refusal to eat are other difficulties which may make family life very trying. They often start when the child is very young and not infrequently begin, as it were, accidentally. On some odd occasion when he shows a lack of appetite the child may find out that an interesting amount of concern is caused. In no time the refusal of food becomes a weapon against his mother. By it he can attract attention, can witness her distress on his behalf, and may obtain the food he most enjoys. The answer to the problem is at the beginning. No child who is not otherwise showing signs of illness will ever come to harm if he is allowed to miss a certain dish or even a meal. He will soon get hungry, and if he is told that he has to wait for the next meal he will have no wish to repeat the performance. Apparent indifference on the part of the mother is not easy, but it is certainly the soundest way of dealing with the child on such occasions.

Many books have been written on the development of children, on their behaviour and their needs, but in this chapter some of the more common milestones and problems have been described and some suggestions made as to how best to deal with them. Only experience in handling children will give a nurse confidence and the more she learns, the more she will understand the great complexity of child behaviour and child care.

Summary of Some Average Milestones

At Birth

Weight 7½ pounds. Length 20 inches. Head circumference 13 inches. Head large in proportion to the body; anterior and posterior fontanelles open. Sutures can be felt, moulding may be present. Face small. Limbs short and thin. Little subcutaneous fat. Hair is a fine down inclined to fall out. Nails soft, inclined to peel off. Eyes lack pigment and appear blue. Reflex reaction to light. Hearing present. Sensitive to hot and cold. Skin red and inelastic, inclined to peel. Mental responses: responds to pain, hunger. Movements, mostly reflex. Reflex response when held out but no control over bladder or bowel sphincters. Bowels act 3 to 4 times daily, meconium at first, changing to soft, sour-smelling stools on about the third day. Passes 3 to 4 ounces of urine per day. Respiration rate 40 per minute, irregular. Pulse rate 120–140 beats per minute. Blood pressure: systolic 60–80, diastolic 50–60 millimetres of mercury. Hæmoglobin 110 per cent. (16·3 grammes/100 millilitres). Sleeps 20–22 hours a day.

At 3 Months

Weight 11¼ pounds. Head now normal shape. Posterior fontanelle closed. Begins to balance head and lift it off the mat-

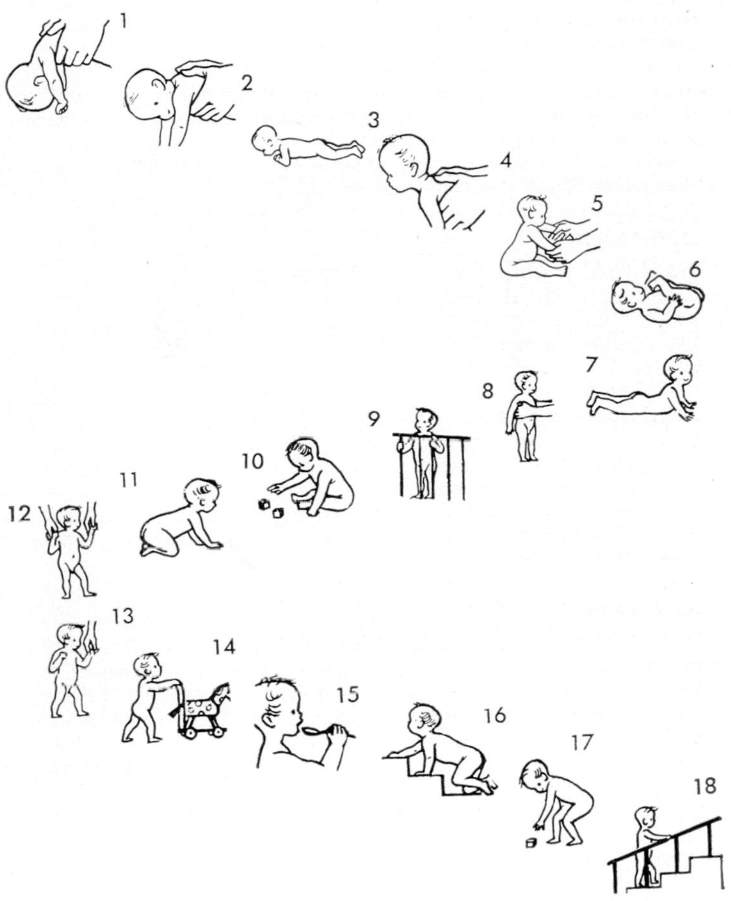

Fig. 1. GROWTH AND MOTOR DEVELOPMENT IN THE AVERAGE CHILD DURING THE FIRST 18 MONTHS.

The figures indicate age in months.

tress. Limbs now well covered, the face round, the skin elastic. Second growth of hair replaces the initial down. Eyes have their permanent colour. Has achieved some coordination of eye movement and is attracted by light. May notice new surroundings. Enjoys music, cooing and soft voices. Will accept or reject new tastes. Mental responses: takes notice, recognizes mother, responds to her smile, smiles with pleasure. Plays with own hands and feet, attempts to grasp rattles and soft toys. Sleeps 18–20 hours a day. Hæmoglobin about 85 per cent. Pulse 110–120. Urine 10–16 ounces daily.

At 6 Months

Weight 16½ pounds. Eyes can follow people around; turns head to increase visual field. Can determine direction of sound. Enjoys new tastes and takes solid food. Begins to masticate. Drinks from a cup. First teeth erupt (usually central lower incisors). Carries everything to his mouth. Can hold objects in both hands. Grasps things deliberately (no longer reflex). Sits up, if supported. Has pleasure in rocking his body. Spine is very straight. Mental responses: smiles back at familiar faces. Is capable of real laughter. Coos and babbles. Makes sounds involving use of lips and tongue. Prepares for speech. Loves repetitive games, e.g. hide and seek by pulling shawl over his head. Blood pressure: systolic 75 millimetres of mercury. Pulse rate 110–120 beats per minute. Sleeps 14–18 hours.

At 1 Year

Weight 23 pounds. Length 29 inches. Head circumference 18 inches. Looks around freely. Crying now accompanied by tears. Eats most foods, masticates well. Beginning to feed himself. Has between 8 and 10 teeth (central incisors 4, lateral incisors 4, premolars 2–4). Hair may need its first cut. Nails are now strong and hard. Sits alone. Can move from one place to another. Can pull himself to standing position. Mental development: can bring thumb and forefinger together and pick up tiny objects. Loves tearing up paper. Can say several monosyllables, two or three proper words. Imitates various sounds. Goes through a negative stage: may be difficult with diet. Blood pressure: systolic 80 millimetres of mercury. Pulse rate 100–110 per minute. Respirations 20–30 per minute. Bowels opened twice a day, stools formed and darker. Passes 15–20 ounces of urine per day. With careful routine is dry and clean in daytime. Shows interest in his body. Sleeps 12–16 hours a day.

At 18 Months

Weight 24–26 pounds. Length 30 inches. Anterior fontanelle closed. Has 12 teeth. Can walk fairly steadily, turns corners, begins to run. Mental development: goes on simple errands, loves fetching and carrying, is full of curiosity, investigates and opens everything within reach. Takes an interest in strangers, enjoys animals and other young children for short periods. May be dry at night time.

At 2 Years

Weight 28 pounds. Length 33 inches. Head circumference 19 inches. First set of teeth almost complete. Central incisors 4, lateral incisors 4, premolars 4, canines 4, second molars 4.

Motor and mental development: can feed himself. Dresses and undresses with help. Says sentences of three to four words, mostly expressing needs and desires. Plays happily on his own. Mothering and affection still very important. Lives entirely in the present. Can build tower of six bricks, folds paper, turns pages of books, enjoys playing with sand, water and clay. Blood pressure: systolic 80–90 millimetres of mercury. Pulse rate 90–100 beats per minute. Respirations 20–30 per minute. Hæmoglobin 75 per cent. (11 grammes/100 millilitres).

Although this summary has been compiled to help the student nurse working with children for a short time only, it is stressed once again that there is no true "norm" and that every child is an individual who develops and responds in his own way. Earlier or later development can be taken as a sign neither that the child is abnormally forward nor that there is necessarily any cause for anxiety.

The section on the normal development of the child and the summary on "milestones" is the result of extensive studies by many experts in the field of pædiatrics, psychology and education. There are many interesting books on these subjects that the student nurse will enjoy reading.

Safeguarding the Child's Health

Even before the birth of a child there are many services available which are designed to promote his health, to prevent disease and to treat defects at the earliest opportunity. Provision is made for the care and education of the physically handicapped and the deprived child. Although in hospital the medical social worker is the expert on these special services, it is of interest to know something of the facilities available and to have an idea of the wide field they cover.

Already before the child is born he is cared for by means of the *antenatal services* for his mother. Maximum health is assured by regular medical examination of the mother and by providing her with additional milk, vitamins and iron. Adequate national insurance enables an expectant mother to cease work 11 weeks before the expected date of delivery and to receive a maternity allowance for a total of 18 weeks. A well-developed midwifery service cares for the mother and baby up to the 14th day after delivery and immediately after this the Health Visitor takes over. It is her function to promote the health and happiness of the whole family, and it is often the newly born infant who brings her into contact with each individual member of the household. Welfare centres in every district hold regular clinics at which the infant's progress can be watched and guidance given. Whenever necessary the clinic doctors are readily available. Vitamins and dried milk are on sale, or are available free of charge under certain circumstances, and vaccinations and immunizations are carried out. Informal talks and demonstrations are given, a good deal of health education is undertaken, and the mother is taught how to live a healthy life and bring up children who too are healthy and contented. She may also be helped with household problems and with her weekly budget.

Mothers who have to go out to work can take their children to *nurseries* where they are cared for both physically and educationally up to the age of 5 years, when they are ready to enter school. Up to school age children are entitled to 1 pint of milk a day at a reduced rate and $\frac{1}{3}$ of a pint is issued free during term time in the schools. Both nurseries and schools provide meals at a low cost. The *school medical service* aims at supervising the child's health throughout school life. The object is to reveal defects which require attention and to refer the child to the family doctor and through him, when necessary, to the specialist for treatment. The *school dental service* supervises the child's teeth and can advise on conservative and corrective treatment. These services constitute a valuable follow-up of the child's health throughout school and right into early adult life.

Special Schools. Handicapped children are also catered for. Those whose sight or hearing is too poor for them to be educated by ordinary means go to schools for the physically handicapped, e.g. those for the deaf and blind run by the local education authorities. Education for these children can start at the age of 2 years. Special arrangements are made for sufferers from cerebral palsy, for hæmophiliacs and for children who are in any way crippled. Debilitated children and those suffering from chronic heart disease or chest infections and nervous illnesses, and children from households in which there is a tendency to tuberculosis, can be sent to open-air schools where extra rest hours, fresh air, physiotherapy and medical supervision are incorporated in the programme. The mentally retarded go to schools for the educationally subnormal. Children who suffer from epileptic fits which either are so severe or occur so frequently that they have to be excluded from ordinary schools, are also sent for special education. Any of these schools may be day or residential ones. Special school buses take these children from their homes to school in the morning and back again in the evenings. Finally child guidance clinics deal with those children who suffer from behaviour or other psychological disorders and schools for the maladjusted are also provided. Chronically sick children can be both nursed and educated in their homes and the deprived or illegitimate child is catered for by foster parents or adoption societies and voluntary agencies such as the Dr. Barnardo's Homes. For the ineducable, occupation centres and mental institutions are provided by the mental health authorities.

While this list is by no means complete, it gives some idea of the many-sided care which assures maximum mental and physical health for our children and helps to produce citizens capable of supporting themselves and living happy and useful lives.

Immunization and Vaccination

In this country all immunization is voluntary and the Government relies on the effect of propaganda and health teaching by posters and through personal contacts from family doctors, health centres and schools. Good knowledge of the advantages and possible dangers of immunization and vaccination and a good personal approach will set the minds of most mothers at rest and convince them of the value of these protective measures for their children.

It is now possible to offer to children a substantial measure of protection against diphtheria, whooping cough, smallpox, tetanus and poliomyelitis.

The necessary injections can be given either at the local Welfare Clinics or by the family doctor. It is usual to give three injections, in the third, fourth and fifth months of the baby's life to protect against diphtheria, tetanus and whooping cough, and to vaccinate against smallpox in the second year. Many clinics now use the oral vaccine for poliomyelitis. This involves giving three doses, each of 3 drops, at intervals of about 4 to 8 weeks. In other centres a combined vaccine for diphtheria, poliomyelitis, whooping cough and tetanus, called Quadrilin, is given. However, it is important to remember that a child who has been vaccinated in this way should still be given 0·5 millilitre of tetanus toxoid in case of an accident.

Smallpox vaccination done in infancy gives protection for some years and lays a foundation on which to build up immunity by further vaccination, usually during the first year at school. Rapid air travel has again made the danger of smallpox, imported from far eastern countries, a very real one. The risk of post-vaccinal encephalitis is extremely slight in the very young infant. Infants with *eczema* are never vaccinated, nor should eczematous babies be allowed to be in contact with others recently vaccinated, as there is a risk that a serious condition, known as generalized vaccinia, may develop.

Diphtheria is now so little known in this country that young mothers, who are ignorant of the terrors of this disease, frequently need some persuasion before they consent to immunization. This has resulted in outbreaks recently, with some tragic results.

It is important to know that there is increased susceptibility to poliomyelitis for several weeks after immunization.

B.C.G. vaccination against tuberculosis is not a routine procedure in this country, but B.C.G. (Bacillus Calmette-Guérin) is now available for selected children at any age and is frequently given just before the child leaves school. It produces a benign type of tuberculosis and a relative immunity in the inoculated child. (For details see page 339.)

2

INFANT FEEDING

Breast Feeding

The nurse in general training is not likely to have much dealing with the encouragement of lactation and the establishment of breast feeding, nor is she likely to have an opportunity for gaining much experience in this field. Emphasis here is therefore laid on methods and principles of artificial feeding, which is more likely to be seen in the sick children's wards. It must be stressed that breast feeding is the natural way of establishing close relationship and secure love between mother and baby. It is nature's way of giving the baby the food especially produced for him, at the right temperature, of the right composition and free from infection.

Modern life and civilization are probably to be blamed for the frequent failure of lactation, for various abnormalities connected with breast feeding, and for the psychological attitude which often causes the mother to reject any thought of feeding her baby in this way. Good teaching, interest and enthusiasm on the part of midwives and health visitors are all important both during pregnancy and in the immediate post-natal period. Both can do much to encourage and support a young mother, and so make breast feeding a success.

Harassed mothers of large families, those dependent on earning wages for one reason or another and those suffering from certain types of ill health should not be urged to breast feed, or the strain caused may be too much for them. Undue stress on the importance of breast feeding would merely cause feelings of guilt if breast feeding could not be carried out successfully. Those advising the newly delivered mother should therefore know her background well and be careful before they take the responsibility of giving advice. But once all serious contra-indications have been considered or excluded, no trouble should be spared in assisting a mother in making breast feeding a complete success. It has been shown beyond doubt that, provided lactation is adequate, breast-fed babies are happier, more resistant to infection and more secure in their emotional development than bottle-fed ones. Even a short period of breast feeding is worth while and if artificial feeding has to be started partly or entirely after some 2 months, the most vital period has probably been passed; breast feeding can then be stopped with a sense of achievement and artificial feeding started with confidence.

Management of Breast Feeding

Aids to breast feeding are often simple and always common sense. Of first importance is a peaceful, confident attitude on the part of the mother. She should, if possible, feel unhurried and relaxed. Her position needs to be completely comfortable, and a low or easy chair and suitable footstool can be of great assistance in achieving this. The mother should hold her baby comfortably in her arm, but support from a pillow may be necessary to avoid fatigue. The baby might be allowed to play with breast and nipple before starting to suck—an excellent stimulus to the flow of milk. A little milk squeezed from the nipple may cause a baby who is slow to realize that he is expected to suck to take the nipple into his mouth and start to feed. He should always be allowed to take the whole nipple and areola into his mouth or sucking may give the mother pain and cause sore nipples. The baby will also obtain less milk if he takes hold of the tip of the nipple only.

Mothers with poor lactation can be helped by stimulating the flow of milk by hot and cold bathings immediately before starting to feed, by breast massage, by adequate support from a good brassière and by drinking extra amounts of fluid; milk with such additions as Lactagol is particularly suitable. Adequate washing and drying of the nipples will prevent them from cracking—a very painful condition liable to cause a mother to dread the next feed and so in turn interfere with successful breast feeding. The mother's general nutrition and state of health may need some attention as conditions such as anæmia or inadequate intake of proteins may cause fatigue and make breast feeding a burden instead of one of the greatest experiences in a mother's life. The close contact between mother and baby during breast feeding is an important factor in the establishment of a happy, secure relationship and contributes greatly to the healthy psychological development of the baby.

Artificial Feeding

Although it is a fact that each baby is an individual with an individual appetite, and fine children are reared all over the world on a great variety of diets, a few basic principles may be useful as a guide to feeding infants. What follows must not be considered to be comprehensive, and the reader is advised to refer to books dealing solely with the subject of infant feeding for more detailed knowledge of the subject.

Artificial feeding should preferably not be started before the age of 2½ or 3 months, unless the mother's milk has failed or there is some contra-indication to breast feeding. By that time some babies may even be ready to start mixed feeding, beginning first with the addition of a little bone and vegetable broth, cereals such as groats, Farex or Twin Pack, purée tomato or apple and special rusks. It should be remembered, that no two babies are alike in their requirements and that some babies are hungrier than others; amounts must therefore be varied. The nurse must also know that occasionally a baby cannot tolerate the usual fat, carbohydrate or protein content of milk as well as others, and that feeds may have to be modified to suit him. Babies get used to certain bottles and teats and they also get used to the person who usually feeds them and to a certain temperature of the feed; any deviation from this routine may cause refusal.

Gaining Weight

A baby loses weight in the first few days after birth, owing to the passage of the first stool (meconium), the drying off of the umbilical cord, and the fact that lactation does not become established until about the third day, but by the end of the first fortnight feeding should have become established and the child should have regained his birth weight. From then until he is 4 to 5 months old he should gain an average of 6 ounces per week and afterwards about 4 ounces a week for the next few months.

For estimating the average requirements for a baby, it is necessary to know the *expected weight*; that is the weight he should be, for an underweight baby fed to his *actual weight* will never achieve his *expected weight*. To estimate the expected weight, it is necessary to know the baby's birth weight and age. The *expected weight* is then calculated by finding what he should have gained and adding it to the birth weight

—always remembering that he does not begin to gain weight for 2 weeks. His gain therefore should be: 6×(weeks of age−2) ounces. An example may make this clearer:

Baby's age	$3\frac{1}{2}$ months (14 weeks)
Birth weight	7 lb. 8 oz.
6 oz. gain per week for 14−2 weeks =6 oz.×12=72 oz.=	4 lb. 8 oz.
Expected weight is therefore	12 lb. 0 oz.

Estimating Average Feed

The average feed of any baby is worked out as follows: $2\frac{1}{2}$ ounces or 50 calories per pound of body weight (or expected weight if he is underweight) per 24 hours. Babies under $5\frac{1}{2}$ pounds birth weight need $3\frac{1}{2}$ ounces or 70 calories per pound in 24 hours until they achieve average weight for their age.

Babies over 10 pounds birth weight need only 2 ounces or 40 calories per pound body weight per 24 hours. If it is found that the baby is not happy and satisfied on this, but wakes hungry before his feed time, it can be assumed that he has a larger appetite and can be offered more.

From the above it will be seen that each ounce of fluid offered to a baby needs to contain 20 calories. In the case of artificially fed babies this can be offered either as:

1. Reconstituted dried milk.
2. Fresh boiled cow's milk, suitably diluted.
3. Evaporated milk, suitably diluted.
4. Other milk substitutes with equivalent proportions of protein, fat and carbohydrate, e.g. Soylac or Vitasoy, for babies who are allergic to milk.

Feeds are made up, with the addition of sugar where necessary, to contain 20 calories per ounce of fluid. Full details of these with comparative proportions can be found in books on infant feeding.

Some Points about Artificial Feeds

In this country there are many types of artificial feeds available, and all except a few derive from cow's milk

The percentage composition of human milk and cow's milk compare as follows:

	Human milk	Cow's milk
Protein	1·5 — Casein 0·5, Lactalbumin 1·0	3·3 — Casein 2·7, Lactalbumin 0·4, Lactoglobulin 0·2
Fat	3·8	3·8
Carbohydrate	7·0 (Lactose)	4·8

When comparing human milk and cow's milk it is as important to consider the qualitative differences in the composition as it is to consider the quantitative ones.

The chief difference lies in the fact that cow's milk contains six times as much casein as human milk. Cow's milk may therefore cause large indigestible curds to form in the infant's stomach. Although this could be at least partially remedied by diluting the milk, it must not be forgotten that other important proteins present (e.g. lactalbumin) are diluted at the same time, thus depriving the infant of a food essential for growth. The same applies to the carbohydrates. Although the percentage of fat is the same in human milk and in cow's milk, the constituents differ and the larger proportion of less easily digested fats in cow's milk must always be considered. This may be of particular importance after an attack of infantile gastro-enteritis, and in very young infants whose powers of fat absorption are still incompletely developed.

In order to make cow's milk suitable for very young babies, the milk should be modified to achieve the following changes:

A reduction in the excessive amount of casein.

A breaking up of the cascin so as to render it more easily digestible.

A reduction in the amount of fat.

An increase in the amount of carbohydrate to the amount contained in human milk.

Special consideration must of course be given to the changes brought about by diluting the milk, e.g. extra amounts of sugar must be added in order to keep the carbohydrate value of the milk as approximately 7 per cent.

The usual methods of modifying are:

Heating to boiling point to make the casein curd more digestible and finer.

Dilution by the addition of water.

Drying the milk to produce a milk powder.

Skimming the milk (up to 80 per cent. of fat can be skimmed off after milk has been allowed to stand some time).

Addition of sugar to increase the carbohydrate content.

Dried Milk

There are certain advantages in using dried rather than fresh cow's milk or condensed milks. These advantages include the easy preparation of feeds, the fact that the drying process has already modified the milk, that liquid milk easily turns sour unless a refrigerator is available, and that in poor or overcrowded homes contamination of liquid milk is almost inevitable. Furthermore, dried milk is easy to obtain and easy to store, simple to handle and make up and constant in composition. There are various types of dried milk, some of which are mentioned here.

1. *Humanized* milk, that is cows' milk altered to make it like human milk, e.g. Trufood; this contains less protein and more sugar than untreated cows' milk, and the protein and fat are modified to make it more digestible.

2. *S.M.A.* This is a skimmed milk with non-milk fat and lactose as basic ingredients.

Both these contain 20 calories to the ounce if they are reconstituted with one level measure to 1 ounce of boiled water; they need no further addition of sugar.

3. *Half cream* milk for babies up to 6 weeks of age who are contented and are gaining weight. When they are no longer satisfied thus, they should be changed gradually over to:

4. *Full cream* milk. If sugar is added to half cream and full cream milks in the proportion of:

Milk powder	3 measures	each reconstituted ounce yields approximately 20 calories
Sugar	1 slightly heaped teaspoonful	
Boiled water	4 ounces	

Fresh Cows' Milk

All cows' milk for babies should be boiled and rapidly cooled. During the first few months the baby should be offered diluted milk in gradually increasing strengths until he is able to digest full strength milk—at approximately 5 to 6 months. In all instances in which liquid cow's milk is given to children under school age it should be scalded or boiled whether it has been pasteurized or not. Brought to the boil in a double saucepan and cooled, the taste alters very little and few children seem to dislike it.

Evaporated Milk

This is either full cream or half cream, and is normally diluted one part milk to two parts boiled water, although it will need to be more diluted for very young babies.

Sugar can be added, one slightly heaped teaspoonful to each 4 ounces of feed for either cows' or evaporated milk mixture, although this proportion should be decreased if the baby has loose stools, and may be increased if he is constipated. Demerara sugar can be used for its aperient value instead of granulated sugar, but it is unnecessary to go to the expense of using glucose, dextrin-maltose, etc., for a baby with normal digestion—although these have their place in the diet of ill babies.

The Basic Principles of Infant Feeding

From the above facts any baby's feed can be calculated, but an example may again make the facts clearer. If the baby has an actual or expected weight of 12 pounds, he needs $2\frac{1}{2} \times 12 =$ 30 ounces of feeds in 24 hours. If he is fed 4 hourly (giving 5 feeds but omitting the middle of the night feed) he will need $\frac{30}{5} = 6$ ounce feeds. These can be made up as either:

	Humanized milk or S.M.A.	6 measures
	Boiled water	6 ounces
or	Any other dried milk	4½ measures
	Sugar	1½ teaspoons
	Boiled water	6 ounces
or	Cow's milk	4 ounces
	Sugar	1½ teaspoons
	Boiled water	2 ounces
or	Evaporated milk	2 ounces
	Sugar	1½ teaspoons
	Boiled water	4 ounces

A level measure, found in tins of dried milk = 1 drachm apothecaries' weight.* Alternatively one fairly heaped teaspoonful of milk powder or a slightly heaped teaspoonful of sugar is equal to 1 drachm apoth. It is usual when dealing with sick infants to *weigh* feeds for greater accuracy. Usually in

* Take care not to confuse the apothecaries' system (8 drachms to 1 ounce, 12 ounces to 1 pound), with the avoirdupois system (16 drams to 1 ounce, 16 ounces to 1 lb). When reconstituting feeds in quantity from dried milk by weighing, apothecaries' ounces must be used.

hospital feeds are made up for 24 hours at a time, but these can be readily calculated from the figures already given.

In hospital nurses are concerned with sick infants whose digestive system is delicate on account of their illness. In addition infants admitted to hospital are exposed to special hazards such as cross infection and lowered resistance to illness and they probably suffer from separation from their mothers and change in their accustomed routine. The method of choice in feeding these infants is consequently a cautious one, though it will still be based on the same principles. Unless there is good reason the infant's feed should not be changed when he is admitted to hospital, but the mother should be advised on discharge, or the diet adjusted when the baby has recovered, should this prove necessary.

Thickened Feeds

Feeds may be thickened or fortified for a number of reasons:

1. To increase the calorie value without increasing the bulk of the feed.
2. To control regurgitations and vomiting.
3. For the treatment of feeding difficulties.

Up to the age of 3 to 4 months, it is usual to add predigested starches for the purpose of thickening. Suitable foods are Bengers, Savory and Moore and Sister Laura, and only later Groats and Farex.

When giving advice to mothers it is wise to tell them that although reconstituted milk powder, Groats and Farex need no cooking, Bengers, Savory and Moore and Sister Laura do need cooking; they should be told to read the exact instructions which may be found on all packings, as the method of preparation varies with different brands of foods.

Other Basic Dietary Needs of Infants

Cows' milk contains virtually no iron. Iron is stored in the liver of the fœtus *in utero* from the 34 to 40th week of pregnancy (one reason why new-born babies have a palpable liver) and is normally sufficient to tide the baby over (with a lowered hæmoglobin) until he takes iron-containing food by mouth. However, in a premature baby, some or all the weeks when iron should have been stored *in utero* are missed, and therefore all premature babies need added iron before the age of 6 months, depending on the degree of prematurity and the hæmoglobin level. This can be administered orally and is best given in the first ounce of feed in a separate bottle, to ensure the full amount of iron is taken, even if some of the feed is left. Many dried milks and some evaporated milks have additional vitamins and iron, and care should be taken not to give added vitamins in excess of the essential daily dose, or a serious state of hypervitaminosis will occur (see page 243).

Basic Daily Dose of Vitamins Required for Normal Baby

Vitamin	A	1,500 I.U.
	C	30–50 mg.
	D	400–800 I.U. until one year, then 400 I.U.

If this is not given in the milk feed vitamins A and D can be given in the form of cod-liver oil, halibut-liver oil, Adexolin, Radiostoleum, etc., and vitamin C as concentrated orange juice (government issue), fresh orange juice, blackcurrant juice, rose hip syrup, etc., or as ascorbic acid tablets.

Vitamins A, C and D should be added in some form by the age of 6 weeks at the latest. If cod-liver oil is given whilst the child is in the bath, this avoids staining the clothes, and the spoon (e.g. a coloured plastic one) should be kept for this purpose. The vitamin A and D preparations in the form of oily drops should be put either directly on the tongue, or on to the outside of the teat before a feed, since, if added to the feed, the oil will coat the bottle and the infant will fail to get the vitamins intended for him.

The Milk Room or Feed Kitchen

In hospitals special rooms are set aside for preparing bottle feeds. Ideally there should be a room for cleaning and sterilizing bottles, which are then passed through a hatch to the room where the feeds are made. However, it is often necessary to incorporate these two rooms, and, if so, the bottles should be cleaned and sterilized and the room thoroughly cleaned and left for some hours before the daily quota of feeds is made up. Efficient ventilation will ensure maximum cleanliness and prevent the entry of flies. Anyone making up feeds should wear an efficient mask, and wash her hands before putting on the gown, and no one else should be allowed in whilst feeds are being prepared.

Sterilization of equipment can be carried out by boiling, autoclaving or immersion in a sterilizing solution, e.g. Milton, 1 in 80, for $1\frac{1}{2}$ hours. A stand should be supplied in which milk tins are placed at an angle. This allows for the scooping out of

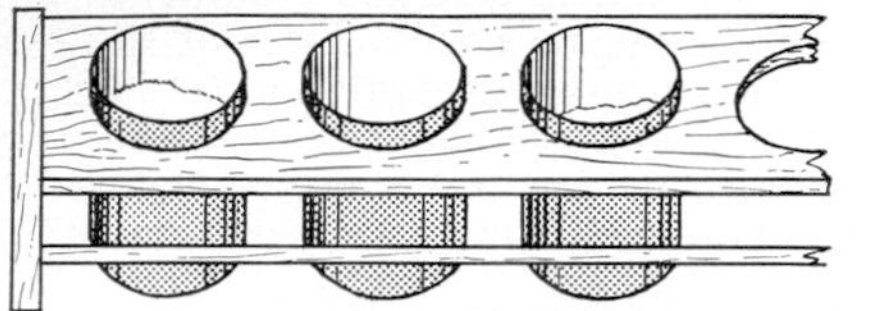
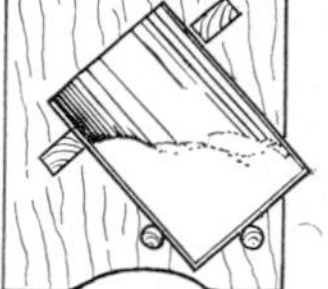

Fig. 2. STAND FOR MILK TINS.

the milk powder without touching the outside of the tin (Fig. 2) once the nurse has finally washed her hands. A rack fixed at eye level can be used to prop up the open feed order book, making it unnecessary for the nurse to touch it whilst making up feeds. The area for making up feeds should be marble, formica or other material easily washed down with soap and water, and covered with a sterile towel before commencing feeds. The utensils required (which should always be kept sterile for an emergency admission) include spoon, whisk, fork or spatula, graded glass measure and jugs, a funnel and small strainer (plastic if sterilized by Milton) and a pair of scales with weights, which are sterilized prior to use.

Preparation of Feeds

After setting out utensils and bottles, putting feed book in position, and removing lids from the tins in the stand, the nurse should wash her hands before starting to make the feeds.

After reading the feed formula for the 24-hour period, the milk powder, sugar, etc., are weighed and put into a jug. Sterile hot water (unless preparations containing lactic acid are being used, when hot water would curdle the feed) is measured in a glass measure held at eye level for accuracy and a little of it is poured on to the powder and sugar and mixed to a smooth paste. The remainder of the water is then added whilst stirring vigorously. The amount of mixture for each bottle is then measured in the glass measure and poured into bottles with the help of a funnel. A strainer may be balanced on the funnel as any small lump allowed into the bottle might block the teat when feeding the baby. A valve is then put on the bottle, the feed adequately labelled, and put into a refrigerator. In some hospitals feeds are made up and then terminally sterilized by autoclaving before being put into the refrigerator. At feeding time the feed bottle is put into a jug of hot water, covered, and taken to the bedside on a tray which also has a container with the individual baby's teats, sterile and ready for use. After feeding, the teat should be removed and the outside washed under running water, the inside of the teat and bottle washed and the teat replaced in the container for resterilizing. The bottle should be filled with cold water and the valve placed on it. The tray should be returned to wherever it is kept between feeds and the bottle placed ready for cleaning and resterilizing. If there is any possibility of the baby having an infection, the tray, jug and teats should stay in the cubicle and the bottle should be disinfected before being put in the feed kitchen. Teats can be cleaned by rubbing with common salt inside and out and can be sterilized by boiling or placing in a container of Milton, 1 in 80, large enough to submerge the teat completely. This need not be rinsed before use. Student nurses should never tamper with the holes in teats, as only an experienced person knows the optimum size of hole and rate of flow for each baby. More than one teat may be kept on each feed tray, as it is sometimes wise to change from a medium to a fast teat when the baby tires towards the end of the feed.

Bottles

Two types of bottles, either made of heat-resistant glass or plastic, are commonly used—the upright (or Soxhlet), and boat-shaped. The upright type is easy to handle and store, but

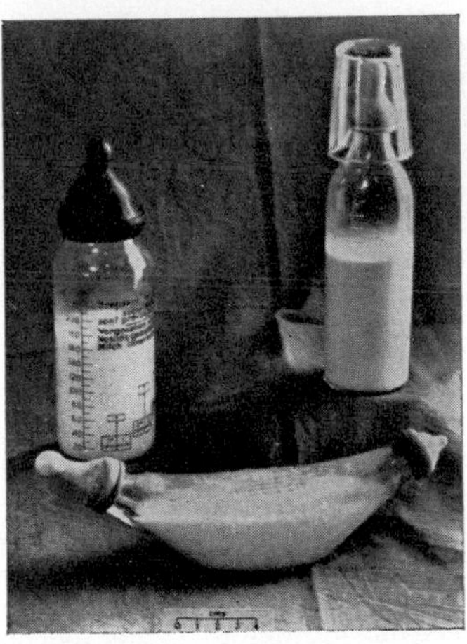

Fig. 3. VARIOUS TYPES OF FEEDING BOTTLES.

Note protective glass cover over teat.

it is not always easy to clean, and inexperienced nurses or poorly feeding babies may have difficulty in keeping an adequate air entry, so avoiding a vacuum. The boat-shaped bottle takes up more storage space but can be flushed through easily in the cleaning process. Since it is open at both ends, air can enter from the distal end, which may be left open or covered by a new or perforated valve. Feeble babies, who suck badly, may feed better from this type of bottle, but the hole in the teat may have to be smaller than with an upright bottle as the milk flows more freely. Bottles, after cleaning with a bottle brush (electrically rotated ones are ideal), washing soda or soap flakes and hot water, are sterilized by boiling, autoclaving or a sterilizing solution. If boiled, or immersed in Milton, or in another solution, it is absolutely essential that there should be no air bubbles in the bottle and that it should be completely full, as any part of the bottle that is not in contact with the fluid remains unsterile. When sterilized, a valve is placed on the bottle until it is needed.

Feeding the Infant

Whenever possible the baby should be taken out of the cot for feeding, and held, comfortably wrapped, in the nurse's arms. He should have been changed recently and the napkin should be taken away and the hands washed before the feed is brought to the bedside. Feeding time should also be used as an opportunity for cuddling and physical contact, so necessary for any baby, particularly when deprived of his mother. The bottle should be held at a sufficiently steep angle to keep the teat constantly filled with milk and so prevent the baby from sucking in air. He should be allowed to sit up and bring up wind at least once during a feed, but many babies need to bring up wind immediately before starting and several times during the feed. The feed should be kept at an even temperature by re-warming it when necessary, as babies are very sensitive to temperature changes, and if part of a feed has become cold, it is often completely refused. If, on medical grounds, sugar cannot be used, artificial sweetening such as saccharin is harmless and should be used; otherwise the baby may refuse the feed altogether. The teat should, if possible, be the one the baby is used to, and the hole should be of a size which allows him to take his feed without much effort and yet does not deliver the milk so quickly that he chokes. It is sometimes a good idea to ask the mother to bring the teat she uses at home. Inadequate holes cause the baby to tire before completing the feed and so he refuses the last ounce or two, or swallows air by sucking hard without effect. Failure to thrive, colic, vomiting and restlessness result. When using an upright bottle it may be necessary to twist the bottle and teat while the baby is sucking, in order to allow air to enter and replace the milk, though many babies will let go from time to time and so prevent a vacuum from forming, thus solving the problem themselves.

Babies who are too eager or underfed tend to gulp the first ounce of feed, a habit which is likely to result in vomiting. An ounce of boiled water, given before the feed, or an increase in the feed, are two ways of solving this problem. Failure to bring up wind, and excess crying on account of hunger or discomfort between feeds may cause air swallowing and distension which may in turn cause vomiting.

Different brands of artificial foods produce different stools and when considering these for any abnormality the feed should always be borne in mind (see Chapter 13 and the table on abnormal stools on page 212).

A blocked nose can cause quite serious difficulty in feeding and can be one of the most commonly missed reasons for refusal of feed. The nasal passages may be cleaned by inserting a wisp of cotton wool into the anterior nares, so inducing sneezing; alternatively nasal drops may be ordered for a short time. Any baby with a blocked nose will take feeds more easily by spoon, as he is unable to breathe adequately with a teat in his mouth.

Premature and weak babies may have to be fed by tube, pipette, Belcroy feeder or spoon. In the case of Belcroy feeder and pipette there is a degree of danger of inhalation of milk introduced into the mouth of a baby who is not sucking adequately and who has a poor swallowing reflex. Tube feeding is probably preferable for that reason. Belcroy feeders are open at both ends. At one end the rubber bulb of a pipette acts as a teat and an unperforated teat is attached to the distal end. As this is squeezed rhythmically it helps the flow of milk into the infant's mouth, by acting like a pair of bellows.

Bringing up the Wind. It is important to help the baby to bring up his wind, if unnecessary regurgitations, vomiting and colic are to be avoided. The baby should be sat up on the nurse's knees, his head and body well supported, or alternatively laid over the nurse's shoulder and his back either rubbed or gently patted. This is comforting to the baby and appears to help in getting the desired effect. The principle is of course that of the air bubble which rises in a bottle. All babies swallow air when crying or feeding, and the nurse should not be satisfied until the baby has had at least one good eructation. Babies who cry a lot should be allowed to bring up wind before starting to feed.

Complementary Feeds. Complementary feeds are feeds offered after breast feeds when these are insufficient. The baby may have been test weighed to estimate the amount to be offered or he may be offered about two-thirds of his requirements and allowed to please himself. The techniques of sucking from the breast and from the bottle are very different and many authorities advocate spoon rather than bottle feeding when complementary feeds have to be given. The feed should not be sweetened as there is a danger of the baby preferring the artificial feed to the less sweet and less readily obtained breast milk.

Supplementary Feeds. Supplementary feeds are given to replace one or several entire breast feeds per day. This may be done to rest the mother's nipples or because the mother is temporarily absent or indisposed. Once more the feed should be unsweetened and given by spoon in preference to a teat.

Some Feeding Difficulties

Vomiting. There are babies who vomit readily and there are babies in whom the vomiting becomes an established habit without any underlying pathological cause. The possible reason should, however, be investigated and often the observant nurse will be able to find it. A wide range of causes may include failure to bring up wind adequately, sucking from a teat with too small a hole, gulping the feed too quickly, frustration (see ruminating), hiatus hernia, congenital pyloric stenosis, atresia of the œsophagus, generalized infection, finger sucking, unsuitable feeds, air swallowing (aerophagy).

When describing a vomit, the nurse should always state whether it was forcible or effortless, and when it occurred in relation to the feeds. She should describe the appearance of the vomit, the presence of curds or mucus and the apparent stage of digestion. Every effort should be made to estimate the amount accurately. In this connection it is useful to experiment by measuring up half an ounce of water in an oil cup and pouring it on to a bib, to give an idea as to how wet this will make the bib. It will come as a surprise to most people to see what a large amount half an ounce of vomit is.

Some babies have what might be described as a "slowly emptying stomach". They are easily treated by sitting the baby up in a special chair so that gravity helps to keep the feed down. The baby eventually outgrows the condition.

Regurgitation and posseting should not be confused with vomiting. In these cases the baby returns a small amount of feed as he brings up his wind or between feeds. It is rarely of importance, but is often a sign that he is having a little too much.

Ruminating. Ruminating is a very tiresome condition which it is difficult to control. The ruminating baby is as a rule 1 to 3 months old, alert, intelligent and overactive. He appears to enjoy the taste of the regurgitated feed which he brings up in mouthfuls and which he moves around his mouth as if "chewing the cud", finally depositing it on his pillow. This habit can be very persistent and considerable amounts of nourishment can be lost by it, though it is a curious fact that few ruminators suffer markedly as far as their weight gain is concerned. In the younger baby there is a danger of inhaling feed. The condition is extremely difficult to cure. Bandaging the jaw, as is sometimes advocated, and sitting the baby up is of little benefit. Sedation is probably the safest and most effective treatment. The feeds should be thickened, and a thickening agent called Nestargel is of particular value. Occasionally the baby is given undiluted condensed milk from a spoon 3-hourly and his fluid requirements as boiled water every alternate 3 hours. This may considerably cut down the ruminating.

Weaning

Although at present there is a vogue for adding extras to milk feeds at a very early age, this is not altogether to be recommended. Increased carbohydrate intake, for instance, is inclined to cause abdominal distension and therefore discomfort to the baby. The baby also becomes overweight, flabby, pale, lethargic and prone to chest infections. It is useful to add a little to the last feed at night if this ensures a peaceful night for baby, mother and (probably) the rest of the household, but often babies thrive well and are contented with very little in addition to milk feeds until 3½ to 4½ months, or until they are about 15 pounds in weight.

Additions to the diet should be tried for 2 to 3 days before a further addition is tried, and if the baby obviously dislikes the taste after a few days, the addition should be omitted and tried again some weeks later. If the baby is unwell, no new foods should be introduced to risk upsetting his digestion until he is fit again.

The additions to the diet should be given with a spoon, and the amounts gradually increased, with a corresponding decrease in the milk feed and with the times of feeds gradually being altered to fit in with meal times, or convenient times for the household routine. All food offered should be sieved, strained, purèed, pulped, or in some way made devoid of lumps, skins and pips. Food should be freshly cooked and never reheated before serving. There is a large selection of tinned baby foods suitable for a weaning diet, but these are no substitute for freshly cooked food when available. If tinned food is used, but the whole tin not consumed at one meal, the food should be kept covered and in a refrigerator. At the age of 5 to 6 months a rusk or crust can be given, and the infant enjoys biting it when teething. Once some teeth are through, the food should cease to be soft or semi-liquid as chewing helps to develop the dental arch and helps to keep the newly erupted teeth healthy.

Suggested diet for baby of 6 months:

On waking.	Orange juice. Rusk.
8.30–9 a.m.	Breakfast. Cereal—Farex, Twinpack. Groats with sugar and milk. Hen's egg very lightly boiled or scrambled or poached. Crisply fried bacon. Bread and butter. Milk feed—4–5 ounces to drink.
12–1 p.m.	Finely minced meat, fish, liver or grated cheese with vegetable purée (made with aid of Turmix machine or Mouli-mixer), a little mashed potato, bone and vegetable broth or nourishing gravy—or white sauce with fish or cheese. Purèed fruit, custard or milk pudding. Water or orange juice.
During the afternoon	Biscuit or rusk, milk if desired.
5–6 p.m.	Farleys Rusk or cereal or custard, jelly. Bread and butter, honey or seedless and skinless jam. Biscuit or sponge cake (sponge cakes made for trifles can be bought and cut into fingers, and are useful as they do not crumble). Full milk feed (including what is put on rusk or cereal).
10–11 p.m.	Feed until baby does not wake for it.

3

NURSING THE NEWBORN

Nursing new-born babies is a great responsibility at all times but even more so when they are premature, feeble or sick. Changes in the infant's condition may be extremely sudden and of urgent importance, and the nurse must be observant and capable of fine judgment and swift action when caring for these babies.

To be a really good baby-ward nurse, considerable knowledge and great experience are essential, coupled with the keenest powers of observation, alertness, integrity and gentleness. Only the nurse who knows the normal, can appreciate the often slight, but always important, deviations from it and she needs to be the kind of person who will always stop and enquire thoroughly into the reason for such a change. Speed may be life-saving in infancy and even an hour's delay in seeking medical aid or advice may entail disaster. Initiative, too, is a great asset in dealing with sick babies and may often save a life. On the other hand an experienced baby nurse knows that masterly inactivity may sometimes be the most appropriate way of dealing with a sick baby. This applies in particular to the immature infant and to cerebral babies. Neatness and toilet routine may be of secondary importance to undisturbed rest and doing too much may be as fatal as neglect.

General Points

For the nursing of sick babies the cot should be large enough to allow for all procedures to be carried out with ease and for adequate observation of the infant without necessarily coming close up to the cot. No baby under the age of one year should be given ordinary pillows on account of the danger of suffocation. Small firm pillows may be built up armchair fashion in special cases where orthopnœa is present. The head of the mattress can also be raised by placing a pillow underneath it, or the head end of the cot can be raised on specially designed hooks. The majority of babies are best nursed lying flat. At the head end the bottom sheet can be protected by a piece of plastic sheeting covered by a small pillowcase. This is neat and allows for easy and frequent change of linen if it becomes soiled by mucus, secretions or vomit. Babies who have to be nursed in an upright position can be helped by a rolled-up napkin placed underneath their thighs like a knee pillow. If this is slipped under the mackintosh and napkin the baby is sitting on, with the distal end doubled around it, the baby will be effectively prevented from slipping. Young babies should always be allowed as much freedom to move around and kick as is compatible with their condition.

Nurses working with sick babies soon learn the significance of their cry. The causes may be manifold, for example hunger and thirst, loneliness, fear of the dark, discomfort from cold or heat, colic, teething, excessive wind, tight clothing or a soiled napkin. The cause should always be found and dealt with. It is erroneous to contend that it is good for a baby to cry for long periods and the danger that a bad habit will be formed if the baby is picked up when he cries, has probably been exaggerated. Some authorities maintain that, if the child is given the security, comfort and love he is asking for at the infant stage, he will grow into an easier, less demanding personality in later life. Research and experiments have also shown that the close bond between mother and child which is necessary to the mental health and happiness of every human being, is established in the first days after birth. The mother has been said "literally to fall in love" with her baby in the first two or three days, a process which cannot be delayed or it will never really take place. The seriousness of having to deprive a baby of this experience for reasons of illness or prematurity cannot be over-estimated. Mothers have been known to be unable to establish the same feelings for their sick or premature infants nursed in special units as for their other children with whom they have been able to have regular physical contact soon after birth. The conclusions to be drawn from these findings are obvious and it is for the nurses to see that such a situation is avoided if at all possible.

Taking an Infant's Temperature

Every infant must have his own thermometer. Infants may have a very low temperature and in these cases special low reading thermometers are used. They record temperatures as low as 29·4° C. (85° F.). Thermometers with short, rounded bulbs are supplied for taking rectal temperatures. Oral and skin temperatures are not usually suitable for infants as they have little subcutaneous tissue and friction from slight movement may give a false reading. If a skin temperature is taken, this is best done in the groin after carefully drying the skin. Occasionally it is convenient to leave the thermometer in the groin while feeding the infant. When taking a rectal temperature the anal region is cleansed and dried with a swab and the bulb of the thermometer carefully inspected and then lubricated with some petroleum jelly applied on a piece of old linen (thermometers should preferably not be dipped into the lubricant). A broken bulb can cause painful abrasions in the rectal mucosa. The baby should be lying on his cot or on the nurse's knee, his legs are raised, the thermometer inserted and the buttocks held together with the thumb and fingers either side, the thermometer being steadied between the first and second fingers as one would hold a cigarette. Alternatively the baby can lie on his side.

Taking the Pulse

Both pulse and respiration are taken while the infant is asleep or resting and before he is disturbed or the cot side lowered. In small infants it is often difficult to feel the radial pulse. Alternative methods, also less likely to rouse the baby, are: feeling the pulse over the temporal artery immediately in front of the ear, counting the pulsating movements of the fontanelle or the external iliac or the femoral artery in the groin.

Bathing a Sick Baby

In the United Kingdom most babies are bathed on the mother's or nurse's lap. Everything should be prepared and conveniently arranged before the baby is disturbed. A rubber and a Turkish towelling apron, reserved for each individual baby, are worn to protect the nurse's gown and uniform.

The bath temperature should always be checked with a thermometer and the water should be approximately 40·6° C. (105° F.) when first prepared. It will have cooled to 37·2°–37·8° C. (99°–100° F.) by the time the baby is ready to be lowered into it. The hot water tap should be movable and should swing to the side to avoid water dripping on to the baby.

After taking the pulse and respirations the baby is lifted from his cot, his clothes taken off and a bath towel securely wrapped around him. After washing her hands the nurse swabs his eyes with sterile cotton wool and boiled water from within outwards, using each swab once only (in cities ordinary tap-water is sufficiently clean). The face is then washed and dried with plain water and cotton wool. None of the orifices, such as mouth, nose or ears, are cleaned. Should special cleansing be necessary this is considered a treatment and not part of the daily toilet. Next the head is washed, holding the baby over the bath water. The scalp should be made thoroughly wet before applying soap and then thoroughly rinsed, as soap left on the hair is a common cause of seborrhœic dermatitis. On account of the wide open fontanelle the washing and drying should be done with great care and gentle-

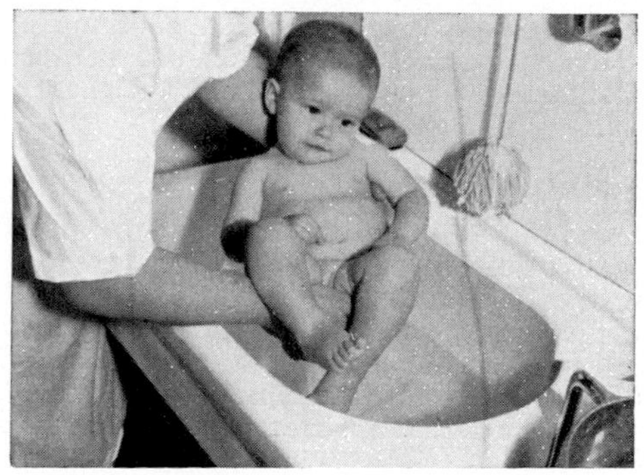

Fig. 4. A Good Way of Holding a Baby while Lowering him into his Bath.

ness. The napkin is next taken off and the infant's buttocks washed. He is placed on a clean square of non-absorbent cotton wool or cellulose while his temperature is taken. Care is taken not to expose the baby unnecessarily. In hospital, babies are frequently weighed daily and this is now done, though the scales will have been tested before disturbing the baby. Returning the baby on to her lap, the nurse now soaps him with her own soapy hands, carefully including all skin folds and the palms of the baby's hands. Weak or sickly babies are best not rolled on to their stomachs too often, as milk is easily regurgitated. The back can be soaped by raising the shoulders and the buttocks in turn. As both the nurse's hands and the baby's body are slippery he must be very securely held when lowering him into the bath (Fig. 4). Care should also be taken not to allow the head to drop backwards. Babies should enjoy their bath and should be allowed a few moments kicking time in the water.

In lifting the baby back on to her lap the nurse may roll him *towards* herself into the prone position. (This is the only time the child should be rolled.) The skin is well dried. Dusting powder may be used, but must never replace thorough drying. A soft towel should be available and dabbing movements are preferable to rubbing the infant down.

The vest and previously folded napkin are now placed over the infant's back before he is turned over. In doing this the

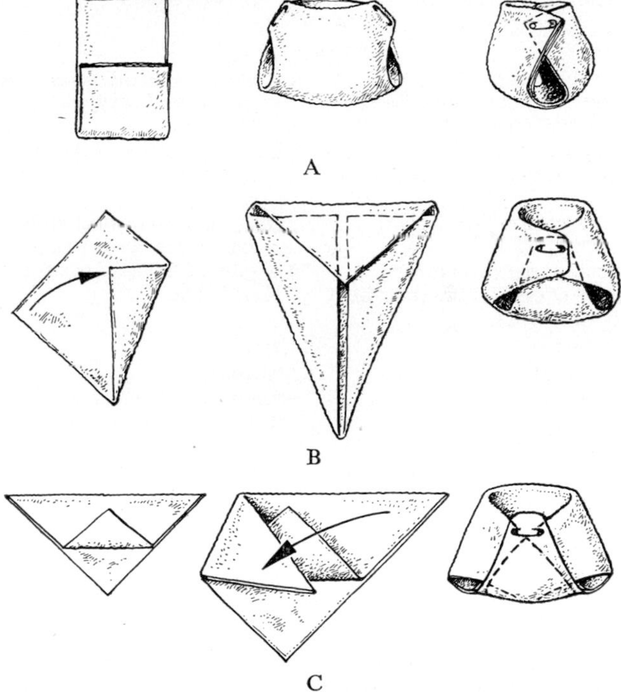

Fig. 5. Various Ways of Folding Napkins.

towel is brought out and the baby comes to lie on the dry apron. The baby is now dried in front and again great care should be taken to dry the skin folds thoroughly. The remaining clothes are then put on and the nails and hair attended to. The total procedure should take no more than 15 minutes.

There are various ways of putting on napkins but in all cases the safety pin should lie horizontally in order to minimize any risk of injury should it accidentally become undone. (Figs. 5a, b, c.)

List of Requirements for Bathing a Sick Baby

For the nurse

Rubber apron. Flannel apron.
Special gown. Face mask.
A table or special trolley for requirements.

For the bath

Bath thermometer.
Water temperature initially 40·6° C. (105° F.).
Pure curd soap.
Boiled water in sterile container.
Sterile cotton wool swabs.
Dusting powder.
Zinc and castor oil cream.
5-inch squares non-absorbent cotton wool.
Rectal thermometer with moist and dry swabs and lubricant.
Two buckets or receivers with lid, for soiled clothes and napkins.
Baby scales protected by tissue paper and a napkin.
A pair of fine nail scissors.
Hair brush.

For the baby

Bath towel.
Vest and open gown.
Woollen jacket.
Bootees.
Mittens.
Napkin and safety pin.
Small blanket or shawl.

For dressing the umbilical cord (*if not left exposed*)

Sterile tray for keyhole dressing
Sterile cord powder and swabs.
Sewing needle and cotton.
A pair of scissors.
Flannel binder or crêpe bandage.

When discharging a baby home the mother can be told that a daily bath is desirable but not essential and that it might well be omitted at her discretion should the only room available not be well heated at times.

Sore buttocks in the newborn may originate from a variety of causes, the most common of which are frequent loose stools, "strong" ammoniacal urine, excessive fat in the feeds, careless or infrequent toilet and change of napkins, inadequate rinsing of napkins after washing them in detergent, and unduly sensitive skin. Frequently the distribution of the rash gives a clue to the cause. A urine-soaked napkin will cause a widely distributed rash not only over the genitalia but spreading up to the abdomen and the sacrum and down to the thighs, while the skin folds and the natal cleft may be left unaffected. On the other hand, loose or fermented stools cause soreness of the perineum, around the anus and the back of the scrotum.

Intertrigo is a variant of napkin rash, which causes much soreness particularly in the groins and flexures. Intertrigo may also appear in the folds of the neck and is as a rule seen in fat and ill-kept babies. The soreness is caused by contact of two moist skin surfaces which are cut off from the air and gradually become infected. Careful hygiene and drying and the use of dusting powder is the only treatment required.

The *treatment of sore buttocks* varies according to the preference of those in charge and to the cause of the soreness. Dietary errors should be investigated and corrected. Ammonia dermatitis may be due either to a low fluid intake which is readily put right, or to decomposition of urine when in contact with stools and intestinal bacteria. Frequent changing and careful toilet is the best remedy. The practice of sprinkling boracic powder on napkins to prevent "burning" from ammonia produced by the decomposition of urine is dangerous. When boracic acid is absorbed, e.g. through broken skin, it is cytotoxic and may cause convulsions, diarrhœa and extensive rashes. More recently "nappy rash" caused by the splitting of urea in the urine through bacterial activity has been successfully prevented and treated by the use of Roccal (benzalkonium chloride). It is used in a solution of 1–5,000 for the final rinse after washing and boiling nappies. The best way both to prevent sore buttocks and also to cure them is by regular washing with plenty of water, adequate drying using a soft towel and dabbing movements, and the use of a good plain dusting powder. Petroleum jelly or zinc oxide cream, either plain or containing castor oil, may be applied. Babies suffering from gastro-enteritis are best protected by the application of tulle gras to prevent contact of the stools with the skin. In many cases it is a good plan to expose the infant's buttocks. The infant should normally wear bootees and may have the feet lightly restrained by ankle restrainers. A small blanket covers the feet, another one the body of the infant, while the buttocks are left exposed, resting on a napkin. Draughts are kept off by the use of a bed cradle. Whenever possible the healing properties of sunlight should be utilized.

The Stools of the New-born Infant. These are at first dark green to black in colour with a shiny appearance and viscid consistency and are known as *meconium.* After one to two days they gradually change to lighter ones and are then called *changing stools.* The stools of breast-fed babies are a golden mustard colour and of soft consistency. They have a characteristic, slightly sour smell. From one to six stools are passed each day.

The stools of infants fed on any type of cow's milk (whether fresh, dried or condensed) are pale yellow, larger in bulk and more formed than those of breast-fed babies. From one to three stools are passed daily. The stools of infants should always be carefully observed for much can be learned from their colour, odour, frequency and consistency. Changes occur readily and the cause may be even the slightest deviation from health, change of the usual feed or the giving of medicines or a little more or less fluid intake. When putting up stools for inspection (see Fig. 6) it must be remembered that they change colour quickly on the surface and to get a true picture a stool may first have to be broken up.

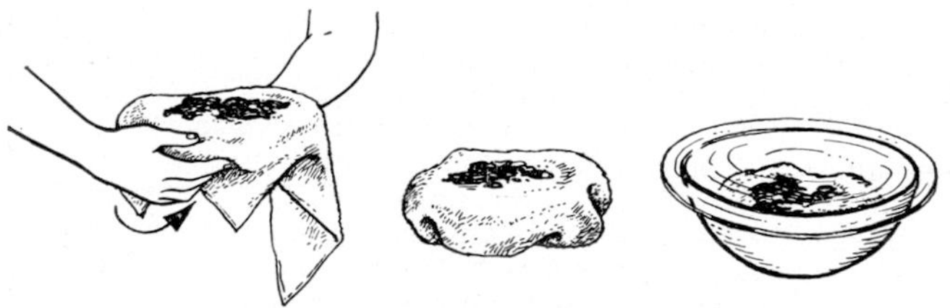

Fig. 6. Preparing a Soiled Napkin for Inspection.

It sometimes happens that a new-born baby fails to pass meconium in the first 24 to 36 hours. This is an important abnormality and must be reported at once as it may be due to a variety of causes such as imperforate anus, meconium ileus and atresia of the bowel.

The Temperature of the New-born Infant. It is often difficult to maintain a stable temperature in the newborn because the heat-regulating mechanism is still poorly developed and the body surface is large in proportion to the body weight. New-born infants may have a low body temperature for some days without coming to any harm, and this applies particularly to premature babies whose temperature may at first not ever exceed 33·8° to 35·5° C. (93° to 96° F.). Special low reading thermometers exist for these cases. On the other hand, during the first days it is not uncommon to find a rise in temperature known as *dehydration fever* in cases where the fluid intake is inadequate owing to the slow establishment of lactation. Boiled, plain water or glucose water should be given. Infants do not always respond to infection with a rise of temperature so that absence of pyrexia need not exclude an acute infective condition.

The Weight of the New-born Infant. Variations in weight are usual and undue importance should not be attached to stationary weight or to slight, occasional losses. A contented baby who sleeps and feeds well, whose colour is good and whose skin looks healthy need not be weighed daily or even

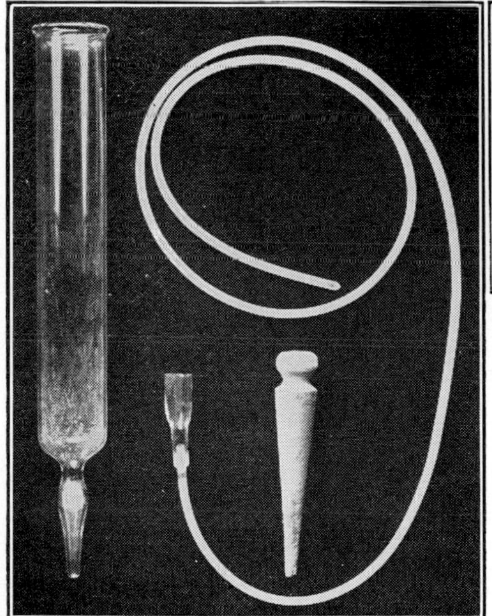

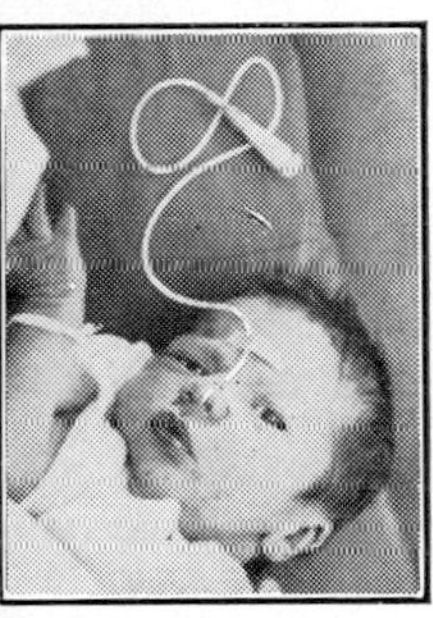

Fig. 7A. *Left:* INFUSSION BARREL, POLYVINYL TUBING AND SPIGOT.
Fig. 7B. *Above:* THE TUBE IN POSITION.

weekly. Much anxiety—one of the causes of poor lactation—could be avoided if scales were less frequently used (see page 1).

Continuous Drip Feeding. Occasionally it is necessary to give babies their feeds in small, continuous amounts. Figs. 7a and 7b show a good way of securing the tubing for this purpose. Polyvinyl is non-irritating and can often be left *in situ* without being changed for 2–3 weeks. This method is as a rule to be preferred to passing a tube repeatedly at frequent intervals.

Prevention of Infection in Neonatal and Sick Infants' Units

General Points

The younger the child the greater is the risk, from infection, to his immediate and subsequent health. Many of the infections prevalent in infant wards have lost some of their terror since the advent of antibiotics. But undue faith in antibiotics and general complacency are never justified where sick children are concerned, and each time infection and cross infection occurs, nurses and others in contact with the children should try to discover where a fault in technique may have occurred. These remarks about the newborn may be taken to apply also to older children, although both technique and dangers are modified as the older child has greater resistance to infection. But barrier nursing and general preventive technique must always be of the highest standard when dealing with children whose resistance is already lowered by illness.

At birth the infant possesses few antibodies and the process of building these up takes several years. Some passive immunity is passed on from the mother, as for instance immunity to measles; on the other hand many antibodies, for instance those of whooping cough, do not cross the placental barrier. Infants have, in addition, a poor heat-regulating mechanism and exposure to cold easily causes chills with an attendant lowering of resistance to attack by pathological organisms.

Staphylococcal infections are a particular danger in the newborn, who easily picks up the infection from adults who are carriers (such as the mother, medical and nursing staffs) or from other infants who act as carriers. A satisfactory way of reducing staphylococcal infections in infants' wards and nurseries is the use of hexachlorophene powder which is applied over the whole trunk, the axillæ, the groins and the perineum. In some units neomycin and chlorhexidine cream is applied to the infants' nostrils twice a day, as well as using the powder.

Cubicle Nursing

Ideally babies under a year old should be nursed in separate rooms or cubicles. These should be light, well ventilated and free from draughts. The temperature and humidity should be even and easily regulated. The flooring should have a smooth, easily washed surface and sweeping and high dusting should be done with an efficient vacuum cleaner, lined with a strong paper bag. If this is not possible the dust should at least be laid with the help of damp tea leaves or damp sawdust. Other dusting should be done with a damp duster and each cubicle or nursery should have separate cleaning materials.

The number of staff allocated to infants' and children's wards is usually high, in order to make a wise allocation of duties, and isolation of infected babies a reality. The number of people in contact with each individual patient should, however, be cut to a minimum, though this should never mean exclusion of the mother. Any person approaching the young, sick child must be free from infection, and the highest standard of personal hygiene, integrity and health is essential for sick children's nurses and medical staff. Where masks are

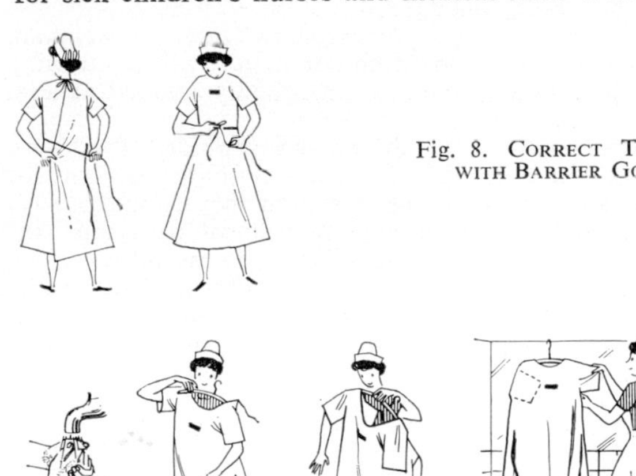

Fig. 8. Correct Technique with Barrier Gowns.

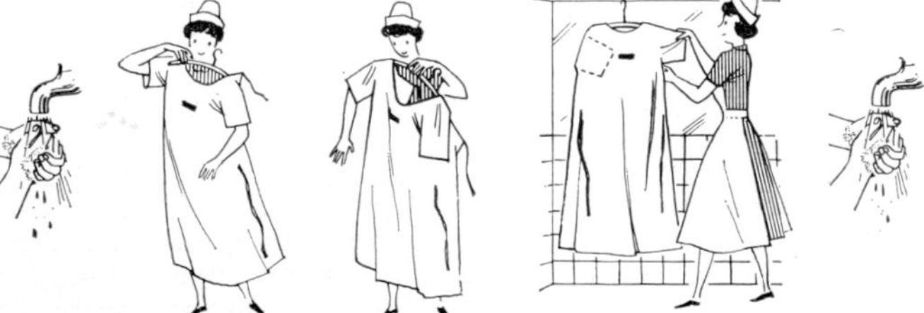

worn, the technique must be absolutely faultless and masks must cover both nose and mouth effectively. They must never be touched. (To take off a mask when talking to a superior is a sign of irresponsibility rather than of courtesy.) When finally taken off, only the strings of the mask should be handled. Masks should be changed every hour and the supply of clean masks should be virtually unlimited. The hands should be washed each time a mask is handled.

Gowns, if worn, should be used properly and there should be two gowns for use with each infant. The gowns should always be worn when more than the nurses' or other persons' hands come into contact with the baby or any part of his equipment and bed linen (Fig. 8).

Equipment required for toilet purposes, cleaning, treatments or feeding should be reserved for the individual infant. Some such articles are thermometers, washing utensils, powder, creams, towels, stethoscope, tape measure, pencils for charting frequent observations (other charts should be kept outside the cubicle), sphygmomanometer cuffs, and pulsometers. Medicine bottles and bottles containing vitamin preparations should either be handled before entering the cubicle or kept for the individual infant and disinfected and returned to the dispensary when he is discharged.

Equipment common to several babies, such as weighing scales and their weights, should be adequately protected using fine tissue paper. They should be thoroughly cleaned at least once a day.

Ideally, three pedal bins should be provided for every cubicle. One for nappies, one for used clothing and one for bed linen. Where removable lids are used they should always be laid down with the inner side uppermost to avoid contamination of the floor by the soiled side of the lid.

Infectious Babies. Cubicles of infants suffering from infections should be supplied with separate brooms, dust pans, dressing drums and feeding utensils. None of these should be returned to the common storage places, kitchen or milk room until they have been thoroughly disinfected. In all children's wards crockery and cutlery are boiled after they have been washed. Occasionally sterilization in a solution of electrolytic sodium hypochlorite (Milton solution 1 in 80 for 1½ hours) can conveniently be substituted for boiling, but, since Milton solution corrodes metal, plastic spoons should be used. Similar precautions are taken with washing bowls, tooth mugs, bed pans and pots. When carrying infected equipment, such as for instance bed pans from a cubicle, one hand should be kept clean to touch door handles.

There should be a liberal supply of soft "paper wipes" for use as handkerchiefs, and paper bags should be available for their safe disposal by burning and for the safe disposal of all dressings.

Children's toys should be passed from one to another as little as possible, and the toys of infants and toddlers should be reserved exclusively for the individual patient and thoroughly washed or disinfected before they are passed on. Children who are liable to drop their toys on the floor should have them tied to the cot sides to prevent the danger of infection. Common dressing gowns, slippers and bath mats have no place in a children's unit.

On the patient's discharge the entire cubicle should be washed down and allowed to air for several hours. Mattresses and pillows unless covered by mackintosh material should be sent for fumigation or aired in the open. Woollen blankets have to be treated in the same way before sending them to the laundry, but cotton blankets which are on the whole more suitable for children's units, can be sent to be boiled.

Napkins and soiled linen should never be allowed to remain in the cubicle or ward. They should be placed in covered receptacles and removed without delay. They should be washed in the laundry or by staff specially engaged for the purpose, not sluiced by nursing or ward staff.

4

THE PREMATURE BABY

Introduction

By international standards a baby weighing $5\frac{1}{2}$ pounds or less (2,500 grammes) is termed premature, irrespective of the time of gestation. But many babies who weigh more than $5\frac{1}{2}$ pounds appear immature at birth and may need the same care as premature ones. Those infants weighing below 2 pounds at birth are unlikely to survive but the chances of survival increase in direct proportion to their weight.

The nursing of premature babies is a responsible and exacting task and only a brief outline can be given in the pages of a small text book. Approximately 40,000 babies are born prematurely each year in Great Britain. Apart from the human aspect, their healthy survival is a national necessity in an age in which the average age of the population is constantly rising. Much research is going on to determine whether prematurely born babies may eventually be expected to reach normal standards and recent reports suggest that past fears may have been greatly exaggerated. It would seem that, all other things being equal, premature infants are likely to have reached satisfactory standards by the age of 4 years.

All human beings need love, physical contact and a sense of security. The premature baby is no exception. As soon as he is independent of continuous oxygen therapy, even if only for a short time, he should be taken out of his cot and nursed. If this is done under first-class nursing conditions the benefit to the infant greatly outweighs the slight risk involved. Nurses caring for premature babies must be exceptionally patient, gentle and observant and should have real devotion and interest for this type of work, for much of the care of these babies falls upon the nursing staff.

Meticulous attention to every detail of observation and technique is essential if a success is to be made of premature baby nursing. The essentials of "cubicle nursing" are set out in Chapter 3, page 41, and these apply also for the nursing of premature babies although in their case any carelessness in technique may lead to even more serious consequences than in the nursing of stronger babies. Hand washing, the use of a disinfectant barrier cream such as chlorhexidine (Hibitane), correct mask technique and absolute integrity with regard to personal hygiene and health are essentials. As few people as possible should be allowed to go near the baby (but those few must include the mother) and the infant should be handled as gently and infrequently as is compatible with reasonable care. Fatigue must be avoided by measures such as tube feeding, and by supplying a constant atmosphere, adequate in oxygen, humidity and temperature.

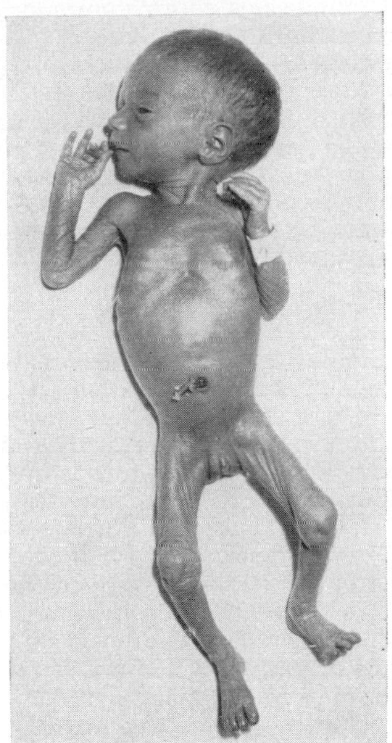

Fig. 9. A PREMATURE BABY AGED 5 DAYS.
Birth weight 4 pounds.

The premature or immature infant presents a number of characteristic features. His head is large in comparison with the body, the skin is wrinkled and the nails are soft and short. Insulation is poor due to the absence of subcutaneous fat and to the fact that the baby's body surface is proportionately large. Both heat-regulating centre and cough reflex are poorly developed. The baby may be so feeble as to be unable to expand his lungs or, if the lungs have been expanded, to keep them adequately inflated (*primary and secondary atelectasis*). The fact that respirations are shallow and irregular and that gas exchange may be inadequate, coupled with a drawing in of the soft chest wall at every breath, contributes to the frequency of cyanotic attacks or periods of apnœa. Exhaustion and asphyxia may eventually prove fatal.

Physiological jaundice is more common in the immature baby than in babies born at term, and is a contributing factor to their already considerable drowsiness. The renal function is poor and aggravates the tendency to retain salts and fluids in the tissues, causing œdema, which is common in these infants. Intracranial bleeding, or bleeding into the intestinal tract and lungs on the slightest provocation is common, probably due to some abnormality in the clotting properties of the blood. Vitamin K therapy, often necessary in premature babies, is also discussed on page 57.

General Care

The general care of premature babies follows the lines indicated by these physiological characteristics and their implications. The infant should be kept warm but must never be overheated. Both oxygen requirements and general metabolism are reduced when the temperature is low and these babies often do very well even when their body temperature is as low as 33·8° to 35·5° C. (93° to 96° F.). A special low reading, 29·4° C. (85° F.) thermometer is used. If they are nursed in an incubator (Fig. 10), the incubator temperature may be kept to 29° to 32·2° C. (84° to 90°F.) or if nursed in a cot, the cot temperature can be maintained at a maximum of 32·2° C. (90° F.) by means of well protected hot-water bottles. A useful routine to achieve this is to have three hot-water bottles suspended in pockets in the canvas cot sling and to change one every hour in rotation. The room is kept at a temperature of 18·2° to 21° C. (65° to 70° F.). Because these infants lose comparatively much moisture from the large skin surface and through rapid breathing, and because their initial fluid intake is likely to be low, the room humidity should be as high as 60 to 80 per cent., checked by means of a special hygrometer. When an incubator is being used this is easy, but if the baby is nursed in an open cot, the room humidity may have to be raised

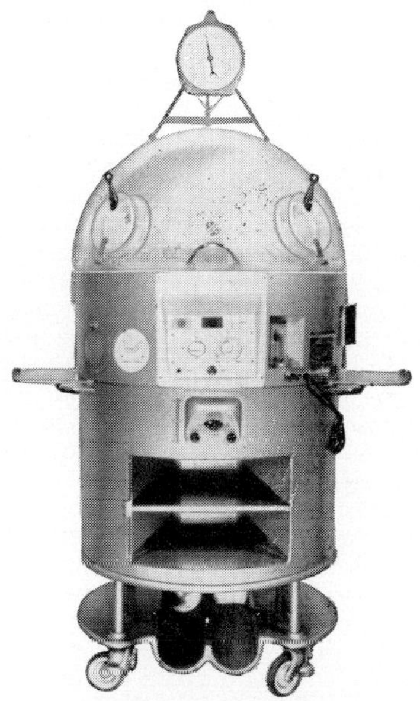

Fig. 10. A Modern (*Oxygenaire*) Incubator.
It illustrates well the complexity of modern, technical nursing.

by using a steam kettle or fine spray nebulizer. Babies who are cyanosed or have repeated periods of apnœa have to be given oxygen. The doctor may intubate the baby and give the oxygen via an endotracheal tube. Alternatively the oxygen may be given intermittently via a mask of the polythene bag type at 0·5 to 1 litre per minute. When oxygen is needed for short periods, until respirations are established after birth, 1 to 2 litres are delivered by means of an incubator. Oxygen must always be given in the minimal effective dosage and for the shortest possible period and if given for any length of time, withdrawn very gradually when no longer needed. The danger of causing blindness from retrolental fibroplasia should always be borne in mind (see page 71).

The feeble respirations of premature infants can be aided by changing their position every three hours, by occasionally slipping a hand beneath the back and gently lifting the thorax so expanding the chest wall, and by nursing the infant naked to avoid impeding the respirations by the weight of clothes. In positioning babies, care must be taken to avoid any kinking of the trachea and no feeble baby should ever be allowed to lie on his back lest he inhale mucus and saliva. The careful use of a mucus extractor is often indicated as both secretions and regurgitated feed are liable to be inhaled. At feeding time the head of the cot is raised but it is lowered during cyanotic attacks and when the airway is being cleared. When a feeble infant requires to be resuscitated, the process should include gentle clearing of the air passages from mucus, feed or liquor and an ordinary mucus catheter may be used to do this. Sometimes the tongue has to be brought forward with a pair of fine tongue forceps of the double pointed type. In severe cases endoscopy is performed and suction carried out under direct vision. A suitable laryngoscope and sucker should always be kept in readiness.

Artificial respiration is sometimes needed after clearing the air passages (see page 71). Nikethamide (Coramine) 0·25 to 0·5 millilitre, given intramuscularly or intravenously, is given as a stimulant. The drug is also effective when given orally as the buccal membrane absorbs it rapidly. A few drops are given by means of a pipette. Another commonly used drug is Vandid, a respiratory stimulant given either orally or by intramuscular injection.

The *daily toilet* is reduced to a minimum, as all handling which is not strictly necessary should be avoided. The infant need be weighed only once or twice a week and unless each baby has a pair of scales of his own, the weights and the scales are carefully protected with tissue paper to prevent any risk of cross infection.

Feeding of the premature infant can often be started 4 hours after birth, but is sometimes delayed for much longer, depending on the size and strength of the infant and the establishment of the swallowing and sucking reflexes. If feeds are given too soon, the danger of regurgitation and aspiration is very great. There is also a danger of the tissues becoming waterlogged due to the inefficiency of the kidneys in these babies. The baby will show signs of thirst as soon as he is ready to commence feeding. Whenever the baby seems sufficiently strong, breast or bottle feeds are given. Babies too weak to suck should be fed by œsophageal tube. This method causes little trauma or exertion and is always safer than feeding by Belcroy feeder, pipette or spoon. The possible danger of inhalation of feed given by these more forcible methods is self-evident. The amount of feed given to premature infants will vary according to the pædiatrician's request and the routine usual in any given department. One such scheme is set out below.

In the cases of very small babies and of babies who have to be tube fed, 2 millilitres may be given every 2 hours, beginning between 24 and 36 hours after birth. The amount is gradually increased until the baby receives approximately:

1 ounce	per pound of birth weight by the	4th day	in every 24 hours.
2 ounces	,, ,, ,, ,, ,, ,, ,,	8th ,,	
2½ ,,	,, ,, ,, ,, ,, ,, ,,	10th ,,	
3 ,,	,, ,, ,, ,, ,, ,, ,,	14th ,,	

The interval between feeds is adjusted according to the size and progress of the baby. Often the first bottle feeds are given at intervals of 6 hours, then at intervals of 4 hours and finally they are established at intervals of three hours. Only the feeblest babies may require very small amounts to be given every 2 hours.

The Choice of Food. Breast milk is as a rule the feed of choice even though it may have to be diluted during the early days of life. Sterilization is undertaken with special care and sometimes extra protein is added. For some curious reason babies often fail to gain weight after being on expressed breast milk for any length of time and temporarily an artificial feed may be more satisfactory. Sweetened condensed milk or Frailac (Cow and Gate) are particularly suitable in these instances. At about three weeks vitamins should be started. Vitamin C is best given as ascorbic acid (25 mg. daily) and vitamin D in the form of one of the concentrated preparations (1,000 international units daily). At 1 month iron should be given. A suitable preparation is ferrous sulphate 75 milligrams (gr. 1¼), given two to three times a day. If the hæmoglobin is low (below 8 g./100 ml.) iron in the form of Imferon may be given by intramuscular injection.

In the case of very small and very immature infants it is necessary to progress from one stage of care to the next in graded phases until a satisfactory point of development has been reached and before discharge home can be achieved. As soon as the baby has reached the stage of gaining weight steadily, when he appears to be making uninterrupted progress and when he weighs about 4½ pounds, steps are taken to wean him from the special care and conditions of the premature baby unit. He will already have been moved from the incubator or Sorrento cot to a normal cot and he may now be moved into a "cooling off" room (temperature 10° C. (50° F.)) or to a sheltered corner of the general nursery. It will then be possible to allow the mother to take a greater part in her baby's care. She may be taught to bath him, to give him his feeds from an ordinary bottle and to nurse him for longer periods than before. If progress remains uneventful and the mother seems competent, the baby can usually be allowed home when he has reached 5 pounds in weight.

5

APPARENT AND TRUE ABNORMALITIES OF THE NEWBORN

In the following section an attempt is made to describe briefly some of the abnormalities which may be seen in an infants' ward of a hospital for sick children or in a maternity unit. In some cases their significance and treatment are discussed in this section; for others, treatment and nursing care are dealt with in more detail in later chapters.

The new-born infant has recently undergone tremendous stress during the process of birth and this may sometimes result in more or less serious damage. Likewise, great changes have taken place in the physiology and mechanism of the body within a short space of time and in some instances the process may have remained incomplete or be faulty. Abnormalities might well be more frequent than they actually are.

The *skin* of the newborn is covered with a wax-like substance, the *vernix caseosa*, which serves as a lubricant, heat preserver and protection for the skin. Left untouched it soon dries off in scaly flakes. For that reason not all authorities favour bathing the baby during the first few days. "*Stork beak marks*" as they are commonly called are areas of red staining on the eyelids, the nape of the neck and the edge of the hair line. They are quite harmless and usually disappear within a few days of birth. Small white spots may cover the nose. These minute, blocked sebaceous glands, known as *milia* are very common and disappear spontaneously after a short time.

The *scalp* tends to be scurfy. Daily toilet includes washing it with a bland soap followed by very thorough rinsing. In some cases the application of sodium bicarbonate (one teaspoonful to a pint of water), gentle massage with olive oil or a shampoo with one per cent. cetrimide solution assists in getting rid of excess scurf. Generally speaking the skin should be left alone as much as possible. When washing or drying any part, gentle, dabbing movements are preferable to rubbing. The oral and nasal orifices should never be cleaned as part of the daily toilet. A wisp of cotton wool touching the margin of the nose suffices to make the baby sneeze and so clear his little nose, should this be necessary.

The *finger nails*, which at first are very soft, should be cut straight across if they grow too long and the infant may also be prevented from scratching himself by little cotton mittens which can be changed and boiled each day. The use of mittens must, however, be considered carefully as it has happened that a loose cotton thread inside the mitten has become wrapped round a finger, resulting in gangrene and loss of a phalanx. The *umbilicus* must be kept dry from the time of birth. A healthy umbilical cord dries up within 24 hours and should fall off within a week. In some units the umbilicus is left exposed, in others the cord is treated with spirit or an antiseptic or a sterilized and astringent cord powder is applied. In the latter case a keyhole dressing is used and kept in position with the help of a crêpe bandage. Whichever method is favoured, it is important to realize that a moist umbilicus is an ideal breeding ground for sepsis and that the direct communication between umbilicus and liver in the newborn may be the path of a most serious spread of infection and generalized septicæmia. *Sweat rashes and "woollie rashes"* are common in infants and should be treated by careful hygiene, and the application of dusting powder. In some cases it is best not to allow wool next to the skin.

The *colour* of the healthy new-born baby is a raw, bright red. Abnormal colouring includes pallor and cyanosis due to neonatal anoxia; a grey, ashen appearance due to severe shock or generalized infection; a yellow tinge due to physiological jaundice and a dark orange tinge caused by hæmolytic disease, obliteration of the bile duct or severe jaundice of the newborn, due to prematurity.

Physiological Jaundice. This occurs in about 50 per cent. of babies and is caused by liver insufficiency and by the liver's inability to metabolize bilirubin broken down at a rapid rate during the first days of life. The condition requires no treatment and can be expected to clear spontaneously within the first week of extra-uterine life. Jaundice due to this cause is never present at birth and jaundice present at that time or appearing during the first two days of life is due to other, more serious causes. The jaundice caused by congenital obliteration of the bile duct appears much later and is of progressive intensity. Another serious condition causing jaundice is hæmolytic disease of the newborn. Both these conditions are discussed in detail later in the text (see index).

Enlarged Breasts. These are seen fairly frequently in newborn babies, and girls may have a vaginal discharge similar in mechanism to menstrual bleeding. Both these conditions are caused by maternal hormones still present in the infant's circulation. They require no treatment, but must be reported to the doctor or sister in charge.

Minor Head Injuries

Cephalhæmatoma is one of these common injuries to the infant's head which may occur in the case of vertex (head first) deliveries. A swelling may appear on the first or second day after birth. It is due to a subperiosteal hæmorrhage caused by birth trauma. As may be expected the swelling is limited by the suture lines to any one of the cranial bones. It should be left alone and requires neither drainage nor aspirating, although it takes some weeks before it disappears. Very occasionally it may be an indication of a bony fracture.

Caput succedaneum is another of these harmless injuries. The presenting part is subjected to severe pressure during delivery. Œdema of the soft tissues may result and is present at the time of birth but will resolve within a matter of days. Unlike the cephalhæmatoma, the swelling is not confined by the suture line, when it occurs on the skull.

Moulding of the head may be marked and may not disappear for some time. It is caused by the overlap of the cranial bones at the suture lines, one of nature's ways of adapting the size and shape of the skull to its passage through the birth canal. Considerable temporary asymmetry may thus be caused.

More Serious Head Injuries

Precipitate, premature or difficult labour may be the cause of intracranial injury.

Intracranial Injury. This is usually serious and may lead to cerebral palsy, hydrocephalus, mental deficiency, epilepsy or death. Infants who have suffered such injuries are limp and apathetic, their colour is ashen grey and their respirations irregular and shallow. They are often restless and have a wrinkled, worried facial expression and seem constantly wide awake. Other important signs include nystagmus, twitching, rigidity, a high-pitched whining cry and an unstable temperature. The fontanelle may be tense and bulging. Occasionally these symptoms are present at birth but improve within the first 24 hours only to reappear with greater severity after a further 24 to 48 hours. Once feeding has started this is often noticed to be slow; the infant sucks feebly and the powers of swallowing are impaired. As a result the baby fails to thrive. Vomiting and cyanosis are not always present but when they do occur are warning signs of severe injury with a poor prognosis.

Treatment. Infants suspected of or known to have sustained intracranial injury need absolute quiet. They are not taken out of their cot, toilet attention is reduced to a minimum, noises and sudden lights must be excluded and medical examinations are as restricted as possible. Inhalation pneumonia is prevented by keeping the air passages clear with the help of a mucus extractor and by raising the head end of the cot. Feeding is not attempted for 48 hours or longer and then tube feeding may be deemed safest and least tiring for the infant.

Sedatives such as chloral hydrate 30 to 60 milligrams ($\frac{1}{2}$ to 1 grain) four-hourly or phenobarbitone 8 milligrams ($\frac{1}{8}$ grain) four-hourly may be prescribed. With care, recovery may be complete but prognosis must always be guarded and a special watch is kept over such children for the first year or 18 months.

Subdural hæmatoma is a somewhat later manifestation of intracranial injury. The baby may at first appear to be normal, but fails to thrive, becomes difficult with feeds, and eventually convulsions and other signs of intracranial pressure, such as a bulging fontanelle or an enlarging head and irregular breathing may become apparent. The hæmatoma is close to the dura and may lie over any part of the brain, though a common site is over the cerebrum. Treatment consists in aspirating the hæmatoma, usually through the coronal sutures lateral to the angle of the fontanelle. The blood-stained fluid obtained varies in appearance according to the length of time it has been present. For the purpose of the treatment the infant's head has to be shaved. He is wrapped securely in a blanket and the head steadied by the two hands of the nurse held over the sides of the face and skull, presenting the fontanelle towards the doctor. Successful treatment carries a hopeful prognosis.

Other Injuries

Local nerve injury may be caused by forceps or by any other abnormal delivery. *Facial paralysis* is clearly seen when the infant's mouth is pulled towards the unaffected side in the act of crying. Nursing measures include careful feeding, keeping the skin around the mouth and in the folds of the neck healthy in spite of the constant dribble of saliva (e.g. by silicone vasogen ointment), placing the child on the affected side to avoid saliva reaching the permanently open eye and protecting the cornea with lubricating eye drops (e.g. castor oil drops). This type of paralysis may be expected to clear within the first month.

Erb's palsy is a nerve injury affecting the brachial plexus. The limp arm is internally rotated with the elbow extended. The hand is partly closed and the palm directed backwards. The arm should be rested in a position which relaxes all the affected muscles. This is easily achieved by pinning the baby's cardigan sleeve to the pillow with the humerus at right angles to the body and the forearm pointing upwards, the hand lying beside the head (Fig. 11). Alternatively a light splint is used to maintain the correct position. Recovery is usually complete though passive movement or massage may be needed for several weeks or months.

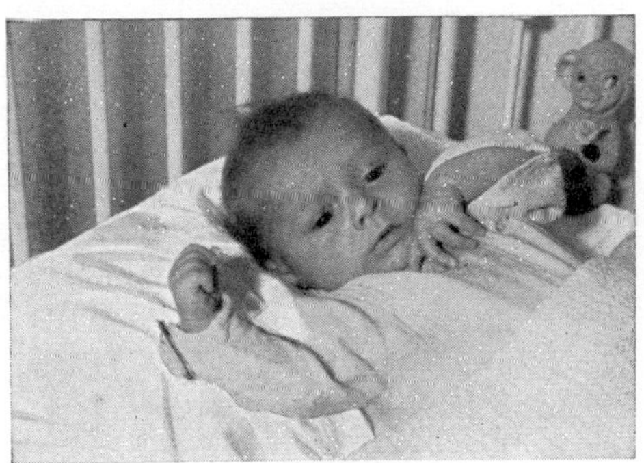

Fig. 11. ERB'S PALSY.

The affected arm can easily be kept in the correct position by pinning the sleeve to the pillow.

Injury to the sternomastoid muscle is occasionally caused by difficult labour. A small tear may result in bleeding and exudate which, after a matter of days, causes a noticeable, firm but painless swelling. The only treatment needed is passive movement of the head to avoid fibrosis and resulting torticollis.

Fractures are as a rule not of a serious nature as the bones unite easily and in a good position with a minimum of treatment. The bones most commonly affected are the clavicle and humerus. A pseudo-paralysis or reluctance to move the arm may be the first sign of such injury.

Infections of the Respiratory System

The respiratory system of the newly born baby is particularly prone to disease, and respiratory failure is by far the most common cause of death in the first few days of life. Inhalation of liquor, meconium, blood or mucus causes aspiration pneumonia, and this is virtually present at birth. Infection is readily caused by contact with anyone carrying a pathological organism or even a common cold. The lungs of the feeble or immature infant do not always expand completely and this causes a condition known as *atelectasis* (see page 46). Atelectasis may also be caused by damage to the respiratory centre during birth; 5 per cent. of all perinatal deaths are due to asphyxia, but many could be saved if intubation were carried out in all cases in which the baby fails to breathe within 4 minutes of birth. Occasionally the lungs expand at first, but extreme weakness, lack of nervous control or inhalation of foreign matter such as mucus, saliva or feed may cause secondary atelectasis. When this occurs, cyanosis and shallow respirations may be marked. Treatment consists in changing the infant's position frequently, clearing the air passages, gentle stimulus to cause crying and by giving oxygen. Rest, warmth and protection from infection are essential. The infant is best nursed in the horizontal position but a small pad may be placed underneath the shoulders to expand the thoracic cage. Care must be taken not to kink the neck and with it the trachea. Babies with respiratory difficulties should never be wrapped tightly, abdominal binders should not be used, and clothes should be reduced to a minimum as even a vest may impede breathing by its weight. Lowering of the infant's head and shoulders causes the abdominal viscera to restrict the diaphragmatic movement and should consequently be avoided. The use of an incubator is often a great advantage.

The newly born baby breathes exclusively through his nose, and nasal obstructions may have to be overcome by gentle cleansing or the instilling of nasal drops. It is frequently sufficient to insert a wisp of cotton wool into the anterior nares, so causing the baby to sneeze. A blocked nose is a common and often missed cause of slow or reluctant feeding even in healthy infants.

Hyaline Membrane Syndrome. This is a serious condition, the cause of which is still unknown. In this condition a gelatinous, waxy membrane lines the alveoli inhibiting oxygen exchange and causing clinical signs similar to those of atelectasis. The condition becomes apparent within hours of birth and carries a high mortality rate; it occurs mostly in premature babies born by Cæsarean section. Steam and oxygen therapy may be tried but are usually of little avail. If the infant survives, absorption of the membrane takes place after a few days, followed by complete recovery. More recently successes have been reported by lowering the temperature of any baby at risk, to 32·8° to 33·4° C. (91° to 92° F.) for 24 or 48 hours. In lowering the metabolism and oxygen requirements in this way, the available oxygen is sufficient to maintain the vital centres until the membrane is absorbed. Alternative experiments are being made by placing the baby in a pressure chamber.

Hæmorrhagic Disease of the Newborn

Occasionally a baby may suddenly vomit blood or pass a melæna stool or blood stained urine, or may be found to be bleeding from the nose, vagina or umbilicus. The bleeding occurs without warning and is most common from the third day onward. The cause is lack of vitamin K, which in turn causes hypothrombinæmia and an abnormally long prothrombin time.

Treatment must not be delayed and consists of giving vitamin K (1 to 2 mg. by intramuscular injection), commonly used preparations being phytonadione (Konakion) and Vikastab. With prompt treatment the prognosis is good, but delay in reporting signs of bleeding may have serious consequences.

Occasionally a small vomit of altered blood or a melæna stool are caused by the baby swallowing blood as, for instance, during birth or from the mother's cracked nipple. It is for the doctor to decide and confirm the cause of any such signs of bleeding and the nurse must report them promptly and save the abnormal stool or vomit for medical inspection.

Hæmolytic Disease of the Newborn

It is possible for the blood of the fœtus to be incompatible with that of his mother. The mother then produces antibodies which pass via the placenta into the fœtal circulation, where they cause the red blood cells to hæmolize. New red cells are produced, at an abnormal speed and reach the circulation while still in an immature stage, when they are known as erythroblasts. After birth the antibodies gradually spend themselves and the condition may rectify itself, though commonly transfusion is required. In serious cases severe jaundice occurs, followed often by much damage to the central nervous system and the baby may even die. The incompatibility described above happens generally when the mother is rhesus negative and the father and infant rhesus positive. There are numbers of complicated variants of this problem and sensitization does not usually occur during a first pregnancy.

There are four principal manifestations of rhesus incompatibility:

1. *Still-birth or death* within a few hours, associated with hydrops fœtalis.
2. *Icterus gravis neonatorum.*
3. *Kernicterus.*
4. *Congenital anæmia.*

Hydrops Fœtalis. Infants with this condition are grossly œdematous and anæmic and the placenta shows pathological changes. The condition cannot be treated once it has occurred.

Icterus Gravis Neonatorum. In the severest form of this condition, the liquor, vernix and umbilical cord are stained yellow at birth, the baby is severely jaundiced and anæmia is marked. In less severe cases the infant becomes seriously jaundiced within 24 hours of birth, but even in the early stages the jaundice can be demonstrated by pulling taut the skin. Liver and spleen are enlarged, œdema may be present and often there are petechiæ on the trunk and limbs. The infant is lethargic and difficult to rouse. Exchange blood transfusion is the usual treatment and doctors are guided by the level of bilirubin in the blood serum which is responsible for the jaundice. With proper treatment recovery is possible.

Kernicterus. Circulating bile pigment (bilirubin) may cause serious complications in the brain. This condition is known as kernicterus and causes staining and degeneration of the brain cells. The infant shows reluctance to feed, has a feeble cry, neck stiffness and opisthotonos, unusually brisk reflexes, impaired respiration and convulsions. If the infant survives, he may suffer from deafness, cerebral palsy or mental deficiency.

Congenital Anæmia of the Newborn. Congenital anæmia may be present at birth and be severe, or it may develop within the first two weeks of life and be of a mild type (see also familial thrombocytopenic purpura, page 194).

The *treatment* for hydrops fœtalis and for severe anæmia is exchange blood transfusion. Some "rhesus babies" respond sufficiently to conservative methods such as iron therapy for anæmia and a small proportion of them do not require treatment of any kind.

Exchange Blood Transfusion

In anticipation of severe disease, a blood specimen is taken from the cord at the time of birth and examined in the laboratory. The cord is not tied in the usual manner but is kept moist by wrapping damp, sterile gauze around it, while tests are carried out. If there is evidence that the bilirubin level is reaching dangerous proportions, or if the cord hæmoglobin is less than 15 g./100 ml. an exchange blood transfusion is given. The umbilical vein, still patent at this stage, is used to introduce a plastic cannula. With the help of a four-way tap and syringe, 20 millilitres of blood at a time are withdrawn and replaced by rhesus negative blood. Alternatively the blood can be of the baby's own group or group "O". It should always be fresh blood. The procedure is continued until approximately 80 millilitres of blood per pound of body weight have been exchanged. (The total volume of blood of a 7-pound baby at birth is approximately 300 millilitres.) The infant is securely immobilized on a "T"-shaped splint and it is important to ensure that he is kept warm throughout the procedure, and allowed to rest when the transfusion has been completed. Penicillin or streptomycin may be ordered after the exchange. Vitamin K, 1 milligram, may be ordered and sometimes calcium gluconate is given to counteract the effect of the citrate in the donor blood. A specimen of the last blood withdrawn is sent to the laboratory for estimation of the hæmoglobin and serum bilirubin levels. To avoid clotting in the apparatus, heparin in saline is syringed through it at each withdrawal and injection of blood. (Saline 100 millilitres to heparin 1,000 units.) Following the transfusion, the level of serum bilirubin is carefully watched in case it should rise again to dangerous levels, necessitating a second transfusion.

Hæmolytic disease of the newborn is in most instances a preventable disease. Special blood tests during pregnancy give an indication of the risk to the baby. If the risk appears to be great, labour may be induced prematurely, or arrangements made for delivery in a hospital where the special blood tests and treatment required can be carried out.

Œdema of the Newborn

Severe anoxia and respiratory distress, infections such as septicæmia, excess chilling, prematurity, congenital heart disease with cardiac failure, and faulty feeding may all cause œdema in the newborn. This is often difficult to assess and the carefully kept weight chart is of great value. The œdema is not necessarily of the pitting type, as in adults, but the fluid accumulation in the tissues causes the extremities to take on a rounded appearance while the skin may be unusually pale and shiny with a rubbery sensation when touched. Œdema is postural and marked in the dependent parts or on the side on which the infant is lying. Treatment is according to the cause. It should be appreciated that salt retention automatically causes fluid retention. Hartmann's and other solutions containing salts are consequently not given unless diluted nor is cow's milk, which has a comparatively high salt content.

Cold Baby Syndrome

This syndrome is one which has only recently been recognized. It occurs as a rule in the first month of life, in premature babies, babies who suffer from severe heart disease, infection or cerebral birth injury, and babies who have been exposed to cold as for instance in an inadequately heated room.

The infant's colour may at first be bright pink and this may give a deceptive impression of excellent health, but the colour

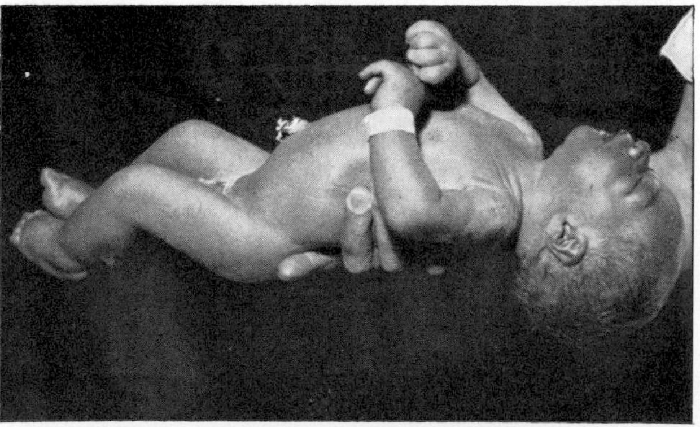

Fig. 12. Baby with "Cold Injury" showing the Generalized Rigidity characteristic of this Syndrome.

soon changes to a grey pallor. He is reluctant to feed, drowsy and slow to react to external stimuli. The entire baby is rigid (Fig. 12). Œdema may be present and urinary output is low. The skin is cold and hard to the touch and the rectal temperature registers between 26·4° and 32·2° C. (80° and 90° F.), or even less. When taking the temperature a special low-reading thermometer should be used. This should be inserted into the rectum for a distance of at least 1 inch (2·5 cm.) and left in position for 2 full minutes.

Treatment. Admission to hospital is usually necessary. The baby is often best nursed in an incubator at a temperature 1–2° above his own. He should be handled as little as possible. Food is not well tolerated and at first glucose 5 per cent. with or without $\frac{1}{2}$-strength saline solution added to it, is given via a tube. During the process of re-warming the baby, metabolism is increased and this in turn increases the need for glucose. Special care should be taken, however, to prevent regurgitation of the concentrated glucose into the lungs. Milk feeds are introduced gradually as the infant's condition improves. An antibiotic is usually prescribed to combat any infection.

Improvement is steady and rapid in the majority of cases and the baby may be expected to recover completely from the cold syndrome although the underlying condition may yet have to be treated.

Infections in the Newborn

Infections occur readily in the newborn as the infant has little resistance and no antibodies. It is often difficult to notice the early signs of infection in the neonate. Frequently there is no rise in temperature, pulse or respiration and only the most experienced nurse would notice a disinterest in feeding or a minor change in colour as being of importance. Sometimes there is merely an unaccountable change in the baby's previously good condition, but this change should be a warning that the pædiatrician should be consulted. Osteomyelitis, pneumonia, urinary tract infections, meningitis and gastro-enteritis are not uncommon and are frequently secondary to a blood stream infection, particularly due to *Escherichia* (*Bacterium*) *coli.* Infection at this age presents rather an atypical picture and can be easily missed if experience is lacking. Often a serious infection is associated with very vague signs. The infant may merely become very reluctant with his feeds or become lethargic and limp. A fall in temperature may be the first sign of an infection and the temperature may even remain subnormal for the first day or two. His colour may be grey and ashen, jaundiced or cyanosed, and every possible irregularity of respiration and pulse rate and volume may be registered.

Meningitis is typically associated with a bulging anterior fontanelle but even this may be absent or possibly reversed if loss of fluid from vomiting or diarrhœa has caused dehydration.

Pneumonia may be present without any sign of dyspnœa or cough, and *convulsions* are common. Alternatively there may be high fever and a hot, flushed skin.

Urinary tract infections are particularly common in the neonatal period and these infections often recur. Investigations are usually carried out to exclude congenital abnormalities of the urinary tract.

Skin Infections. These, however slight, should be treated with care in order to avoid a spread of the infection or generalized septicæmia. With the advent of modern drugs many skin infections have lost their severity but occasionally a particularly resistant strain may still cause serious disease. The skin is easily damaged in young babies and small pustules and paronychia should be treated immediately and the patient isolated at once. For instance pemphigus, a bullous septic skin eruption, caused by *Staphylococcus aureus*, continues to carry a poor prognosis, despite treatment with penicillin, antibiotics and cortisone.

Mongolism (Down's Disease)

Mongol children are usually delightful little people. Totally unaware of their mental and physical handicaps, they are as a rule good-natured, affectionate and happy. They enjoy learning simple tasks and delight in repeating them again and again. Although mentally subnormal and ineducable, the high grade ones can sometimes be taught to earn a simple living.

Mongols account for about 25 per cent. of all mentally defective children born in the United Kingdom but many do not survive to adult life. Congenital heart disease and a tendency to intercurrent infections play a part in shortening life.

The mongol's characteristics include a small head, flat at the back and resting on a short neck; small ears and a round small nose; adenoids are common and cause even very young babies to have grunting respirations. The tongue is often long and pointed and known as scrotal tongue owing to its fissured surface. Eyesight is frequently poor and the narrow, slanting openings and epicanthic folds give the face its mongoloid look. The hair is scanty but soft to the touch. The shoulders are round, the chest flat and the abdomen protuberant. Many have an umbilical hernia. There is generalized hypotonicity. The hands are broad and short with a deep palmar crease, short thumb and a short, curved fourth finger. There may be a wide gap between the first and second toes. Syndactyly (webbing) occurs frequently. A longitudinal deep fissure runs down the sole of the foot. Dentition is usually delayed.

Most mongol children love music even more than ordinary children do, and, in spite of a croaking voice, love to sing simple songs and tunes. They are often excellent mimics and very entertaining.

As they are clean in their habits they are usually pleasant children to care for, although their dependency on adults has a profound influence on the life of their families.

A good deal of research is at present being done to find the cause and possible treatment of this congenital abnormality. So far at least one interesting fact has come to light, namely that mongol children have 47 instead of the usual 46 chromosomes in their cells.

Congenital Anatomical Abnormalities

Many congenital abnormalities can nowadays be treated surgically. A list of the more common types is of interest and some knowledge of them may lead to keener observation even in a maternity or medical pædiatric ward.

The Head. Microcephaly, hydrocephaly, oxycephaly, nævi.

The Eye. Buphthalmos, congenital cataract, strabismus, microphthalmia.

Ears. Absence of the pinna or meatus. Congenital deafness. Bat ears.

Mouth. Cleft lip (hare lip), cleft palate, micrognathia (congenital smallness of the lower jaw).

Alimentary Tract. Pyloric stenosis, œsophageal atresia, tracheo-œsophageal fistula, hiatus hernia, Hirschsprung's disease, imperforate anus, congenital obliteration of the bile duct, meconium ileus, rectovaginal fistula.

Bones. Osteogenesis imperfecta, spina bifida, achondroplasia, syndactyly, talipes, congenital dislocation of the hip joint, missing bones.

Thorax. Diaphragmatic hernia, congenital heart disease (with or without cyanosis).

Abdomen. Varieties of hernia, exomphalos.

Genito-urinary Tract. Horse-shoe kidney, double ureters, hypospadias, epispadias, rectovaginal fistula, pseudo-hermaphroditism, hydrocele, undescended testicles, ectopia vesicæ.

Central Nervous System. Cystic spina bifida (meningocele, myelomeningocele), anencephaly, microcephaly, hydrocephaly and a variety of conditions which may be responsible for cerebral palsy.

Nævi or Birth Marks

Nævi (singular: nævus) consist of a localized cluster of dilated blood vessels. There are various types of nævi, some of which are present at birth, others appear some months later. Of the different types most disappear spontaneously but others persist. Some nævi are very extensive and may disfigure an entire side of the face or cause considerable enlargement of the tongue associated with difficulty of speech, eating and breathing.

Treatment. This is by means of radium, application of thorium-X, injection with necrosing agents, and surgical excision.

The nursing care of patients treated by deep X-ray therapy or radium is given in Chapter 16 (Wilms's tumour).

One type of nævus which can be expected to disappear spontaneously is known as strawberry or cavernous nævus. This type of nævus is liable to grow considerably but rarely causes serious trouble or hæmorrhage. After the first year of life the nævus tends to shrink and gradually regresses completely leaving a flat, paper-like scar by the age of about 5 years. No treatment should be given for such a nævus but much tact will be needed in persuading the mother to accept conservative treatment for her disfigured child. In contrast to this nævus, those known as "portwine nævi" stay for life. Excision and grafting is usually the treatment of choice.

Diaphragmatic Hernia

Some babies are born with a defect in the diaphragm (usually on the left side). As a result abdominal organs such as stomach and intestines, and sometimes even the liver, rise into the thoracic cavity. The heart is then displaced to the right and, since the lungs cannot expand normally, cyanotic attacks occur. If an attempt is made to relieve these by giving oxygen via a mask, the oxygen enters the stomach causing further distension. The procedure is therefore a dangerous one and must be avoided. Early and accurate diagnosis is life saving and must never be delayed.

Treatment consists of intubating the baby and giving oxygen via an endotracheal tube. Emergency operation is carried out without delay. Thoracotomy is performed, the organs returned to the abdominal cavity and the defect in the diaphragm repaired. A gastric tube is left in position and for the first 2 or 3 days the stomach is aspirated at frequent intervals. After-care is similar to that for any other cases recovering from thoracic surgery, but the baby is often sat up in a "hiatus hernia chair" to maintain an upright position for several weeks following operation.

Hiatus Hernia

Hiatus hernia is a special type of diaphragmatic hernia. The abnormality is caused by a defect in the muscles forming the diaphragm so that these do not fit closely around the distal end of the œsophagus and part of the stomach is pulled through the opening into the thoracic cavity. Sphincter control is impaired and there is a constant reflux of gastric secretions and food into the œsophagus. As a result the baby starts regurgitations within a week of birth. He fails to gain weight as much food is lost in this way and if the condition is not corrected, ulceration

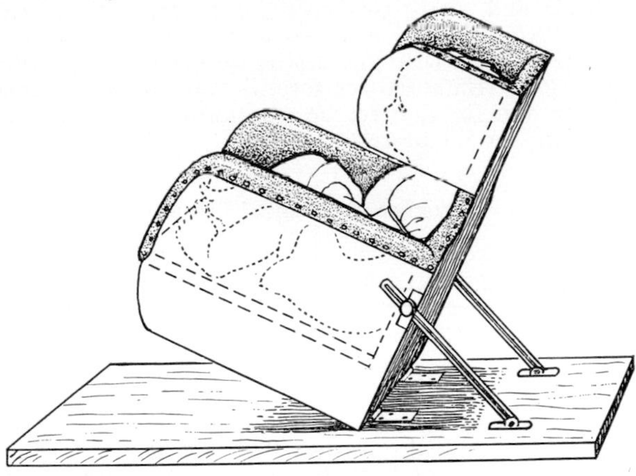

Fig. 13. Hiatus Hernia Chair.

This can also be used for the collection of a specimen of urine or fæces. In this case part of the seat is removed and a receiver placed underneath the seat.

of the lining of the œsophagus results. The milky vomit may become streaked with blood. In time the œsophagus becomes scarred, and stenosis, shortening and fixation develop at the distal end. Regurgitation is worst when the baby is laid down in his cot.

The diagnosis is confirmed by a barium swallow and X-ray but sometimes this procedure has to be repeated once or twice before the condition is proved. In some cases œsophagoscopy is performed.

Treatment in mild cases consists of keeping the baby constantly in an upright position and this position should be maintained day and night and even when the baby is bathed or nursed (Fig. 13). In this way the stomach is kept below the diaphragm and vomiting made more difficult by force of gravity. It may help to thicken feeds with Nestargel or with Benger's and mild cases are likely to improve when a solid diet can be started. Severe cases which are not likely to respond to postural therapy are best treated by surgery.

Operation for Repair of Hiatus Hernia. Thoracotomy is performed and the stomach reached through the left side of the chest. The organ is replaced in the abdominal cavity below the diaphragm, the hiatus stitched closely around the œsophagus and the defect in the muscle repaired. The chest is then closed and after-care is similar to that of any case of thoracic surgery. As soon as his condition permits the child is, however, returned to his hiatus hernia chair and the upright position maintained for several more weeks. Recurrence is common and for that reason optimism with regard to permanent cure should be restrained.

Tracheo-œsophageal Fistula

Tracheo-œsophageal fistula (also termed *atresia of the œsophagus*) is a congenital abnormality in which there is both an atresia and an associated fistula. There are several common variants of this condition.

1. The distal end of the œsophagus opens into the trachea near its bifurcation.
2. The œsophagus is not continuous, but neither of the blind ends open into the trachea (there is no fistula).
3. The proximal end of the œsophagus opens into the trachea.

Symptoms vary according to the abnormality but in the main they cause regurgitation and inhalation of food and

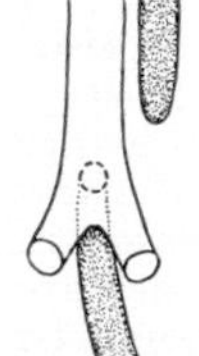
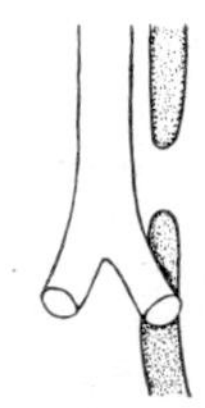
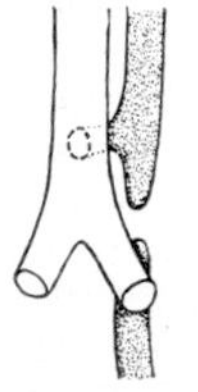

Fig. 14. Common Varieties of Tracheo-Œsophageal abnormalities.

secretions and regurgitation of hydrochloric acid from the stomach. Aspiration pneumonia and ulceration of the lining of the œsophagus result. Coughing and choking occur from birth, as saliva accumulates and spills into the lungs. It is vitally important that this should be reported at once since, if feeds are started, the baby will literally drown from inhalation of feed. In those cases in which there is a communication between trachea and œsophagus air enters the stomach and the intestinal tract becomes distended with air.

The diagnosis is confirmed by attempting to pass a fine catheter. Occasionally X-rays are taken, after giving a few drops of a radio-opaque substance, but this procedure is not without risk.

Treatment. This is carried out within a few hours of birth and consists of anastamosis of the two ends of the œsophagus and closure of the tracheal fistula. Occasionally a graft is necessary to bridge the gap between the two blind ends of the œsophagus. The graft may consist of some inert plastic material or may be taken from the patient's own intestinal tract. Occasionally it is necessary to do the repair in two stages. In that event the proximal end of the œsophagus is brought on to the surface at the base of the neck and through it secretions are discharged. It also makes it possible to give the child a certain amount of food so as not to deprive him completely of oral feeding and in order to develop a normal swallowing reflex. A gastrostomy is established through which the baby can be fed. Later, when the structures are larger and the infant stronger, extensive surgery is undertaken. Even the simplest repair of such a severe abnormality is a serious matter within hours of birth and very careful and experienced nursing care is required. The usual points which apply to the nursing of any case of thoracotomy are described in Chapter 9.

Post-operative shock is usually severe. The baby should be handled as little as possible and it is convenient to use an incubator in which the temperature and humidity can easily be adjusted, oxygen given and the plane tipped so that the foot end can be raised to treat shock and the head end raised during feeding, without disturbing the baby. If a one-stage repair has been possible a gastric tube may be left *in situ* for several days and the first oral feed given consists of a few drops of sterile water, to test the adequacy of the anastamosis. If feeds have to be given through a gastrostomy tube they are given very slowly to avoid distension. The funnel should be held 1 inch above the chest when lying flat so that gas can escape if necessary. Special attention is given to the surrounding skin and to the care of the mouth.

Both before and after operation excess saliva may have to be aspirated by means of a sucker. An intravenous infusion will be set up as soon as diagnosis has been confirmed and by this means hydration is maintained and the electrolytes regulated. Penicillin is given to prevent chest infection. Gentle vibration of chest and back and postural drainage are started as soon as the condition is recognized and continued postoperatively.

Duodenal Atresia

Duodenal atresia causes vomiting soon after birth. At first the vomit is merely milky but soon it changes to bile-stained or clear fluid and later to a fæculent vomit. There is obvious distension and visible peristalsis. On X-ray the distal part of the gut is free of gas.

Treatment. Even though intestinal obstruction calls for emergency treatment the infant has to be carefully prepared. A Ryle's tube is passed and any gastric contents aspirated, an intravenous infusion is set up, blood taken for grouping in readiness for transfusion and the urine tested for chlorides. The patient is likely to be shocked and handling should be gentle and reduced to essentials and he should be protected from exposure to cold and draughts.

At Operation. The site of the obstruction is sought and a short-circuit gastro-enterostomy or resection of the stenosis and anastamosis of the normal segments performed.

Postoperatively. The infant requires the usual care given after any major operation. The intravenous infusion is continued until hydration and electrolyte balance are satisfactory and oral feeding has been established. Gastric aspirations with a syringe are continued until only a few millilitres are aspirated every few hours. Any strain from distension on the anastamosis should be avoided. The prognosis is as a rule a good one. Feeding is commenced when the aspirate has almost stopped and bowel sounds can be heard. Bland fluids are given at first and when milk is introduced expressed breast milk is the food of choice and this is at first given in dilution; strength and amount are increased on the same principle as for a pyloric schedule.

Imperforate Anus

Every baby should be examined to exclude an imperforate anus at the time of the first toilet, but even if this is omitted, failure to pass meconium will soon arouse suspicion that an abnormality may be present. The deformity may be superficial or deep and it may involve the genito-urinary tract as well as the rectum (see page 284). On examination the anus may appear as a dimple or there may be a minute hole through which a small amount of meconium is discharged. The anus may be merely hidden by skin which covers a normal rectum and sphincter. More commonly there is a gap between the anal dimple and the blind end of the intestine.

Signs and Symptoms. Within 48 hours of birth at the latest, the three typical signs of complete obstruction will develop: vomiting, abdominal distension and complete constipation.

In order to determine the distance between the blind end of intestine and the perineum the infant is held upside down under the X-ray screen. Intestinal gas thus rises to the apex of the blind pouch. A marker is placed over the anal dimple and the distance between the marker and the apex measured.

Surgical Treatment. In the most favourable cases the superficial skin can be pierced and the underlying anus dilated. At other times it is possible to pull the rectum through and create a normal anus with good sphincter control. A colostomy is often done as a first measure until the baby is bigger and surgical reconstruction more easily carried out. In some cases there is either no sphincter or the distance between the end of the gut and the anus is so great as to make anastamosis impossible. In either instance a permanent colostomy will be necessary.

Congenital Obliteration of the Bile Duct

In spite of the fact that obliteration of the bile duct is congenital, symptoms may be at first either missed or mistaken for physiological jaundice. Contrary to the jaundice in the physiological variety the jaundice in case of obliteration of the bile duct fails to improve and the baby becomes more deeply jaundiced until he is almost olive colour. The urine and saliva are stained with bile and the stools are grey, clay coloured or white. The obstruction to the normal flow of bile is due to a complete block or absence of a segment of the common bile duct, so that bile cannot pass through it, although a small amount of bile can escape together with the succus entericus.

If left untreated, jaundice gradually deepens, liver and spleen enlarge and cirrhosis of the liver develops. The abdomen becomes grossly distended, the veins of the abdominal wall are engorged and ascites develops. Death takes place within 2 years.

Treatment. As the prognosis is hopeless if the condition is left untreated, operation is as a rule attempted but at the present time it carries a high rate of failure. The aim is to anastamose the common bile duct to the stomach or intestine: cholecystgastrostomy or cholecystduodenostomy. There are many complications such as breakdown of the anastamosis, leakage of bile and attendant excoriation of skin and post-operative bleeding due to delayed clotting time. This is not easily controlled even if prophylactic vitamin K has been given.

Nursing Care. This is largely symptomatic and aims at keeping a seriously ill baby as comfortable as possible.

Ophthalmia Neonatorum

Any purulent discharge from the eye within 21 days of birth is notifiable, irrespective of the cause.

Ophthalmia neonatorum once accounted for a high proportion of blindness in children, but nowadays owing to adequate prophylaxis and treatment with antibiotics, eye infections rarely have serious consequences. Symptoms vary from slight œdema of the eyelids, inability to open the eyes and presence of frank pus, to changes in the eye itself.

Infants with "sticky eyes" should be nursed with strict precautions against spread of infection and should be carefully isolated from other babies. In severe cases sterile normal saline irrigations are carried out every half hour with tube and funnel, to remove accumulated pus. Sulphonamide or penicillin drops (for example Albucid 10 per cent. solution, or penicillin in a 1 in 10,000 saline solution) are then instilled. 2½ per cent. Albucid eye ointment is used as an alternative. The following routine may be ordered: One drop is instilled every minute for the first half-hour, then every five minutes until all discharge disappears (usually a further hour) then half-hourly until the swelling subsides (usually another 8 to 12 hours) then every hour for 12 hours, and every 2 hours for another 24 hours after that. This treatment is modified according to the wishes of the doctor. If one eye only is affected, the infant should be nursed on the affected side to prevent discharge from running over the bridge of the nose into the healthy eye. His arms must be effectively restrained to prevent him from touching his eyes and so spreading the infection.

Retrolental Fibroplasia

Retrolental fiboplasia is caused by excessive oxygen therapy which may result in vascular and retinal changes and the formation of an opaque membrane behind the lens. There is no known cure for the condition. Prematurely born infants are most likely to be at risk. Now that the cause of this kind of blindness is known, it is possible to prevent it by limiting the use of oxygen to strict necessity. The concentration should not be allowed to exceed 40 per cent. The oxygen should be given for the shortest period for which it is essential. Some doctors order it to be given intermittently and when it is withdrawn the concentration should be lowered gradually until withdrawal is complete.

Methods of giving Oxygen to Infants

Methods of giving oxygen to infants include polythene mask, incubator and oxygen tent. The advantage of incubators lies in the ease with which infants can be observed and nursed, the easy adjustment of the flow of oxygen, humidity and temperature, and the adjustment of posture by tipping the plane on which the infant is lying. One to two litres of oxygen should be given per minute.

Artificial Respiration

For feeble infants artificial respiration should as a rule be carried out by merely slipping a hand underneath the baby and lifting and lowering the thorax, thus expanding the chest and lungs. Alternatively gentle pressure and release may be used on the thoracic wall. The Eve rocking method is favoured by some authorities. The baby is lifted out of his cot and at each movement the head and feet are inclined 45 degrees to the horizontal and the long axis of the body moved through a curve of 90 degrees at a rate between 15 and 20 times per minute. By alternate pressure and traction on the undersurface of the diaphragm the lungs are caused in turn to expand and empty. Another effective method of giving artificial respiration is to take hold of the baby's legs by the ankles and firmly lift the legs, bending them at the knees until they are doubled up onto the abdomen. In this way again, the pressure of the viscera moves the diaphragm up and down. Perhaps the most efficient and safest method is that which was originally used some 150 years ago and has recently come into favour again following extensive research. This method is inflation of the lungs and oxygenation by mouth to mouth breathing. When using this method it is of paramount importance to clear the airway from mucus and vomitus and to prevent air from escaping via the nose by the operator placing her cheek over the patient's nostrils. The patient's position must ensure full extension of his head, neck and trachea. The method has been found to be most effective and any considerations against this method seem paltry when compared with its life-saving potentialities.

Intravenous and Blood Transfusion

The reasons for which intravenous fluids and blood are given to children are essentially the same as for adults, but the technique varies and the responsibility of looking after the patient during intravenous therapy is far greater owing to the small amounts and structures involved.

Splinting

When a limb is used adequate splinting is essential and this is a highly skilled procedure, as immobility must be achieved without compressing important blood vessels. The splint should be well padded and covered with jaconet to make it waterproof. For an infant, the splint need be only about 3 inches wide but the length should be sufficient to allow for it to support a loop of rubber tubing. This takes the weight off the tubing and makes it possible to adjust the position of the needle in the vein by suitable padding (see Fig. 15). This method also minimizes the vibrations caused by restlessness or movement of the bottle, which in turn helps to cut down inflammation within the vein. If the internal saphenous vein is used, the splint should reach from the fold of the buttock to some 10 inches beyond the toes or if a vein in the arm is used, from the head of the humerus to some 10 inches beyond the fingers. The foot and ankle are rotated externally and immobilized on the splint by lengths of 1-inch adhesive

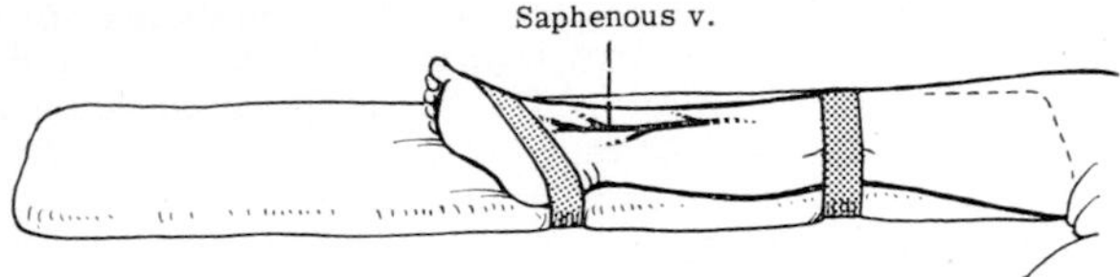

Fig. 15A. Correct Splinting of Leg for Intravenous Therapy.
Note that any strapping used must be taken over a bony prominence to prevent constriction of blood vessels.

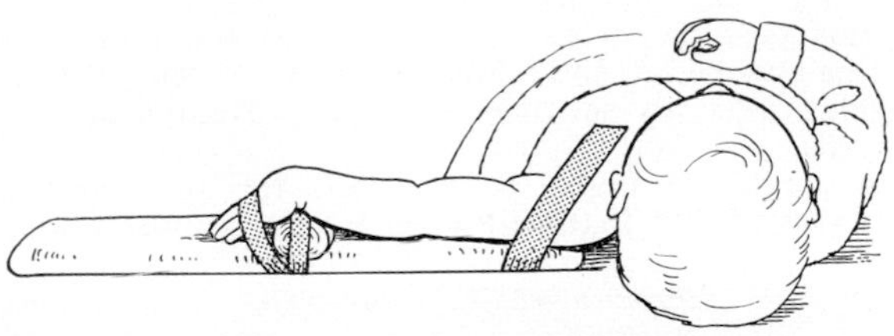

Fig. 15B. Correct Splinting of Arm for Intravenous Therapy into a Vein on the Dorsum of the Hand.
Note roll of cotton wool to prevent wrist drop.

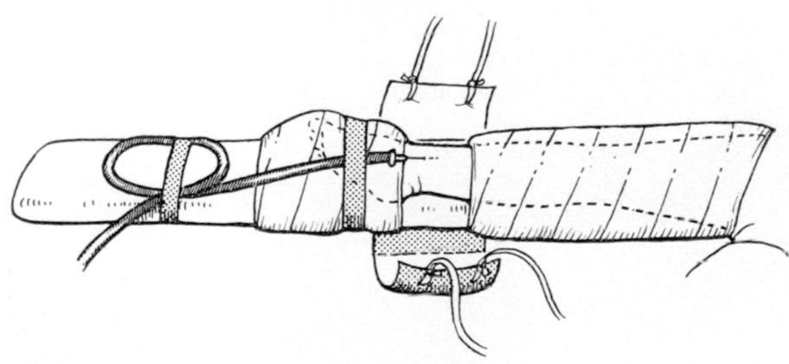

Fig. 15C. A Space is Left between Bandages for Convenient and Frequent Inspection.
The rubber tubing is stabilized on the extra length of splint. This minimizes the movement and vibration and reduces risk of thrombosis or spasm of the vein.

strapping passing across the heel just below the internal malleolus and across the bony prominence of the knee. In this way pressure on important blood vessels is avoided. If the antecubital vein is used, the arm is rotated externally and three lengths of strapping applied: one across the palm of the hand, one just below the antecubital fossa and the third high up on the arm and across the bony prominence of the shoulder. In either case a firm bandage and cotton wool are applied to give added immobility, but a space of some 2 to 3 inches is left uncovered so that the condition of the limb can be watched. A roll of cotton wool can be used to prevent foot-drop or an over-extension of the elbow. The splint should be firmly tied to the bed to ensure immobility.

Good splinting is essential, not only for the successful running of the intravenous drip infusion, but also because it enables the nursing staff to move the patient up and down the cot or to lift him out for feeding or weighing. In order to make this possible an extra length of sterile tubing should always be attached to the adult giving set. Moving the patient at regular intervals is one way of preventing hypostatic pneumonia.

Care should be taken to see that the limb and splint are not twisted and that neither groin nor rubber tubing are

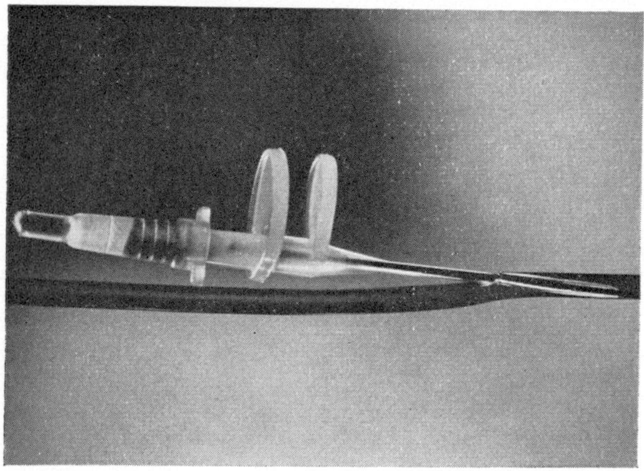

Fig. 16. A "BRAUNULA" NEEDLE.

A sterile disposable plastic cannula designed to facilitate intravenous infusion and to minimize irritation within the vein.

kinked or constricted. It is a good plan to have a bed cradle over the limb, to facilitate inspection and to support the weight of the bed clothes.

The veins most commonly used with young children are the internal saphenous and the antecubital veins, but with infants the superficial scalp veins or the veins on the back of the hand are often very satisfactory (Fig. 15B).

Procedure

Unless a superficial vein can be used, it will probably be necessary to cut down to a vein. The instruments are similar to those used for adults, but mosquito forceps and fairy Spencer Wells artery forceps and scissors replace the larger instruments. As the operator's slightest movement may prejudice his success in entering the vein, it is often wise to place the instruments on a sterile mackintosh and towel, on the patient's bed, in front of the doctor. The patient may be given a sedative and a local anæsthetic, such as procaine in a 1 or 2 per cent. solution.

The usual needles or cannulæ are often replaced by a Braunula or similar intravenous needle. The needle can be inserted into the vein unhandicapped by the weight and movement of the rubber tubing. With a child's small veins this can be of considerable advantage. Once the Braunula needle is tied into position, the tubing and adaptor, with the fluid dripping through it, can be inserted into the cannula without difficulty. The junctures may be made watertight by the application of a little sterile petroleum jelly.

Polythene tubing with a special needle and adaptor is used in some hospitals and often makes it unnecessary to cut down, even with very young infants. Alternatively, there is special polythene tubing which can be introduced into an open vein up to a considerable length without using a needle or splinting. For exchange transfusions the new-born infant is bandaged to a T-splint and the umbilical vein is used for transfusing by means of polythene tubing.

In most hospitals intravenous and subcutaneous infusion sets are of the disposable type. They are made of polythene or portex and a second chamber is incorporated which can be filled with the amount of fluid which is intended for the following hour. This is a valuable safety device. It may be useful to know that 100 millilitres/hour is 1 drop/minute, equalling 2,400 millilitres/24 hours. It is usual to give 150 millilitres/kilogram of body weight per day for the ages 1 to 3 years (2·2 pounds=1 kilogram).

Children's veins easily go into spasm when manipulated and circulation is slowed down if the infant is cold. It is important to keep the child and especially the limb warm. Even if the doctor is certain that the needle is securely in the

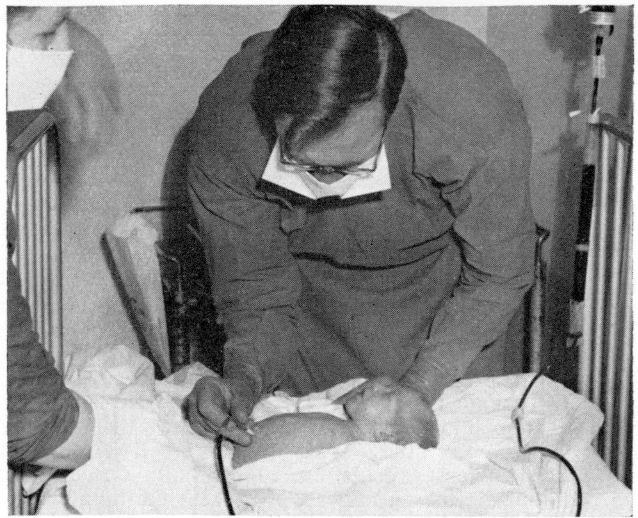

Fig. 17. Intra-peritoneal Infusion of Blood.

vein, a little time may elapse before the flow becomes established and the nurse can assist by applying warmed cotton wool to the limb. Sometimes the clip regulating the drip is left open for a while to encourage the flow. Great vigilance is then required. As the vein relaxes and the circulation improves the fluid may commence to flow freely and too large amounts of fluid may reach the patient. A nurse should remain with the patient until a regular flow has been established.

Young children and infants need constant nursing attention while intravenous therapy is in progress. The rate of the drip in the drip chamber should be checked with a watch every quarter of an hour and the amount given and absorbed should be charted. As the amounts given are very small, accuracy is essential and, for this reason, graduated paper strips are affixed to the flask and the readings are always taken at eye level. In all other respects charting is the same as that in adult wards.

In children's wards intravenous infusions may be difficult to maintain but it should be possible to have the same infusion running for four to six days. The following points may help in maintaining a regular flow.

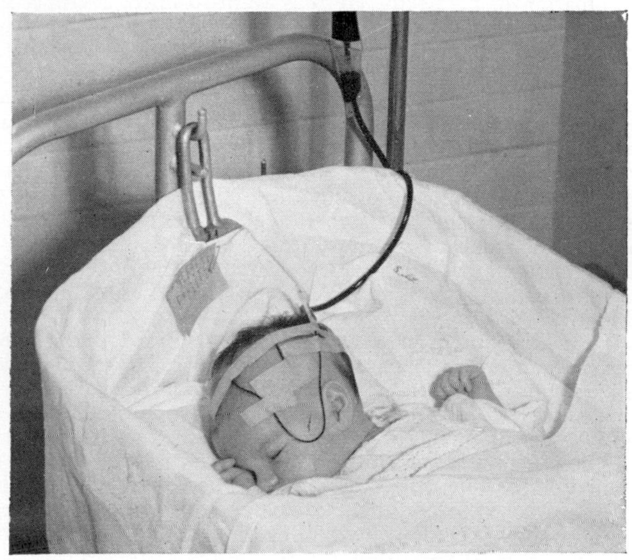

Fig. 18. INTRAVENOUS INFUSION VIA A SCALP VEIN.

Note the special chamber incorporated in the giving set for infants to assist in accuracy in adjusting quantities, and to act as a safety measure should the drip accelerate unexpectedly.

If the flow slows down, the nurse should make sure that there is no kink in either the limb or the tubing. She may take off the bandage to make sure it has not become too tight on account of œdema. The limb should be warmed with warm cotton wool or bottles filled with hot tap water and each protected by two covers. The limb may be moved or elevated and the nurse should ensure that the patient is not restless. Gentle massage of the limb may improve both warmth and circulation. Occasionally it helps to raise the intravenous flask on its stand.

If these procedures fail, a senior nurse or sister may take down the dressing and make sure that the needle is still in the vein and that its tip is not pressing against the vein wall. A slight twist of the needle may start the flow once more. If none of these measures prove effective, the House Officer should be informed and in the meantime a tray prepared in anticipation of his needs. He may want to inject a saline, procaine 1 per cent. or sodium citrate 3·8 per cent. solution into the vein and the necessary equipment should be ready for him. The injection is intended to relax the vein.

If blood is to be given, it will have been cross-matched and grouped in the laboratory, but the doctor with the nurse should check the label against the patient's record sheet. At the termination of the transfusion a few millilitres of blood will remain in the bottle and these should be saved in the refrigerator for several days to be available for laboratory tests in case of an untoward reaction. The amounts to be given in a specified time will be stated by the doctor but will rarely exceed 10 to 15 millilitres per 600 grammes of body weight.

Intravenous therapy is never without hazard. Vigilance is necessary to notice signs of pain in the chest or renal region, sudden shivering or rigor, restlessness or pyrexia, at the onset. The nurse should tighten the clip at once and stop the intravenous drip before informing the doctor. The reaction may be due to a blood clot, an air embolus, overloading of the circulation, or blood incompatibility. Phenergan or adrenaline may be ordered to counteract transfusion reaction. Long-term complications include wound infection, deep vein inflammation and transfusion jaundice.

Scalp Vein Infusion. For a scalp vein infusion, the infant's head is shaved over the parietal bone and an assistant holds the head securely. Once the needle is in position, it may be secured by strapping or by plaster of Paris approximately 3 inches in width. (Fig. 18.)

Intraperitoneal Transfusion

Intraperitoneal transfusion of blood is favoured by some pædiatricians. The procedure is simpler than intravenous infusion, quicker, safe and effective. It is usual to give heparinized blood and amounts of 50 to 100 millilitres are given at a time, the procedure being repeated if necessary.

Subcutaneous Infusion

Fluids are given by the subcutaneous route when there is an urgent need to re-hydrate a patient or to restore the electrolyte balance of the body in cases where it is expected that the patient will soon be capable of taking adequate fluids by mouth or while a difficult intravenous infusion is being set up. This procedure may be used with pyloric stenosis, with patients suffering from shock, when there is pre- or post-operative need for re-hydration, and sometimes when the apparatus and skilled care needed for giving fluids by the intravenous route are not available.

Two methods are commonly used:

(*a*) the fluid is given by syringe and needle (when the amounts given are limited to approximately 30 ml. at a time);

(*b*) the fluid is given over a period of hours by the drip method (when up to 600 ml. can be given in 24 hours).

Isotonic solution of saline or Hartmann's solution are commonly used. Hyaluronidase (Hyalase) is given to assist absorption.

Hyalase is supplied in ampoules of 1,500 units per vial. This is mixed with saline 2 ml. ampoule and one vial each injected into the rubber tubing about 1 inch above the needle, or given as a subcutaneous injection. The hyalase may be repeated after 6 hours if absorption is unsatisfactory.

The usual sites for giving subcutaneous fluids are: the outer aspects of the thigh; the abdominal wall; and the chest wall over the pectoralis muscle. The procedure is a strictly sterile one and is usually carried out by the nursing staff.

Subcutaneous Infusion by the Drip Method into the Thighs

The apparatus needed includes a sterile dressing trolley, a syringe and needle, a flask containing the sterile fluid standing in a jug of warm tap water, the subcutaneous set, ankle restrainers, bootees, a mackintosh and a napkin, and a light, newly laundered blanket or shawl. The subcutaneous set consists of rubber tubing, a Y connection, three gate clips, a drip chamber, two needles 2·5 centimetres, narrow strapping, a bed cradle and two vials of Hyalase. Occasionally a light sedative is given.

When the apparatus has been assembled the air is expelled from it and the drip (approximately 60 drops per minute) is adjusted with the help of the clip on the centre piece of tubing. The infusion sites are cleaned and the needles are inserted subcutaneously. They are secured with strapping and covered with a small dressing.

During the procedure it may be necessary to discontinue the infusion on one side or the other by adjusting the clip on that side. Although the site is bound to swell, the area must never be allowed to become cold, white, shiny or hard and for this reason frequent inspection is essential. A drip record chart must be kept.

6

CHILDREN IN HOSPITAL

In this chapter particular reference is made to the pre-school child of approximately 9 months to 5 years admitted to hospital, as the problems arising here are of a special nature, while those concerning the older child are less complex and more akin to problems of adults with which the reader will already be familiar.

Young nurses dealing with children for the first time may well be puzzled by the problems arising from their behaviour. They will understand them far better if they consider them in relation to the child's family and social background. Children, in the same way as adults, are the product of their country, their district, their educational and social environment, their daily pursuits and contacts; but what applies to the adult applies to children in a far greater degree. The younger the child, the more dependent will he be on his mother or his mother substitute. It is important to realize that in many families the grandmother means as much to the young child as his mother, and that she often looks after him during the mother's absence at work. (NOTE. This should never be forgotten when visiting is considered.) In addition, the pre-school child is defenceless and immature both in body and mind. He cannot express himself clearly. He has not yet learned to be adaptable and to make easy social contacts, and he misses his usual routine, his diet, familiar streets and familiar faces, occasionally beyond endurance. His emotional development is still immature and he lives in the present, incapable of understanding a tomorrow. He has a lively imagination and readily interprets what he sees and hears into frightening fantasies. He is very sensitive to the tone of people's voices, to their gestures and to the expressions on their faces and may read fearful and alarming things into them. Doctors and nurses should always bear this in mind when talking about a child in a ward or out-patient department.

Hospital routine may be particularly disturbing to children. To many of them being put to bed in the daytime implies punishment. This should be considered particularly with children admitted from a waiting list or merely for investigations. They do not feel ill and to put them to bed on admission can only add insult to injury and serves no useful purpose. Many children share a bed at home and few are used to cot sides after the age of 2 or 3 years. To sleep alone in a high, white bed, surrounded by bars can in itself be a disturbing experience.

The *newly-admitted child* may never have seen people dressed in nurses' uniform and to some, hospital, doctors and nurses have in the past been used as threats. (It frequently happens that children are drawn to the ward cleaners, presumably because they wear less unfamiliar clothes and, in the case of a local hospital, talk the dialect to which the child is used.)

Children are very dependent on a familiar routine, and no other person can imitate precisely the way in which the mother would set about the daily toilet or the dressing and undressing routine. This may lead to distress as well as protest. Children are readily labelled as having food fads. But here again, the child is used to certain foods, cooked and served in the way favoured by his mother at home. Family menus are very repetitive and only rarely will hospital diet be anything like the meals to which the child has been used.

Using a pot may be a worrying experience to a child who at home is used to going to the lavatory. Occasionally children fail to use the pot when given one, only to wet or soil themselves a few moments after it has been taken away. This is rarely due to naughtiness and should be treated with understanding. It is often helpful to place the pot on a piece of mackintosh on the floor where it is easier to balance than in bed, and where the child may feel more secure. To balance the pot in bed requires some skill and the child will inevitably tighten up his muscles including those of the bladder and anal sphincters. For that reason the child may be unable to use the pot but as soon as he comes off it and is able to relax, he wets and soils himself.

The nurse should try to appreciate fully what this new experience of coming into hospital means to both mother and child and, whenever possible, should have a chat with the parents of the child she will be caring for and find out as much as she can about his habits and his home background. The following questionnaire is designed to assist nurses in finding out as much as possible about the newly admitted child and is particularly helpful in hospitals where "patient assignment nursing" is practised, and for children below the age of five years.

Patient Assignment Nursing

Questionnaire used for children under 5 years of age

Name of patient ....
Age last birthday .... Birthday ....
By what name is the child known? ....

Names of other children in the family:

Brothers	....	Ages	....
	....		....
Sisters	....		....
	....		....

By what name does he call his granny? ....

Milestones:

Does he sit up without support? ....
Can he feed himself without help? ....(does he use spoon, fork, knife) ....
Does he drink from a bottle or cup? ....
Does he go to a nursery school? ....
„ „ „ „ „ day school? ....
„ „ „ „ an ordinary or special school? ....

What is his usual bedtime? ....
Does he sleep alone? (*a*) in a pram? ....
(*b*) in a cot? ....
(*c*) in a bed? ....

With whom does he share a bed? ....
Does he take a favourite toy, dummy or "Bye-Byes" to bed with him? ....
Has the child brought this article with him? ....

Toilet Training:

Does he wear a napkin? .... by day? ....
by night? ....
Are his toilet habits well established? .... still very new?......
Does he use a pot? ....
What does he say if he wants to pass water? ....
„ „ „ „ „ „ „ „ have his bowels open? ....

Diet:

Is his appetite good? ....
Is his appetite capricious? ....
What is his favourite dish? ....
„ „ „ „ beverage? ....

Occupation:

What types of toys does he like best? ....
Does he watch television regularly? ....
What is his favourite T.V. programme? ....

Has he ever been away from home? ....
Has he ever been separated from his mother? ....
state reason ....

Has he ever been to hospital ?........ state reason ....
at what age was this? ....

Any special points of interest:

What is the child complaining of? ....
(any pains, deformities, etc.) ....
....

Does he know why he has come to hospital? ....
....

Does he know how long he is likely to stay?........

Note for the child's "own" nurse:

Admission to hospital and separation from the family (the mother in particular) may be a frightening and even harmful experience to young children. By knowing as much as possible about your patient you can help to minimize the trauma and give a feeling of security to both child and mother. If you wish, you may take further case notes on your patient and keep this questionnaire for your personal files after the child has been discharged.

Almoner and Health Visitor can do much to give added information and they are always happy to be called in to help. It is often possible to adjust hospital routine and procedures in certain ways and an imaginative, interested nursing staff can do much to mitigate the trauma of a hospital admission. Those nurses who are used to dealing with adults will have to take particular trouble in adapting themselves to the nursing of sick children.

Children admitted to a surgical ward may need particular consideration. It often happens that they have been on the waiting list for some time and that they feel perfectly fit and are unaware of any abnormality which requires surgery and treatment. In these cases it is always important to take some time over explaining to the child in simple words that a certain treatment or operation will be undertaken. If the result is likely to be painful, such as a sore throat following tonsillectomy, or immobility, such as may follow an orthopædic procedure, the child should be carefully warned. Truthfulness towards children is always rewarded by trust and co-operation.

Elective surgery should be carefully planned so that admission at periods when the child is already under stress from other causes may be avoided. Whenever possible such operations should not be planned between the ages of 9 months and 3 years, at a time when the child starts schooling, when a new baby is expected while the child would be in hospital, or when there has been recent serious illness or a death in the home.

Children, like adults, are inclined to associate their own illness with illnesses they have heard discussed by adults and it is not uncommon for a child to have serious fears and fantasies for that reason. Children also resent and fear the loss of organs or parts of their bodies and can be seriously disturbed by the thought that a part of their body such as the tonsils have been "thrown in the dustbin". It is often a good plan to reassure the child by saying something to the effect that this part of his body was no longer needed and that he would get on without it even better than before. Fears of this kind are rarely expressed, but a good nurse should recognize the child who is in need of such reassurance.

Children are sometimes told that the operation will take place while they are asleep. Unless careful distinction is made between the usual sleep and this special one "which is quite different from any other" a child may try to keep awake at night in self-defence, as it were, against the operation.

Long periods of starvation and the giving of enemata or purgatives before operation are quite unnecessary and may even be harmful. Any routine of this kind is outmoded and should not be carried out unless there is a specific reason for it.

The premedication should preferably be given to the child by his own nurse, whom he knows and trusts. He should go to the theatre asleep or at least in a state of drowsiness. He should be allowed to hold his favourite toy, even if this has to be protected by a polythene bag for the sake of hygiene. It is often possible to give the drug which will send the patient to sleep some time before giving the atropine. Even though the injection may rouse the child, it is rarely remembered and in the majority of cases the child settles off to sleep again almost at once.

Surgical after-care in children calls for acute powers of observation and for fine judgment. Changes occur rapidly and delay in taking action or seeking advice may be serious. Changes in the blood chemistry, loss of blood, lack of oxygen and dehydration are all badly tolerated and young children become very toxic and disturbances in the renal function occur easily. On the other hand children recover more rapidly than adults. They rarely need to maintain a special position and can usually be allowed to adopt whatever position they find most comfortable. The absence of anxiety about themselves usually causes children to relax better than adults and muscular pain and tension rarely prevent a child from free movement, as they might do in the adult. Most small children will be ready to run around the ward the day after such operations as herniotomy or mastoidectomy.

Bandages and splints require careful watching and it may be necessary to restrain the patient's hands to prevent him from removing them. Bandages should be secured with adhesive tape or with a few stitches with needle and cotton rather than with safety pins.

A good nurse should never forget the parents' anxiety. She should see that they get the most accurate information they are able to understand about the child, the operation and the length of stay in hospital. Whenever possible the sister or staff nurse should personally speak to the parents the first time they enquire after the operation and so give them the maximum of reassurance about their child. In some hospitals the mother is allowed to stay with her child when the premedication is given and until he goes to sleep, and to be by the bedside when he regains consciousness.

The acutely ill child admitted to hospital is especially pathetic. He is not only feeling ill or in pain and incapable of understanding why all this is happening but, also, at a time when he would most need her, he is deprived of his mother and everything that is familiar to him. A great deal can be done to lessen the distress.

Some hospitals have delightful little books or comics which tell mother and child about the hospital and what is going to happen there. Ignorance is one of the greatest causes of fear and the better informed the mother, the more she can help her child and impart her own confidence to him.

Free visiting is another way in which separation can be made more bearable. Some parents are reluctant to visit because they think their child will cry when they have to leave. The nurse can explain to them that this is only to be expected, and that it is quite natural and far less harmful for the child that he should cry and be comforted than to feel abandoned because the parents do not visit. Visiting can be made flexible so that fathers can slip in on their way to work and mothers come when the other children can be cared for by a kindly neighbour. The freer and the more extensive visiting can be made, the happier the ward. Occasionally, too, visitors other than the parents should be allowed. This applies particularly to a well-loved grandmother and to the child's own parish priest. Ward-prayers and Sunday school are other links with a familiar routine which are appreciated.

Many mothers are eager to help with the nursing care of their child and enjoy giving him his bottle feed or a meal. Thus the mother gains in confidence and understands what is being done so that it is often possible to discharge the child far sooner than used to be the case when visiting was restricted to once a week. It should be the aim of every sick children's nurse to achieve early discharge rather than to keep a child in hospital unnecessarily. Some hospitals make it possible for the mother to be admitted with her young child and, though this arrangement is not without problems, it should be considered in many individual cases.

Not infrequently nurses themselves are tempted to become possessive and to assume the mother-role with their young patients. The nurse's wisdom, tact and skill are needed in handling this kind of situation, and the more mature the nurse, the more likely is she to succeed in striking the right balance for the good of all.

Contact with Home

Occasionally children cannot be visited, perhaps because they have come from a considerable distance. Arrangements should be made to keep up contact with home in every possible way. Examples of this are: daily postcards or parcels from home, telephone calls between mother and child, photographs of members of the family to be kept on the child's locker, Sunday school and evening prayers. Any such link with home will make the stay in hospital less traumatic.

Children of 18 months or older may still be used to a *dummy* or a bottle feed last thing at night. However much a nurse may disapprove, she must resist the temptation to criticize the mother or to break the child of the habit at this particular time. The time of sickness and separation is not the one for breaking a habit which may give much needed comfort. On the contrary, a good nurse who is unable to comfort a toddler, might try bottle or dummy on her own initiative. Sick children regress, and mothers sometimes do not disclose that their child is still used to a dummy or bottle feed, as they fear criticism from the doctor or nurse. The same applies to the child's favourite toy. It is a link with home and however dirty and worn or unattractive, the child should be encouraged to bring it with him and to keep it while in hospital. Hurry is always misplaced in a children's ward; the nurse who picks up a baby abruptly, or forgets to talk to an infant during feeding time, or leaves him crying merely because it is not changing time, is not a good nurse.

Patient Assignment

Whenever possible the child should be handled by as few people as practicable. Each nurse should be allowed to become really familiar with a small number of children, rather than work all over the ward, knowing none of them intimately. She should stand by her patient when he is examined by the doctor and carry out any treatment for him herself. He will take his diet better from the nurse he knows to be his friend who has found out his favourite dish or arranges his food in a certain way. The nurse herself will get greater satisfaction from "mothering" a few children and getting to know them really well, and she will put herself out to please the child and to win his cooperation and love. A good-night kiss from his "own" nurse can make a great difference to a homesick little child.

Nurses used to the nursing of adults often fail to realize that a few minutes spent in play or in reading to a child are as important as some complicated nursing procedure. They should never "feel guilty" if found doing so by matron or a consultant. The accompanying chart is a case in point. The child allowed to draw a picture every time he has had a drink will be willing to take the extra fluids, particularly if crayons can be supplied for the purpose (Fig. 19). The gifted sick children's nurse can think of many such means of gaining the child's co-operation. Incidentally, mothers enjoy bringing a variety of drinks for their children and are grateful for suggestions of this kind from the child's special nurse.

Well occupied, happy children get better more quickly than those who are bored or miserable. Toys are essential in a children's ward and it is desirable that nurses should know what toys are suitable at any given age. Some hospitals are

Name and Age *Rosemary Brown 6 yrs* Ward and Bed No. *Charlotte Ward – 3* Chart No. *5*.

Date and Time	Nature of Fluid	Amount of Fluid	Urine Volume	Remarks
30·10·59 4 a.m.	Orange juice	4 oz.	6 oz.	
7.30 a.m.	Cereal, Toast and Butter			FLAKES
	Milk	6 oz.	N.P.U	
9.30 a.m.	Orange juice Fruit	8 oz.	6 oz.	
11 a.m.	Orange juice	6 oz.		
12.30 p.m.	Fish, potato and peas			POTATOES
	Pudding refused		8 oz.	
	Water	8 oz.		
2 pm	Orange	4 oz.		
3.30 pm.	Tea	6 oz.		
	Boiled egg			
	Bread and butter			
	Ice cream			
6 pm.	Milk	6 oz.	6 oz.	
9 pm	Water	4 oz.		x 2
12 m.n	Water	4 oz.	4 oz.	

Fig. 19. Example of a Chart that a Child can Draw Himself.

fortunate in having a hospital school or nursery nurses who help to occupy the children and assist in keeping the ward play materials complete and in good repair.

Nurses should not be afraid of spoiling children in hospital. It is often quite reasonable to pick up a child, to comfort and to rock him for a while. This applies especially to night time when five minutes comforting may be far more effective and kinder than giving the child a sedative.

Children have a way of asking very direct questions. In some it is a phase of their development, and in others it is anxiety breaking through and needing immediate reassurance. A child's questions should always be answered simply but truthfully. Children are sensitive to dishonesty or trickery. They respond far better if they are told the truth, though this can be done in a sympathetic way and encouragement given at the same time: "this prick will hurt but if you are a brave boy it will not be for long and afterwards we will find you a nice sweet". Questions about going home should again be answered truthfully. The young child may have no conception of time and be satisfied with "it won't be long now" while his mind can be taken off the subject by drawing his attention to a toy. The older child may be helped by making a little calendar on which he himself can tick off the days or fill in a space with a small drawing. It is surprising how much discomfort or disappointment a child can tolerate if he has confidence in his nurse and is treated with courtesy and respect by her.

Kindness and tact also achieve far more than threats and no child should ever be told that his bad behaviour might prolong his stay in hospital or make further painful treatment necessary. Adults should be careful of what they say in front of the child, since he may misinterpret what he has heard.

Some children may experience a *death in the ward*. The nurse should not be evasive or mysterious when asked about this, but give a simple, straightforward answer according to the child's age. "Michael has gone back to heaven" is often all that is needed to stop a child from brooding about the incident. But at the same time it is sometimes wise to add "but this is not going to happen to you for a long time yet".

Emotional Reactions to Hospital

Many children take the experience of going into hospital in their stride. Others suffer disturbances and emotional trauma in varying degrees. Some of these are set out below and should serve as a warning to hospital staffs. Extra visiting, early discharge or admission of the mother may be desirable to minimize the emotional hazards of hospitalization.

Here are some possible reactions which should be understood and treated promptly and with sympathy: Undue and persistent crying coupled with a refusal to be comforted. Regression to more immature behaviour than would be expected at the child's age, for instance bed wetting and thumb sucking. Exceptionally good behaviour or an abnormally cooperative child. The child may be very quiet and subdued and at first glance pass for a very "good" little child, but start to cry when approached. Some children turn away from their parents when visited, others adopt aggressive or boisterous behaviour. Very young infants often fail to thrive and do not gain weight.

For some children a stay in hospital may actually be beneficial, prove an important stage in their social and emotional development and play a valuable part in the inevitable process of growing up.

The problems which arise when children of school age are admitted to hospital are far more allied to those of adults and, with some modifications, nurses in general training should not have serious difficulties in caring for them as long as they remember that kindness and sympathy, consistency, imagination and integrity are needed in a very high degree.

Giving Medicines

The medicine round in a children's ward rarely presents much difficulty as children follow each other's example and the willingness of one readily infects the others. The key-note should always be a matter-of-fact attitude on the part of the nurse giving the medicine. To approach a child with an attitude of apology and a look of disgust, coupled with elaborate promises that it will not taste bad, is likely to court disaster. The child will feel that he is, as it were, expected to dislike the taste and to make a fuss. It is far better to carry on an ordinary conversation and so take the child's mind off the subject.

Medicines for children should be camouflaged to make them palatable. This is often done in the dispensary where brightly coloured syrups of various kinds are available. Medicines are usually taken better in solution than in tablet form. Both should be placed as far back on the tongue as possible and followed by a pleasant drink or a sweet chosen by the child himself from the ward sweet tin. Sometimes it is necessary to mix a drug with a drink or some semi-solid food such as a mashed banana or jam, but even if this is done, the child should be told that the medicine is there. In these cases it is important that the food chosen is not an essential one, in case the child becomes permanently suspicious of its taste. This applies, for instance, to milk, orange juice, mince and custard. Pre-operative drugs are often bitter. If they have to be camouflaged, syrup or honey are best, as they are quickly digested and the danger of vomiting and inhalation during anæsthesia does not arise.

Some children co-operate best if they are allowed to take the medicine from a coloured spoon, through a straw or polythene tube or from a dolls' tea set. The nurse should be adaptable and use her imagination to the full. The trouble taken will be richly repaid. Drugs and medicines are best given at times not closely related to meals in case the child should vomit the feed or meal with the drug.

On the occasions where there is difficulty, it is sometimes best to take the child out of his cot and sit him on the nurse's knee safely wrapped in a small blanket. She may have to shape his mouth with one hand and pour the medicine in, but it should be remembered that this method is not without danger as a screaming, struggling child may well inhale some of the medicine thus forced into his mouth. Some medicines are best given by placing the spoon at the back of the tongue and letting the medicine go down by gravity. It is, as a rule, better to leave the child for a while and to return again later when his mood may have changed and he may be more co-operative. At all times, care must be taken to see that the whole dose is taken and that none is spat out or allowed to run down the chin or bib. Certain drugs are best followed by a small drink of water.

The effect of the drug given should be watched and recorded carefully and signs of intolerance reported at once. Punctuality in the giving is essential, as in many cases the efficacy depends on the concentration reached in the blood and a certain level may have to be maintained throughout the 24 hours. Children also get used to a certain routine and co-operate more readily if the medicine times follow a familiar pattern.

Dosage of Drugs. Children's tolerance of drugs differs from that of adults; large dosages are often well tolerated. The dosage of drugs is often based on the child's body weight. Accurate weight charts and the checking of weights by a state-registered nurse are consequently important. Occasionally the dosage is worked out as a fraction of the adult dose.

Young's rule is one that commonly used:

$$\frac{\text{age of child in years}}{\text{age + twelve}} = \text{fraction of adult dose.}$$

For example, for a child of 3 years, the dose should be:

$$\frac{3}{3 + 12} \text{ of adult dose} = \frac{3}{15} = \frac{1}{5} \text{ of the adult dose.}$$

Safety Measures in Hospital

Restrainers and Cot Sides. In hospital special precautions have to be taken for the child's safety. This is not only for the child's sake, but also because hospital authorities can be held responsible for any accident and considerable compensation may have to be paid by the Ministry of Health. From a psychological point of view, however, both restrainers and cot sides are undesirable and should be avoided whenever possible. Restrainers should never be applied routinely but only used as the result of a deliberate decision of the ward sister or of an experienced pædiatrician (or their deputies). If used, restrainers should be put on with the child's cooperation as part of the process of being dressed. When put on for the first time, the mother may be asked to be present and the cooperation of both mother and child enlisted. The right approach will allay feelings of anger and frustration and will avoid psychological trauma to the young patient.

Where the visiting hours are liberal the mother's presence may help to make the use of restrainers unnecessary, but it is important that the nursing staff should watch carefully lest the mother leaves a toddler unattended while the cot sides are still down.

Restrainers may sometimes have to be applied when there is no other method of managing the child while undergoing some form of investigation or treatment.

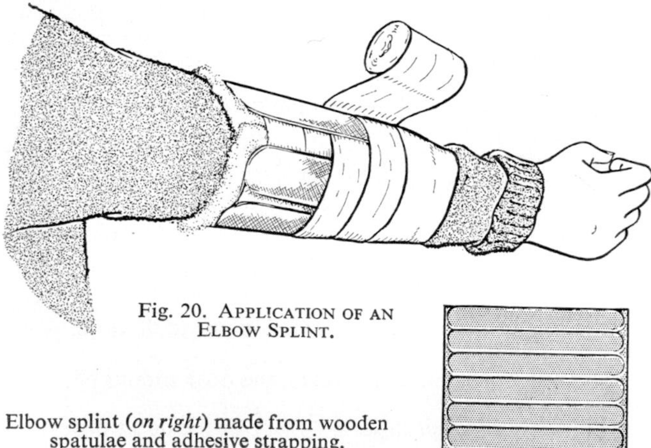

Fig. 20. Application of an Elbow Splint.

Elbow splint (*on right*) made from wooden spatulae and adhesive strapping.

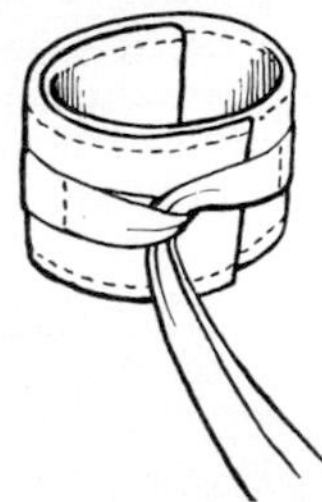

Fig. 21. RESTRAINER FOR WRISTS AND ANKLES.

Improvised restrainers must never be used (e.g. a harness made from bandages). The best restrainers consist of a close-fitting waistcoat which fastens down the back. The ties, made of webbing, should be secured to the rigid, horizontal part of the cot frame and never to the movable cot sides. The ties should be released when the child is asleep to exclude danger from strangulation and should be long enough to allow for a change of position.

In certain cases it is necessary to prevent children from touching their mouth or face as, for instance, after operation for hare-lip or strabismus. Simple splints can be made from wooden tongue depressors (Fig. 20). These restrainers are known as *elbow splints* and are applied with light, open-woven bandages. The bandage should first be carried round the child's arm, preferably over a sleeve, and then the well padded splint is incorporated in the following turns of the bandage. If this is not done, bandage and splint are liable to slip off like a cylinder. For *wrists and ankles* special restrainers can be made (Fig. 21). Alternatively a crêpe bandage tied with a clove hitch may be used. Infants are sometimes wrapped firmly in a blanket to avoid movement during procedures such as subdural tap or taking of venous blood (Fig. 22).

Accidents in Hospital

Whenever possible children should be allowed to be up and about, rather than kept in bed. This places an extra burden of responsibility on the hospital staff.

The children who present the greatest problem are the toddlers. No equipment left standing about is safe from their urge for adventure. They enjoy opening and closing doors, and easily get their fingers caught. Any unguarded electrical point lends itself to investigation, and milk and other drinks are upset for the mere fun of it.

Children's wards should be as homely as possible and untidiness will never worry an understanding ward sister. But she must be able to anticipate danger and prevent accidents by wise precautions. Some of these are mentioned below but many more could be added and others need only be put into effect when circumstances warrant them.

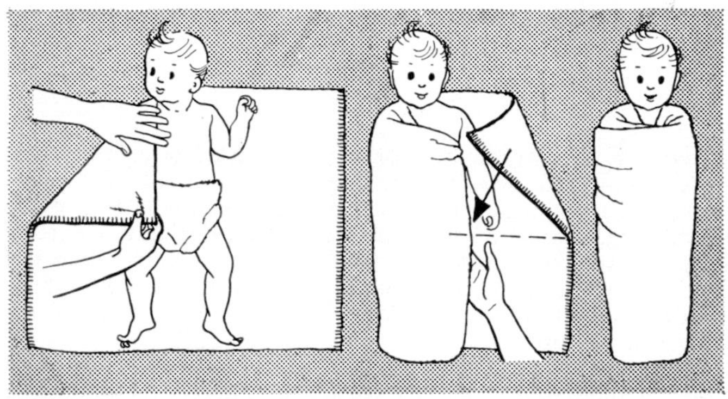

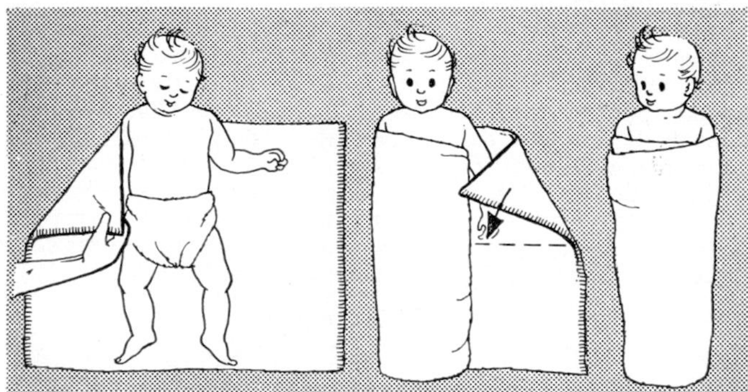

Fig. 22. RESTRAINING THE PATIENT.

Very young children should never be allowed out of sight and objects which may cause accidents should be removed or suitably guarded. These include: sterilizers, radiators, lamps and light switches, thermometers, pots and bottles containing pills, lotions or medicines. All windows should have window guards and the hot water taps in the bathrooms should be detachable and hung out of the children's reach. Children should never be left unaccompanied in the bathroom and neither bathrooms nor lavatories should have bolts or keys. Drinking glasses and sharp feeding utensils are unsuitable for the very young, and no chipped equipment must ever be allowed in a children's ward. Drinks should be just the right temperature, for a toddler will not wait to test a drink set before him but will eagerly immerse his entire face in a cup. Infants under a year should never be given a soft pillow and are usually best left without any pillows at all. If pillows have to be used they should be small, firm ones or the mattress should be raised, by placing a pillow underneath it. Hot water bottles should never be left in the bed unless by express order and even then they should be protected by two separate flannel bags covering the entire bottle. The water is best taken from the hot water tap rather than from a kettle. Electrical equipment should never be used unless a nurse can remain with the child for the entire time. Toys should be chosen for their safety and sharp, protruding corners or wires removed. *Mechanical toys which give off sparks are as dangerous in an oxygen tent as the striking of a match,* and watch must be kept on the type of toy given to children nursed in a tent.

Before taking a rectal temperature the bulb of the thermometer should be inspected and the nurse should keep a firm, restraining hand on the child to avoid sudden movement. When making the bed of a young child he is best lifted out or else a nurse should be on either side of the cot while the sides are down, or only one side let down at a time. A toddler can roll over with amazing rapidity and fall out on the far side. Bed trays left in position invite the child to climb on to them and make an otherwise adequate cot side low enough for him to fall over. Lotion-thermometers and bath-thermometers must always be used and no reliance placed on the nurse's sense of touch. Plastic bibs should never be left on a child during sleep, as there is danger of asphyxia if the bib falls over his face. Small toys and beads are unsuitable for the under-3-year-old as they may be swallowed or inhaled. Safety pins should be used only where absolutely necessary and should always be left closed, when not in use. In many instances a piece of strapping, a tape or a stitch with needle and thread replace safety pins very satisfactorily. Finally, two nurses must always be present when injections are given, as even an apparently reliable 10-year-old may suddenly loose control of himself and move, or grasp a nurse's hand, thus breaking the needle.

Any accident that occurs should be reported at once and all details recorded. The parents should be told about it when they next visit, even if the accident has been a trivial one.

Admission to Hospital

The section dealing with admission to hospital has been intentionally left to the end of this chapter. So far, an attempt has been made to describe some of the problems which hospitalization presents to both parents and children and some ways in which such difficulties can be overcome or made more easily acceptable. If these are understood a good admission routine will come almost automatically to an imaginative and sympathetic staff.

If admission is advised, the nurse should remember that what has become so familiar to her may be strange and frightening to mother and child. A few words about the hospital, about visiting and making enquiries, and about the ward and its staff will give a mother comfort and will make her feel that her worries are understood. Her child will sense her confidence, and in turn will be easier to handle and happier and more content. The nurse welcoming the new arrival should act as a hostess would do in her own home. Professional bearing and a kind and understanding attitude will give confidence to the parents and this will quickly reflect itself in the child. In some hospitals it is customary for the nurse who will be looking after the patient, to come to the admission room and meet the new arrival. She should never go there wearing a mask and gown but should put them on in front of the child if his condition demands this. It is a good idea for her to take a toy for her young patient with her.

Once in the ward mother and child should be allowed to look round, meet the other patients and see the child's bed together. As she is taking the mother round, the nurse can learn something about the new patient, such as his nickname or any of his particular interests or fears. Some hospitals have a questionnaire which the nurse fills in and which gives her much interesting information (see page 82).

Only after such a round should the nurse suggest leaving the mother to talk to the ward sister and take the child to "find some pretty clothes". Some hospitals arrange for the children to wear their own clothes. Where this is not possible, nurse and child can play at going to the clothes cupboard on a shopping expedition. The change to strange clothes is thus made easy and is not resented. A bath is not always necessary on admission and children rightly object when submitted to one at such an unusual time and in strange surroundings. If it is essential, the mother should be allowed to be present. In a children's unit it is always wise to examine the child's head to ensure that it is clean. Infestation spreads quickly to other children; it may also be the cause of scratching, leading to infection, such as impetigo and cervical adenitis. Treatment is simple with preparations such as DDT emulsion or special shampoos such as Esoderm.

Since the new patient will already have had one examination in the outpatient or admission unit, the first examination by the house doctor can be delayed for a while, until the child has got used to the ward. If the child is an emergency admission or a seriously ill child, the admission routine will have to be adapted accordingly, but in fundamentals the above points will still apply.

Examining the Child Patient

The physical examination of a child should include every part and system of the body. The technique adopted will have to vary according to the age of the child and the degree of cooperation to be expected. Once again, there should be an *atmosphere of leisure* and confidence and the child should be quiet and happy during the examination. A good children's physician will talk to the child first—no matter how young—for a quiet, pleasant voice can soothe even a very young baby. While doing so, he can observe many points of interest, among them the child's general attitude, e.g. whether he is relaxed or frightened. He can note the general standard of nutrition, physical care and cleanliness, the colour of the skin and the texture of the hair, and also muscle tone and general posture. Occasionally there may be a typical smell, or a certain typical facial expression may help in the diagnosis. The doctor may notice that the child's fingers are sore from sucking or that the finger nails look as if he were in the habit of biting them. The attitude towards the mother may likewise tell an important tale.

If the child is lying on the examination couch the position he adopts may be significant. He may draw up his knees to relieve abdominal colic or immobilize a limb to avoid pain on movement. His head may be thrown back and general opisthotonos be present, or he may turn away from the light on account of photophobia. He may be quiet and unresponsive or restless and anxious looking and his respirations may be characteristic of a certain disease. Some toddlers will roll or bang their heads if they have earache, or stuff their fingers in their mouths when they are teething.

All these details are of significance to an experienced pædiatrician or sick children's nurse, and further observations on these lines will continue after admission to the ward.

Every doctor will have his own routine in examining children but all will leave the more unpleasant or alarming procedures to the last. This applies, for instance, to inspection of the throat which few children will tolerate without protest.

Any instruments needed should be kept out of sight till the last moment and they should be warmed before placing them on the child's skin or tongue. It often pays to allow a child to handle an instrument first and to assure himself of its harmless nature before using it. Alternatively the doctor might listen to "Teddy's chest" before he proceeds to the examination of the patient.

Very young children do not understand instructions given and some little game may have to be employed to get them to do what is required. A mural on the wall or ceiling may for instance induce a child to move his eyes in the desired direction as he is told to look for a certain animal or familiar television figure. Telling a story may absorb the child's interest and so make him relax a previously rigid abdomen and, finally, a good technique in supporting or restraining children can make a great deal of difference to the success of an examination (Fig. 32).

7

SICK CHILDREN AT HOME

Whenever possible, sick children under the age of 10 should be nursed in their own homes. Chapter 6 on "Children in Hospital" will have made clear the possible dangers of admitting children to hospital and separating them from their mother and their familiar surroundings. Not every child will react unhappily to the experience of hospitalization, but some few may show disturbances for life, some serious, some of a minor nature. The pre-school child is the one most at risk in this respect.

Nursing the child at home, however, may tax a busy mother and housewife considerably. This chapter does not deal with special techniques of isolation, special diets or general nursing care. Where these are more complex than an average mother can be expected to manage, the doctor will call in the District Nurse to advise and help. In some areas there are specialized pædiatric District Nurses and well-developed Pædiatric Home Nursing services (those of Paddington, Birmingham and Rotherham are well known). Where these exist, quite difficult nursing procedures and investigations can be carried out in the home. The good family doctor will also arrange for other types of relief such as Home Helps, special laundry services and help with other children in the family. In long-term illnesses Home Teachers are available.

This chapter will give a few hints on keeping the sick child happy and occupied. Few children feel ill enough to want to be quiet and inactive for any length of time. Most will want to do things, see what is going on and demand constant company. The mother's work will probably be much reduced if she brings the sick child into the living room adjoining the kitchen, where she herself has to spend a good deal of time. Often this also means a ground-floor room with a more interesting view out of the window, a saving in heating and far less expenditure on her energy by avoiding constant journeys up and down the stairs.

There is no need to spend money on toys or books. Indeed there is the obvious danger of spoiling the child who may come to expect gifts every time he is off colour. Here are a few suggestions, inexpensive, and yet perfectly capable of serving their purpose admirably.

Ages 9–18 Months

Magazines and comics to tear up, as well as to look at; simple toys that can be taken apart; balloons, teddy-bears or dolls with various rags to dress and undress; simple rattles made from well-sealed tins filled with pieces of wood (this will make just enough noise without deafening the family); wireless and record players if available with children's records of music and stories.

18 Months to 3 Years

Old Christmas cards and magazines; large beads to string; crayons; hollow blocks and other building bricks; a small aquarium or a budgerigar. A bird table just outside the window that can easily be seen by the little patient; jig-saw puzzles or picture trays, bought or home made; conkers, daisies and other flowers to play with and examine; percussion instruments.

3 to 5 Years

Girls. Beads, conkers (through which father has made a hole); sewing cards with large, blunt needles and coloured thread; rags and bandages to dress and nurse dolls; a nurse's outfit; a doll's tea or cookery set; glove puppets (home made).

Boys. Dinkie toys, match boxes with which to build; simple construction toys; interlocking bricks.

Both sexes. Blunt, round-ended scissors; coloured paper; gummed shapes; a scribbling pad; crayons.

5 to 8 Years

Girls. Mother's button box to tidy (have a supply of match-boxes); cut-out dolls; dish-cloth yarn and thick needles for knitting dish-cloths for favourite aunts; loosely woven dish-cloths as a foundation for weaving with coloured wools and bodkin. Cotton-reels with 4 nails at one end for french knitting and coloured wool and blunt knitting needle.

Boys. A book of trains and engines, old motoring and fishing journals.

Both sexes. Tracing paper and pencils; a magnet; an old watch; a kaleidoscope; milk bottle tops to make mosaic patterns, mould or string up into "mobiles".

Match boxes to build or cover in coloured paper; paints and colouring books; bits of felt or dyed lint and scissors to cut out shapes and for picture making; Plasticine; letter and number cards; toy money. Small squares of lint stuck to figures cut out of magazines, fluffy side outwards, can be made to adhere to a board covered with lint or felt.

Pipe cleaners and large beads can be made into animals and other figures. A thick notebook can be used to make into a diary (words and drawings).

8 to 12 Years

Girls. A mirror may give hours of entertainment, either together with a few ribbons, scarves and old hats for dressing up and creating hair styles or to enable the patient to "converse" with her own image in the mirror. Scissors and thin paper for cutting out strips of people or animals and doilies by folding the paper before cutting and leaving a small piece of the contour uncut to form the link after unfolding.

Boys: Marbles; packets of inexpensive stamps, a geographical atlas and a notebook for starting a stamp collection. A mirror to play with reflections of light or sunshine; playing cards; an encyclopædia.

A few points should be remembered:

Protective sheets or mackintosh may be necessary to prevent undue soiling of the top sheet and blankets.

Supply a good steady surface such as a tray.

Sick children tire quickly, and toys and occupation will need frequent changing.

Big or complex toys tire a child more easily than small, simple toys which can easily be changed.

A toy enjoyed to-day may be boring to-morrow.

Needless to say the toys given for the various age groups will please older or younger children. It is usually possible to ask friends or neighbours for the loan of books, jigsaws or other toys no longer needed by their own children (some will be only too glad to pass them on for good). The same applies to magazines, scraps of material and gramophone records.

The charm of any of these toys and occupations will fade quickly if all are left lying around all the time. Their value is greatly enhanced and their interest doubled if they are tidied away regularly, to be brought out again another time.

After infectious fevers toys should be burned or disinfected. The local health authority will advise about this.

8

DISEASES OF THE RESPIRATORY SYSTEM

Young children are very prone to diseases of the respiratory tract, mainly due to the small lumen of the air passages and to their poorly developed immunity to infection.

During infancy and early childhood respirations are often shallow, rapid and irregular in rhythm. At birth the baby breathes about 30 to 40 times per minute, by the end of the first year the respiratory rate at rest decreases to approximately 24 to 30 respirations per minute, by the age of two it is 20 to 24 and by the age of 5 years the respiratory rate is the same as that of an adult.

Respirations

Changes in the rate and depth of respiration occur easily in children and the cause is not always in the respiratory system. Abdominal pain may cause shallow breathing while any increase in the metabolic rate, such as fever, will send the respirations up. One can learn much from the careful observation of a child's breathing. In cases of obstruction it is often important to expose the neck and chest wall and to watch for sucking in of intercostal spaces or the suprasternal notch.

The respirations are best taken when the child is asleep.

Points to notice:

The patient's colour.

Whether the chest wall expands symmetrically on inspiration.

Whether the breathing causes restlessness or distress or is merely rapid.

Whether the child breathes through his mouth or nose, and whether the accessory muscles of respiration are being used. Posture is important. For example, children whose breathing is obstructed may throw their heads back or their arms outwards in an attempt to get more air.

Examination of the Child

It is usual for a nurse to assist the physician in his examination. It is her duty to see that the patient is comfortable and well supported, and to have a small chest blanket at hand to avoid unnecessary exposure. The child who is old enough to understand should be told what is going to happen and it is usually well worth while to allow a few moments in which to gain his confidence. He might be allowed to handle the stethoscope or to listen to his own or his Teddy's chest. The stethoscope should always be warmed as the touch of the cold object will frighten the child and cause him to protest.

The physician will first watch the child's breathing for depth, regularity, complete and symmetrical expansion of the chest wall, any undue wasting and any drawing in of the intercostal spaces. He will note whether the respirations are abdominal or thoracic, and determine the position of the apex beat. By now the child will have gained confidence and only then will the physician use his stethoscope.

Special Point. When using the stethoscope on the back of a young child it is often a good plan for the doctor to hold the patient in his arms for he will know from experience that, as so often when dealing with sick children, orthodox methods are not always the most suitable ones.

X-ray Examination

It is often difficult to obtain good X-ray pictures of young children, but it will help a great deal if someone with whom the patient is familiar can accompany him to the department. With a little forethought, it is often possible to arrange for the patient's mother to be present and to assist. It is well to remember the fear a child may feel when confronted with a dark, unknown room or with the enormous structure of the X-ray apparatus. The X-ray plates and the table should be covered with a soft, warm material or protesting screams may well make the procedure both difficult and unsuccessful.

Position may be a problem in babies and toddlers, particularly when they are feeble and limp. Fig. 23 shows a simple device for supporting young infants during X-ray of the chest. Further problems arise if the child is crying. Nor can the child be expected to hold his breath during exposure. Often therefore more than one picture has to be taken and both lateral and antero-posterior pictures are required.

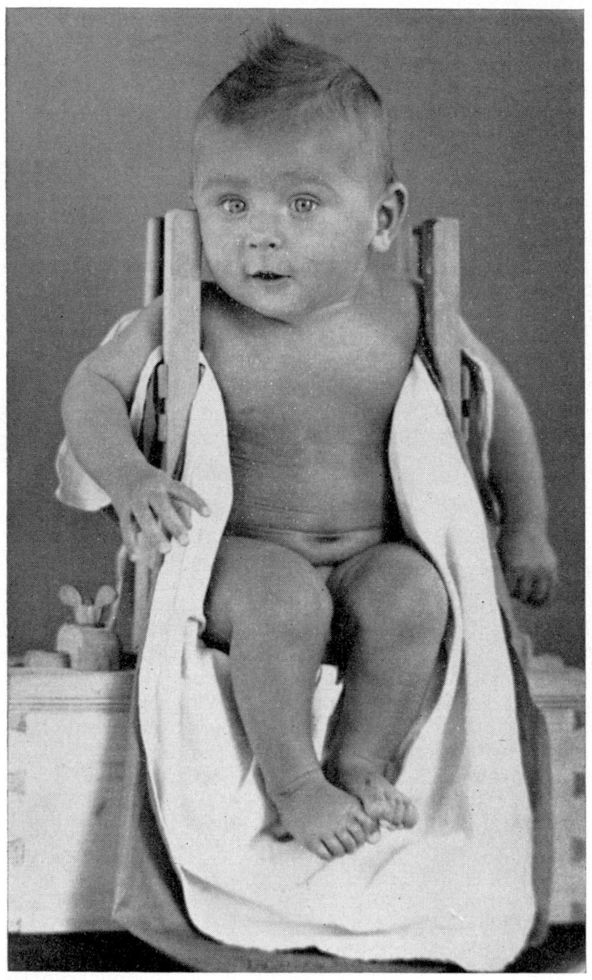

Fig. 23. A Simple Device for Supporting Young Infants for X-ray of Chest.

Special Investigations

Bronchoscopy

Bronchoscopy may be done for various reasons. At times it may be performed in order to suck out pus or viscous secretions; at other times to determine and if possible remove the cause of collapse of a lobe of the lung as for instance a foreign body or a tuberculous gland. Occasionally some tissue is removed for biopsy.

The procedure is the same as for adults, but children are usually given an anæsthetic and preparation is done accordingly. In addition the throat may be made insensitive by means of a cocaine or Decicain spray. Bronchoscopy is not entirely without danger. The small air passages may go into spasm during the bronchoscopy and cause asphyxia. A drink, given before a good swallowing reflex has returned and the effect of the local anæsthetic has worn off, may have serious consequences. Approximately four hours should elapse between spraying the throat and giving the first drink, and the nurse has a special responsibility in this respect. A test drink of a quarter of an ounce of plain water should always be given.

Bronchography

In preparing the patient for bronchography postural drainage should be carried out at night and by a physiotherapist or nurse immediately before the child goes to the X-ray department, in order to empty the bronchial tree of as much stagnant pus or mucus as possible.

Bronchograms are usually done in the X-ray department under a general anæsthetic and, again, the throat may be cocainized. Good premedication will ensure that the child is fast asleep before being moved from the familiar surroundings of the ward. Before taking the X-ray, a radio-opaque substance, usually iodized oil, is introduced into the main bronchus. This is either done by passing a fine catheter over the back of the tongue into the trachea or by inserting a needle through the cricoid membrane into the trachea. The radio-opaque substance e.g. Dionosil with sulphanilamide powder is then injected by means of a syringe and allowed to outline the bronchial tree. According to the positioning of the patient the X-ray picture will show the bronchial tree in the selected lobes of the lung. Irregular filling will be proof of abnormalities which were suspected on clinical grounds and from straight X-ray.

On return to the ward, postural drainage is started almost at once. Thus, the danger of the iodized oil, pus or secretions spilling into the healthy parts of the lung is reduced. Frequently the patient may complain of a sore throat after bronchogram and there may be a productive cough for some days.

Dionosil with sulphanilamide powder, or any other oily substance used for bronchograms, may set up sensitivity reactions due to its iodine content, and it is important first to carry out a simple sensitivity test.

Chest Aspiration

The requirements for chest aspiration are similar to those needed for adults.

The procedure is not really a painful one but it is very uncomfortable and may prove alarming to a young child. He should be told as much about what is going to happen as he is likely to understand and a sedative should always be given.

The patient is made comfortable lying over a pillow, or sitting up and resting on a bed table and pillow. He should be kept warm and, if he is awake, the nurse should distract his attention by reading to or playing with him while the aspiration is carried out. Warning of any injection should be given immediately before the prick and care taken not to let the child see anything of the preparations. Occasionally it is useful for the nurse to have the patient on her lap and to comfort and restrain him in this position.

A warm, sweet drink at the end will often help to settle a somewhat agitated patient and may induce a restful sleep.

Steam Tents

Various types of steam tents (Fig. 24) are in use, but the aim should always be to achieve maximum benefit from the warmed air while allowing for a clear view of the child, as well as for free circulation of moistened air within the tent.

The usual precautions are taken, such as not directing the steam towards the patient's face, but in addition children should wear a loose safety bodice and some sisters like them to wear cotton mittens as well. The spout of the kettle may be protected by bandages as an extra safety measure. A steam kettle may also be a danger to other children running around

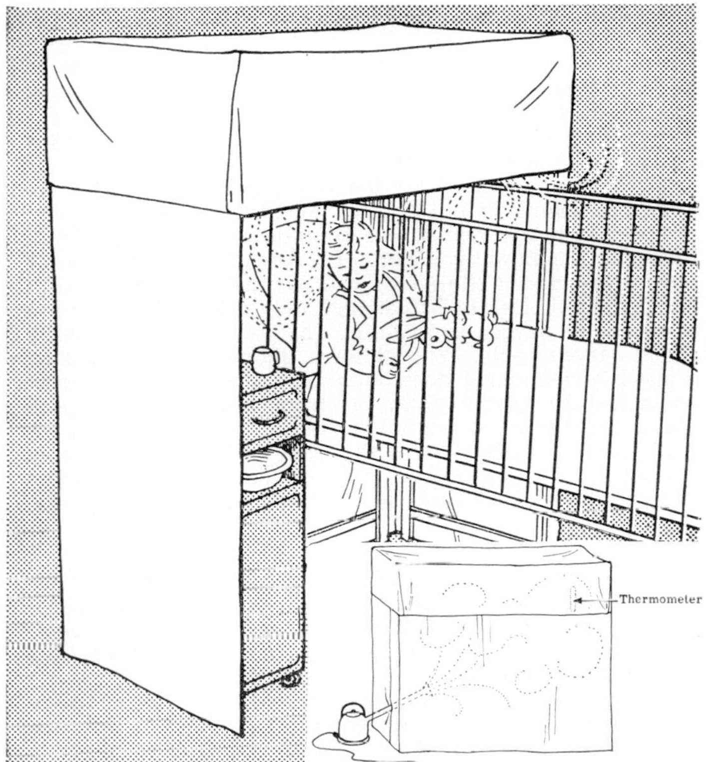

Fig. 24. General View of Steam Tent.
Note restrainers, full face position of patient, and steam circulating in from the back. *Inset*. Rear view, showing good circulation of steam and position of thermometer.

in an open ward and suitable precautions should be taken to avoid accidents.

Whenever possible, a special nurse or the child's mother should stay with the patient while steam therapy is in progress. Alternative methods of humidifying air are steam cubicles and Croupaire, a cool-vapour humidifier, or a Humidaire tent. As soon as the acute stage of the illness is over, plenty of occupation will help to keep the child at rest and this will also help to avoid accidents.

Oxygen Therapy

Up to a short time ago, oxygen therapy was thought to be free of hazard to the patient. More recently, a warning against indiscriminate use has been sounded. A particular danger is the use of too high a concentration of oxygen in the care of premature infants (see page 47).

When oxygen is used for the sick child *the amount to be given* per minute should be ascertained from the doctor and mentioned on any report. An accurate flowmeter is needed. To count the flow by means of a *Woulfe's bottle* is rarely satisfactory, and it should be realized that a speed at which individual bubbles can be counted, only delivers 0·5 of a litre of moistened oxygen per minute. The precautions usual when giving oxygen apply. With children the danger from striking a match and smoking does not exist, but explosions can also be caused by sparks given off from mechanical toys and visitors need to be warned about this.

Children soon show signs that they lack oxygen by being restless and looking anxious. The respirations become rapid and gasping, and the lips and extremities cyanosed.

Methods of giving Oxygen

Not all methods used for giving oxygen to adults are suitable for children. In newly-born infants oxygen given in an endotracheal tube or oxygen via an *incubator* are the most commonly used. Later there are various models of oxygen tents for use at different ages.

Patients having a tracheostomy may have to be given oxygen. In these cases the oxygen can sometimes be delivered directly into the tracheostomy tube by means of a rubber or polythene catheter, or a specially designed perspex collar and fittings.

Acute Bronchitis

Acute bronchitis most frequently attacks children from overcrowded homes who are ill-nourished and debilitated. It is a common complication of measles or influenza, and children suffering from fibrocystic disease of the pancreas, mongolism or congenital heart defects are particularly prone to this and other chest infections. In young children the illness remains a serious one.

Signs and Symptoms. The child suffering from acute bronchitis looks and feels ill. His cheeks are flushed and his skin and mouth are dry due to a fever of 39·4° to 40·6° C. (103° to 105° F.) or more. Respiratory difficulties make him restless and irritable. The accessory muscles of respiration come into play and the alæ nasi may be working. The respiratory rate is increased and the respirations may be shallow due to pleural pain. A cough, harsh and dry at first but later productive, is present throughout the 24 hours and is both an early and an exhausting feature of the illness.

In young children the sputum is swallowed and this may at times lead to gastric irritation and vomiting. Occasionally the mucous secretions form a plug in one of the bronchial tubes causing collapse of a lobe or segment of the lung.

Specific Treatment. Oxygen therapy may be of use, provided the atmosphere is kept moist during the early, dry stage of the illness. Steam may be used to warm and moisten the atmosphere of the room but the high concentration achieved by putting up a steam tent is not as a rule suitable for patients with acute bronchitis.

Drugs. Appropriate drugs, such as penicillin, sulphonamides and antibiotics are given to combat the infection. Antispasmodic drugs are used in selected cases. Cough mixtures and expectorants are rarely of value for children, particularly if the patient is very young.

Complications. Collapse of one or more sections of the lung, anæmia, tuberculosis and general debility may follow the acute stages of the illness, while in young babies diarrhœa and vomiting are frequently associated with it.

Nursing Care. Children suffering from acute bronchitis are best nursed in warm, well-ventilated rooms and should be allowed to adopt any position they find comfortable, though several pillows arranged to give maximum support are usually needed. Alternatively the foot end of the bed may be raised and all pillows removed to promote drainage by gravity. Unless the patient does so himself, the position should be changed frequently so as to move the secretions and to avoid the formation of mucous plugs. When secretions are profuse and the patient too weak to cough them up, the use of a sucker and occasionally even of bronchoscopy may become essential. For the relief of pain warmed Gamgee applied to the chest may be very comforting though care should be taken not to overheat the child. Poultices are heavy and consequently not suitable for young patients.

For the relief of coughing, warm drinks should be given and often warm milk and honey are enjoyed and very effective. Fluids should be given freely, but sore throat, tracheitis and cough may cause the patient to be reluctant and difficult. For bottle-fed babies the feeds are best given diluted during the acute phase and spoon feeding may prove less exhausting than sucking. The feeds should be small and frequent so as to avoid distension of the stomach and resulting pressure on the diaphragm.

Temperature, pulse and respirations are taken 4-hourly and any changes reported at once. The pulse volume should be watched with special care. Intake and output charts should be kept well up to date as intake may be small. As the illness is as a rule an acute one, and of short duration, mouth toilet, treatment of pressure areas and the care of the bowels present few problems.

Young infants may show signs of intolerance to certain antibiotics, such as achromycin (Tetracycline). A preparation of vitamin B is given at the same time to try and prevent diarrhœa and thrush. If diarrhœa should develop it can often be improved by adding Arobon or arrowroot to the bottle-feeds. For the treatment of thrush see page 199.

Bronchiectasis

Children who have had several attacks of bronchitis may develop bronchiectasis in a form which differs very little from that seen in adults. Children so affected are pale, under-nourished, under-developed and generally suffer from poor health. They usually have chronic upper respiratory tract infections and frequently the mother gives a history of several attacks of otitis media, sinusitis and chronic cough. The teeth may be carious and the tongue coated. Halitosis is common and these children usually breathe through their mouths on account of the chronic nasal obstruction which is present. Hearing is frequently impaired. The chest wall may be deformed, there is shortness of breath and often a low-grade fever. Sputum is profuse, purulent and very offensive in advanced cases. The younger children are inclined to swallow the sputum, which causes gastric irritation and loss of appetite. Interrupted schooling, the result of frequent admissions to hospital, adds to the impression of dullness so often seen in these children.

Straight X-rays and bronchograms are done to confirm the clinical diagnosis. The sputum is sent for culture and for tests to determine the sensitivity to various drugs of any organisms present. White blood counts, blood sedimentation rate, Mantoux test, and sinus X-ray are done. Antrum wash-out may be necessary for the frequently associated sinus infection, and dental treatment should be given when indicated.

Medical Treatment

In mild cases, or in those in which the disease is scattered through several lobes of the lung, postural drainage, physiotherapy and disinfectant inhalations remain the treatment of

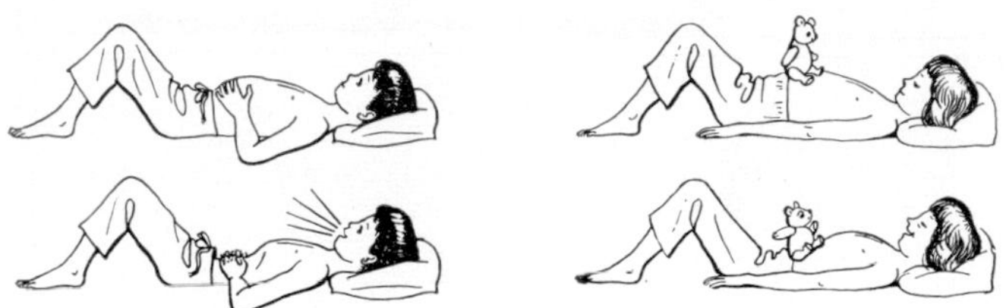

Fig. 25. Breathing Exercises can be Made to be Fun.

choice. In cases in which the diseased areas are well defined, lobectomy gives very good results.

In either case, the patient should have intensive physiotherapy and should be taught breathing exercises to develop his chest (Fig. 25) and the correct position to encourage drainage at night. Special frames are available and ordinary beds can be adapted for the purpose (Figs. 26 and 27). From the physiotherapist, nurses and parents can learn to understand the positions which allow for maximum drainage of the affected lobe. The child should be allowed up and should have plenty of fresh air and exercise to improve the general tone as well as the finicky appetite. Activities such as hospital school or occupational therapy improve morale, and nurses should treat these children with sympathy and kindness, remembering the tedious nature of the treatment and the repeated admissions to hospital. Morning and evening temperatures are taken and observations are made on the nature of the respirations and the type and persistence of cough. The sputum must be accurately measured and its appearance noted. The child should be encouraged to expectorate, particularly on waking in the morning, and a warm drink given first thing may help him to do so. A teaspoonful of compound mixture of sodium chloride in hot water, sipped slowly and given three times a

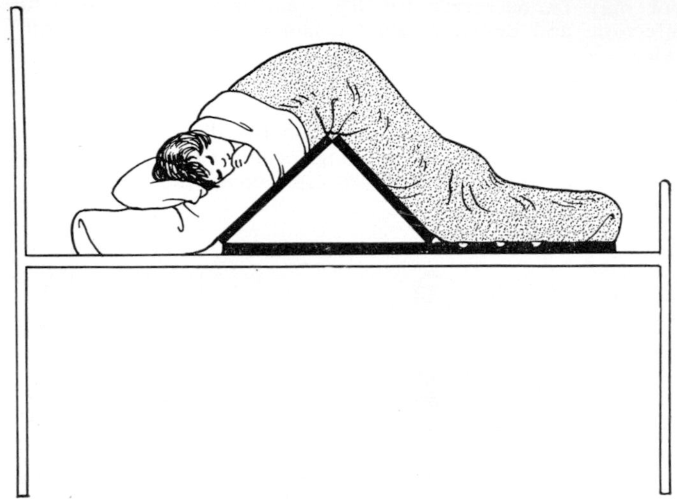

Fig. 26. Postural Drainage for Bronchiectasis.
Children soon get used to sleeping in this position.

day before meals is also helpful. Disinfectants should never be placed in a sputum mug in a children's ward but chlorophyll tablets added to the sputum will combat offensive smells.

Inhalations may help to loosen secretions. When giving inhalations the nurse must remain with her patient throughout the treatment to ensure his safety and to see that the treatment is efficient. She should encourage both coughing and expectoration. Paper handkerchiefs should be provided and the child taught to clear his nose thoroughly on waking and frequently during the course of the day. It often helps to allow the child to hang head downwards over the edge of the bed for a moment or two before blowing his nose, in order to drain the sinuses.

The diet should be nutritious and the addition of protein often helps to build up general strength.

Almoner and school medical officer can arrange for the child's admission to an open-air school where regular medical supervision, additional rest periods and physiotherapy are available during school hours.

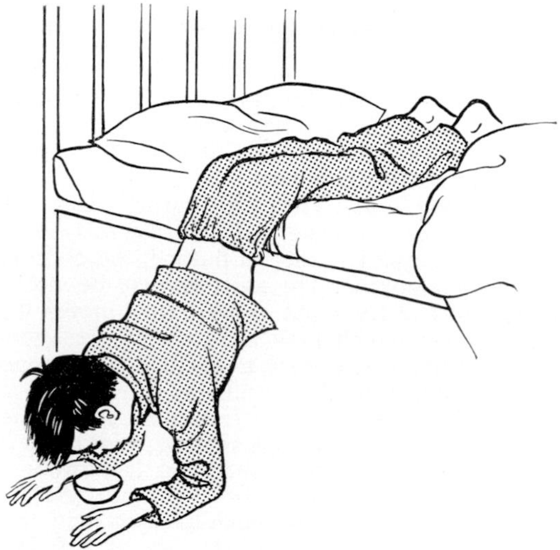

Fig. 27. A HOT DRINK ON WAKING, FOLLOWED BY POSTURAL DRAINAGE MAY HELP TO DISLODGE STAGNANT SECRETIONS AND CLEAR THE LUNGS.

Surgical Treatment

In cases in which the disease process has become irreversible and in those cases in which the changes are confined to one lobe or one side of the lung, segmental resection, or operative removal of the diseased lung or lobe may be considered.

Pre-operative preparation aims at eliminating all septic foci and carious teeth, septic tonsils and infected ears should receive attention. Fresh-air therapy, antibiotics, postural drainage and intensive physiotherapy coupled with attempts at improving the patient's health generally, are all important if the operation is to be successful. The general management of all cases of thoracic surgery are similar and details can be found in Chapter 10.

The improvement in the child's condition is often dramatic, once the septic organ has been removed. The physical handicap following lobectomy is minimal. The child is allowed up two or three days after the operation and in the majority of cases a full, active existence can be resumed within six weeks of lobectomy.

Lobar Pneumonia

Lobar pneumonia rarely affects young infants. The patients are as a rule otherwise healthy, active children who are taken ill with great suddenness. They appear very ill with little warning though occasionally an attack of vomiting or a convulsion may herald the illness.

Signs and Symptoms. The temperature rises rapidly to 39·4° C. (103° F.) or more and may continue to swing at a high level for several days. The face is flushed, the child is bright-eyed and anxious-looking. The alæ nasi may be working. The cough is painful and the child appears to suppress it in order to reduce the pain which may radiate into the abdomen, so that at first it is not always easy to exclude acute appendicitis. The child may hold himself so stiffly as to resemble a case of meningitis and the pain in the region of the kidneys may suggest pyelitis. The breathing is shallow, rapid and inverted, that is to say, a pause occurs between inspiration and expiration instead of normally after expiration. As a rule the rise in the respiration rate is much greater than the rise in the pulse rate. Even at an early stage the skin feels hot and dry and herpes frequently develops around the lips. As the cough becomes productive, the patient brings up sputum, which the younger children are likely to swallow rather than expectorate. Older children should be given a sputum carton and observations of the sputum may show it to be rust coloured and frothy.

As the illness progresses the patient may become drowsy and, if response to treatment is delayed, delirium may set in. Sometimes oxygen needs to be given and the congestive stage is quickly followed by formation of exudate which soon becomes absorbed. This is called resolution. The white cell and polymorph counts are high and the urine may contain albumin. Typical changes in the affected lobe show up on X-ray.

Drugs. With modern drug therapy lobar pneumonia is as a rule an illness of short duration. The infection responds well to sulphonamides, penicillin, broad spectrum antibiotics or a combination of two of these.

Recovery is as a rule complete, though sudden collapse, herpes, pleurisy and occasionally convulsions may complicate the illness.

Nursing Care. The patient is best nursed sitting up, supported by firm pillows but otherwise allowed to find the position which gives him greatest ease in breathing and maximum comfort. Alternatively the special harness used in cardiac failure (Fig. 36) or a special chair, the "Baby Sitta" made by Ekco, may be used.

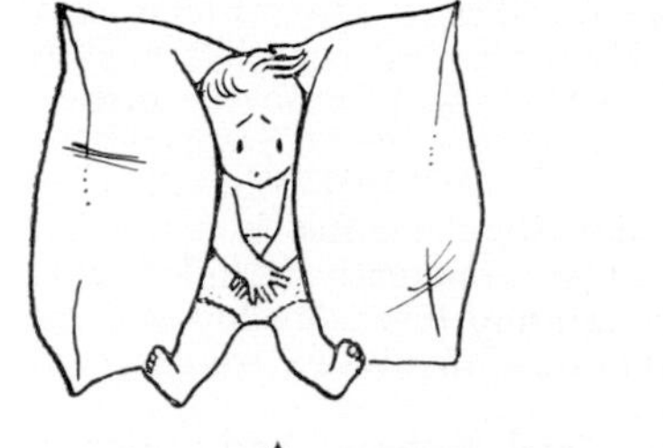

A

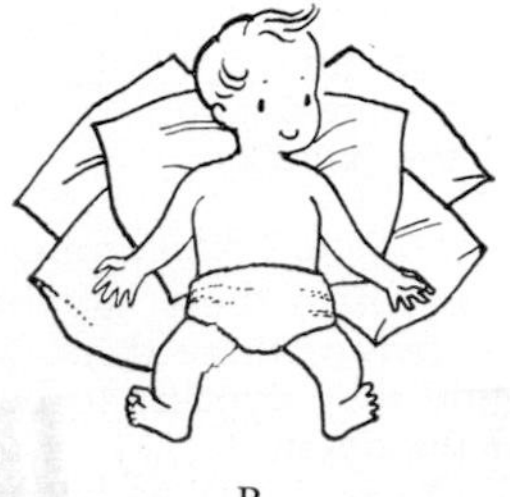

B

Fig. 28. CORRECT USE OF PILLOWS IN UPPER RESPIRATORY TRACT INFECTIONS.

A. *Wrong.* Young children should never be given large, soft pillows as there is danger of suffocation and of overheating.
B. *Right.* The pillows are so arranged as to (1) allow for air to circulate, important in cases with pyrexia, (2) allow for full expansion of the chest on inspiration.

The colour of the child's face should be watched and pallor or cyanosis reported. The mouth must be treated carefully and the lips should be kept supple with petroleum jelly. Herpes, if present, is best treated with dusting powder.

The nasal passages should be kept clear, using pledgets of cotton wool if necessary.

On account of the high fever, the urinary output will be low and the urine concentrated, and special care should be given to the buttocks of incontinent children. Constipation is common but opinions vary as to whether or not this should be treated. It will help both these conditions if copious fluids are given.

The bedclothes should be cradled and an electric fan can be used to assist in bringing down the temperature. Cool sponging of hands and face may do the same and also induce rest and sleep. The room should be of even temperature, but well ventilated.

Four-hourly temperature and fluid charts are kept up and during the acute stage observations should be recorded frequently and fully. Glucose drinks and diluted milk feeds are suitable in the early stage of the illness but when improvement sets in, a normal diet can soon be adopted.

Bronchopneumonia

In contrast to lobar pneumonia, bronchopneumonia most commonly affects babies and children who are already weak and debilitated and this is one of the reasons why it is by far the more severe of the two illnesses. It often affects very young infants and is a fairly common complication of whooping cough, measles, severe burns and fibrocystic disease of the pancreas.

Signs and Symptoms. Occasionally the onset is acute but more often there is a history of an apparently harmless cold for two or three days. Then cough and fever develop and the child soon appears to be severely ill. Convulsions are common at the onset.

The respirations become rapid and distressed and are often of the inverted type with an expiratory grunt. The accessory muscles of respiration are brought into action, and the child may throw his arms above his head in an attempt to increase the air entry. His colour is often ashen grey or cyanosed, and the eyes are dull in contrast to the hectic flush and the bright eyes seen in lobar pneumonia.

Prostration is marked and becomes aggravated by the exhausting nature of the attending cough. The temperature is raised, though less so than in lobar pneumonia, and both respiratory and pulse rate are so high that they are at times uncountable.

The X-ray shows a mottled appearance with small, widely scattered areas of consolidation over both lungs.

Treatment is similar to that for lobar pneumonia but in addition to sulphonamides or antibiotics, digitalis preparations may have to be given. Steam or oxygen therapy are commonly employed. Occasionally the oxygen in the tent is moistened with a fine water or Alevaire spray by means of an atomizer connected to a cylinder of compressed air. As oxygen must be given in constant concentration nursing care and medical examinations should be reduced to a minimum and carried out with speed and efficiency.

Complications. In spite of modern therapy bronchopneumonia continues to be a serious illness. As large areas of the lung are congested, pulmonary circulation is restricted causing considerable strain on the infant's heart. Other complications include convulsions, diarrhœa and vomiting, and pleurisy. The child may be left with a tendency to further lung infections including tuberculosis.

Nursing Care. Most of the nursing points applicable to lobar pneumonia are the same for bronchopneumonia. It is, however, important that all necessary medical examinations, treatment and nursing attention be so co-ordinated as to make any disturbance of the patient as infrequent and brief as is compatible with efficiency. The acutely ill child usually resents being touched and every movement or struggle sets off a new bout of coughing. Long periods of rest and sleep are an essential to recovery. If the child is being nursed in an oxygen tent only a minimum of clothing is needed. In the later stages fresh air is good for the child provided he is kept warm and well covered. During the acute stage glucose fluids or milk and Bengers are very suitable foods. Tube feeding is often less exhausting than sucking and care should be taken not to embarrass respirations further by giving large feeds which distend the stomach. Warm, diluted honey is readily digested and is soothing to the cough. In cases where exhaustion gives cause for anxiety five to thirty drops of brandy (according to age) may be given 4-hourly with the drinks.

Convalescence. A long period of convalescence in the country is highly desirable and, during that time, every attempt should be made to achieve an increase in weight and to build up general health and resistance. Medical supervision should continue until the doctor is satisfied that the lungs are once more fully expanded.

Pleurisy

Pleurisy frequently arises from an attack of pneumonia. As the inflammation spreads from the lungs, the two layers of pleura rub against each other and cause severe pain. The child restricts both breathing and coughing to a minimum on account of the pain, and this causes both rapid and shallow respirations. He may also lean towards the affected side in an attempt to splint and immobilize it. Sometimes the pain is referred to the iliac fossa and may cause the doctor to suspect acute appendicitis. As an effusion forms, the inflamed surfaces are separated and the pain subsides.

A Mantoux test (see page 347) and chest X-ray must be done to exclude tuberculosis and, if an effusion is present, some fluid should be sent for examination and culture.

Treatment of the underlying cause is often all that is required. In mild cases the effusion is absorbed spontaneously but when it causes respiratory distress or displaces the heart and mediastinum, chest aspiration must be performed. In either case fibrous adhesions form and often show up on routine X-rays throughout the patient's life. Apart from this, recovery can be complete but a good follow-up and prolonged convalescence are desirable.

The *nursing care* is described in detail in the chapter on Tuberculosis.

Thoracic Empyema

Occasionally, instead of being absorbed, a pleural effusion becomes purulent. Pus in the pleural cavity remains a serious, debilitating condition and in very young infants it has a low recovery rate.

Signs and Symptoms. The patient with empyema looks toxic, his colour is grey and he is apathetic and anæmic. The appetite is poor, the tongue coated and the temperature swings at a high level.

Medical Treatment. The usual treatment consists in daily chest aspirations, and at the same time an appropriate antibiotic is introduced into the pleural cavity. Antibiotics are also given orally or by injection. Iron and extra vitamins are prescribed and the patient should have as much fresh air and rest as possible.

The *nursing care* is largely symptomatic and at the same time aims at building up the child's strength and weight. The illness may be a long and tedious one, and extra visiting and plenty of occupation should be arranged in order to help keep the patient happy and at rest. Good general nursing routine is obviously called for. The nurse should always remember the uncomfortable and alarming nature of repeated chest aspirations and do all in her power to make the procedure a tolerable one (see page 106).

Occasionally empyema does not respond to the above treatment and surgical drainage becomes necessary.

Surgical drainage of empyema may be done either through a wide-bore tube into a dressing (open drainage) or, if the pus is sufficiently thin, by means of closed drainage through a narrow-bore catheter connected to an under-water seal. In order to insert the narrow drainage tube it may be sufficient to introduce the catheter by means of a trochar and cannula. If a wider tube is used for the drainage of thick pus, rib resection is necessary and the empyema cavity is widely opened. In that case the dressings are changed at least twice a day at first and the tube may be removed and reinserted on alternate days.

In either case intensive physiotherapy is important to achieve full expansion of the underlying lung and obliterate the empyema cavity. The nurse should encourage her patient to cough effectively and may play games with him which encourage deep breathing and lung expansion. As soon as the condition permits and the temperature has settled, the patient is allowed to get up as this will encourage deep breathing and good posture.

Drugs. Hand in hand with drainage, the empyema is treated by antibiotics, given orally, by injection or into the empyema cavity by instillation through the drainage tube.

General Treatment. Fresh air, a high calorie diet, adequate vitamins and iron to correct the anæmia which is usually present are all important adjuncts to surgery. Whatever the treatment adopted, the young patient is likely to be frightened by the various procedures and the drainage tubes and sympathetic handling by his nurses will be needed to reassure him and to restore his confidence.

Asthma

Asthmatic children are very frequently seen in pædiatric departments and, during the course of an attack, may present an alarming and pathetic picture. The first attack may occur as early as the first year of life and the cause is not always easy to determine though, in many cases there is a family history of eczema, hay fever or migraine. Infantile eczema may be replaced by asthma in the older child.

Signs and Symptoms. The following is a typical picture of an acute attack of asthma: After several hours of peaceful sleep the child awakes suddenly with a feeling of suffocation and in great terror. By the time the parents are roused he looks grey or cyanosed, his pyjamas are damp with perspiration, the breathing is laboured and wheezing, and expiration appears to be more difficult than inspiration. The accessory muscles of respiration are working. If the temperature is taken it is found to be only slightly raised or even normal, while the rise in the pulse rate is in keeping with the impression of an acute emergency. The respiratory rate is increased. At other times the attack may start during the day and would sometimes seem to be associated with over-excitement or frustration. In young babies the early signs of the disease may be noisy, harsh breathing and a cough. These attacks are usually diagnosed as teething or acute bronchitis and, though they may clear in one to two weeks, will gradually change to wheezing or obvious asthma. The *duration* of an attack may vary from a quarter of an hour to several hours and the patient may be shocked and exhausted by the time the attack subsides.

On examination, chronically asthmatic children appear pale, underweight and undersized. Their posture is often poor. A slight expiratory wheeze can be heard, as there is a constant, mild degree of bronchial spasm. In the majority of cases the patient is alert and intelligent, but at the same time highly strung and nervy. On closer acquaintance he may be found to be rather anxious, insecure and aggressive in his relationship to others. Very often the parents are over-protective and managing, or there seems to be emotional trouble or discord in the home. It is interesting to note that in many cases children known as established asthmatics never have an attack while in hospital or away at school.

Investigations include X-ray of chest, bacteriological examination of sputum, blood sedimentation rate, sensitivity tests, and inspection of teeth and tonsils. As hypochlorhydria is at times associated with asthma, a test meal is sometimes done. The possibility that psychological factors may bring on attacks must always be borne in mind.

Treatment. Various anti-spasmodic drugs in common use include aminophylline given by mouth, intramuscular or intravenous injection, or as a suppository, pethidine, ephedrine and antihistamine drugs. Occasionally antispasmodic drugs are given in the form of a spray or via an oxygen tent. A sedative is often ordered at the same time. In addition to these drugs the following are now coming into common use, although they are frequently reserved for severe or resistant cases: isoprenaline (10 milligram tablet dissolved under the tongue), by inhalation as a 1 per cent. hand spray, or through an aerosol propellant; adrenocorticotrophic hormone (ACTH) in an intravenous drip infusion, cortisone or prednisone by mouth. Dosage of the last two drugs is usually high at the start and gradually reduced to the smallest dose which will control the asthma. Cortisone therapy is not without danger and is reserved for status asthmaticus. After the attack has subsided, attempts are made to determine the factor which produced it.

Common Causes of Asthma

Causes include cold winds, damp or changeable weather. Possible social or psychological factors include over-ambitious or over-protective parents, insecurity in the home caused by a broken marriage, or inadequate outlet for the child's intelligence and activities. Dietary errors, contact with certain pollens, horsehair and dust from the pelt of some household pet are other possible factors. The constant, faulty respiratory mechanism aggravates the condition but there is often good response to breathing exercises. Classes in correct breathing technique may be a valuable adjunct to treatment.

Successful treatment may depend on close team work between pædiatrician, psychologist, social worker and school authorities. Residential or open-air day schools are often of great benefit, and this applies sometimes also to a spell away from home. Frequently the parents need help and advice in handling the situation. They should understand that, while asthma is often incapacitating and very troublesome, it is rarely serious or fatal.

Wisely handled, some children grow out of these attacks; others have to be taught how to come to grips with their handicap. Attacks should always be arrested before they develop fully or permanent changes, chronic bronchitis and emphysema may result.

Nursing Care. By and large, nursing care is symptomatic and consists in carrying out the doctor's orders, and reassuring the patient and his parents. The patient may get relief from sitting up well supported. (Dunlopillows are very suitable). Cotton blankets should be used in lieu of woollen ones. Fresh air is often helpful and the room should be evenly warm but not stuffy, nor should the atmosphere be too dry. As soon as the condition permits, the child should be offered occupation and diversion. Though the attitude should be sympathetic, a degree of firmness is often essential.

Status Asthmaticus

When one attack of acute, spasmodic asthma virtually runs into the next attack, the patient is said to suffer from status asthmaticus.

Treatment and management are similar to that in ordinary attacks but, as this state may persist for many hours, exhaustion may be extreme. *Stimulants* should be kept by the bedside. Relaxation and rest must be achieved by any means available, and this may tax the nurse's ingenuity severely. Sponging the face and hands, changing and turning the pillows and gentle massage of the patient's scalp with a hair brush can be very soothing. Quiet reassurance by speaking to the child may do much to calm his fears, and hot drinks, given in small amounts often help as much as drugs, in getting the patient off to sleep.

Asthmatic Bronchitis

Attacks of asthmatic bronchitis usually affect children over 3 years of age who are debilitated and underweight and who have infected tonsils, sinuses, or teeth.

The attack may follow a common cold, and bronchial spasm, cyanosis, pyrexia and a troublesome cough may continue for several days. The same drugs as those used for spasmodic asthma are usually effective and the nursing treatment too is the same. Any infected focus should be cleared up as soon as the patient's condition permits.

9

DISEASES OF THE EAR, NOSE AND THROAT

Ear, nose and throat conditions are very common in childhood, and may account for much minor illness and frequent admissions to hospital or visits to the out-patient clinic. Repeated attacks of catarrh, otitis media, obstructed breathing and sinusitis may contribute to poor general development and diminish mental alertness; loss of schooling may affect the child psychologically as well as educationally.

For children prone to ear, nose and throat infections and congestion there are some simple measures which are well worth trying in an attempt at improving the tendency to recurrent infections. Among these are simple but thorough education in nose blowing and encouragement at breathing through the nose. Occasionally simple practices such as allowing the child to sleep with the head lower than the rest of the body may encourage drainage and parents should be made to realize that plenty of fresh air both day and night is as a rule more beneficial than keeping the child indoors for fear of his catching cold.

The Common Cold

Owing to an infant's small air passages, *a cold in infancy can be a serious illness*. Nurses must always remember this and avoid going near babies when they themselves have a cold; they should realize that a day off duty may prove a greater degree of conscientiousness than being on duty while they are a source of danger. The importance of meticulous care in hand washing and attention to every detail of hygiene is evident. Taps should always be manipulated with the elbows, and the hands thoroughly dried. A liberal supply of suitable towels and a hand cream are usually provided to prevent the hands from getting sore or chapped from frequent washing. Fingernails must be kept short and neither rings nor watches must be worn on duty. Masks and gowns, if used, should be put on and taken off as described in Chapter 3, page 41. If a nurse herself has to use a handkerchief, this must be done away from the baby's cot and should be followed by handwashing and a change of mask.

Very young babies breathe wholly through the nose and find mouth-breathing difficult. Nasal obstruction may therefore interfere considerably with feeding as sucking is made almost impossible.

Complications which may arise from a common cold in infancy include otitis media, pneumonia and gastro-enteritis.

Laryngoscopy

When a doctor wants to inspect the larynx, trachea or the vocal cords, or if he wishes to remove secretions such as blood, mucus or vomitus by suction, laryngoscopy is performed. With very young infants laryngoscopy can often be done without an anæsthetic; with older children, except in dire emergency, a full anæsthetic is given.

Before being placed on the table the child is securely wrapped in a blanket leaving the neck and upper chest exposed. In other respects there is little difference from the procedure for adults. Laryngoscopy may have to be performed in the neonatal period and for some of the conditions described below.

Choanal Atresia

Choanal atresia is a congenital abnormality in which the openings at the back of the nose are blocked by plates of tissue. Since the new-born infant has not yet adapted himself to breathing through the mouth, the condition has to be corrected as an urgent surgical measure or the baby will die. An airway is introduced and the obstructing plates pierced by means of a probe. If the condition is unilateral treatment can be delayed until the baby is stronger and the structures involved less minute. In this case babies should always lie on the affected side to ensure an adequate airway.

Congenital Laryngeal Stridor

Congenital laryngeal stridor is not a dangerous condition and children usually outgrow it by the age of 1 year or 18 months. Parents, however, are concerned about the noise the child makes on inspiration and about the sucking in of the intercostal spaces. The condition is best observed when the child is crying or when asleep. Congenital abnormalities have to be excluded but in the majority of cases the parents can be reassured that no treatment is needed.

Laryngismus Stridulus

Laryngismus stridulus is a rare condition, associated with severe rickets. The cause is complete closure of the glottis by muscle spasm followed by a crowing inspiration and lasting only a matter of seconds. The condition is not a dangerous one in itself, and clears as the underlying disease is cured.

Croup

Laryngitis stridulosa or croup affects children of 3 to 5 years who are of a nervous disposition. The stridor usually occurs in connection with a cold. In a typical case the child awakens in the middle of the night, apparently struggling for air, sweating profusely and in a state of acute anxiety. The attack may last as long as an hour and is followed by normal sleep. Often the child has no recollection of the episode on wakening in the morning. While the attacks are very frightening to the parents, they can be reassured about their harmless nature. A warm drink and a sedative may be helpful and late, heavy meals should be avoided. Occasionally unhealthy tonsils are a contributory cause.

Laryngotracheitis

Laryngotracheitis is often caused by a virus or by the *Hæmophilus influenzæ*. It is most prevalent during the autumn and winter months and carries a high mortality rate.

The chief manifestations of the disease are respiratory obstruction and inspiratory stridor caused by inflammation and congestion of the respiratory tract. The whole of the larynx and trachea are coated with thick, viscous secretions so that the air passages are narrowed. Adequate oxygen exchange becomes impossible and this leads to serious respiratory difficulties and general exhaustion.

Although pyrexia is occasionally absent, the temperature is usually 39·4° to 40° C. (103° to 104° F.). The child looks anxious, grey and collapsed, the pulse rate is rapid and the volume poor. An almost incessant cough adds to the exhaustion and leads to extreme restlessness. Respirations rise to 60 or more per minute as the child struggles for air, and the intercostal spaces and supraclavicular region are drawn in and the stridor increases.

Treatment is urgent. A *steam tent* is invaluable as the moisture prevents the secretions from drying up, but care must be taken not to overheat an already feverish patient. An *oxygen tent* may be beneficial provided that the atmosphere is kept moist by means of a vaporizer. Plain water or some preparation such as Alevaire, or a Humidaire tent or a Croupette are used. Occasionally an *emergency tracheostomy* may have to be performed as a life-saving measure, and fine judgment and careful observation are needed when caring for these patients as sudden deterioration is common. All necessary equipment for tracheostomy should be at hand, including an *electric sucker* for the extraction of the viscid mucus.

Drugs. Penicillin often proves useless for this condition and chlortetracycline (Aureomycin), chloramphenicol and streptomycin are the drugs of choice. A stimulant, e.g. nikethamide, should be kept ready. Sedatives may be tried but are rarely of much value in the acute stages. If an aerosol is used the margins of the eyelids frequently become inflamed, but this is of little importance since the inflammation clears as soon as treatment is stopped.

Nursing Care. To procure rest should be one of the prime concerns of the nurse. Well positioned pillows, frequently turned, loose, comfortable clothing (sometimes nothing beyond a napkin if the child is being nursed in a tent) sponging of hands and face, frequent, small sips of water or a glucose drink and even soothing stroking of the head may help to induce rest and so to preserve the strength of these children. Brandy 5 to 10 minims hourly given in warm, sweet water may be useful. Occasionally fluids have to be given parenterally but the restlessness makes any such procedure very difficult.

Tracheostomy

Tracheostomy has to be performed whenever the lumen of the larynx has been so narrowed by disease as to make adequate air entry impossible. This may happen for several reasons, including:

Congenital abnormalities such as papilloma, laryngeal web, or cysts.

Trauma, e.g. œdema following intubation or scalding.

Infections such as diphtheria or laryngotracheitis.

Paralysis, e.g. in anterior poliomyelitis.

Signs of obstruction are:

Distressed respirations, wheezing inspiratory stridor. Restlessness.

An anxious expression.

Sucking in of the intercostal spaces, the diaphragm, neck muscle, sternal notch and the lower end of the sternum.

An increasing pulse and respiratory rate.

Cyanosis (in most, but not all, cases).

With the above signs in mind it should normally be possible to appreciate the impending need for this life-saving procedure and only rarely is an unprepared tracheostomy required. Occasionally a bronchoscopy is done before the tracheostomy and as a rule an endotracheal tube is also passed.

When tracheostomy is to be performed the position of the patient is very important. He should be placed on his back with a sandbag under his shoulders so as to achieve full extension of head and neck (Fig. 29). Spine and neck must be absolutely straight in order to have the trachea in midline and unless a general anæsthetic is given he should be wrapped in a drawsheet or thin blanket with the arms securely fixed to make any struggling impossible. One nurse should control the child's body and another assistant steady the head. In every other respect the operation is similar to that done in adults.

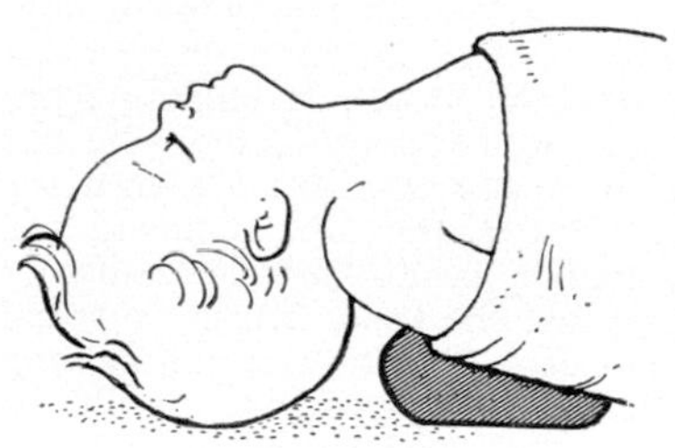

Fig. 29. TRACHEOSTOMY.
Note the position of the sandbag, extending the neck fully. The patient is securely restrained in a blanket, but upper chest and neck have been left well exposed.

At the conclusion of the operation the tube is fastened securely round the neck by means of tapes and the inner tube inserted. It is wise to use coloured tape or to colour white tape with ink, in order to avoid any confusion with the tapes of the child's bib or nightgown and, for the same reason, to tie the tapes at the side of the neck. Improvement in the patient's condition is dramatic. Cyanosis is instantly relieved, breathing becomes normal and quiet and if he is conscious, the patient relaxes and falls into a deep, restful sleep.

Nursing Care. The patient is received back into a warm room and the air should be humidified. Barrier precautions may be carried out if indicated by the primary disease.

The patient's position should be a restful one and as a rule it is best to have him sitting up, well supported by pillows except in the case of diphtheria, when the heart may be affected by toxins. Care must be taken to keep the chin off the opening of the tube, and this is of special importance with young infants as they have very short necks. This may present a problem, which is one of the responsibilities of the special nurse who will have to be with the child all the time. She may achieve this by placing pillows in such a way that the baby's head falls back slightly, so exposing the neck, or even by holding up the chin herself.

It must be remembered that speech is impossible, that the patient is often seriously ill and that he may be frightened and nervous. Wrist restrainers or elbow splints will be necessary for young children and for delirious or uncooperative older ones. While with the patient the nurse must keep a careful watch on his general condition, his colour, the quality of his pulse and the ease of his respirations. Any bleeding from the wound must be reported. It may happen that the tube slips out of the trachea while still remaining in the tissues. A deterioration in the patient's colour, respiratory distress and restlessness are all indications this may have happened (Fig. 30). If there is any doubt a mirror held in front of the tube will soon show whether breath is coming from it. No time must be lost in sending for help if the tube has actually slipped. If it cannot be made to slip back into the trachea the tapes may have to be cut, the tube removed and the tracheal dilators used to make an airway. Occasionally air may leak into the tissues around the tube, causing surgical emphysema. As long as the tube is in the trachea and as long as it is kept well cleaned, the patient's breathing should be inaudible. An electric suction pump may be used to keep the tube free from secretions. Some surgeons allow a few millilitres of a 5 per cent. solution of sodium bicarbonate to be instilled into the tube to help clear it. The electric sucker must be ready to suck the tube out at once, if this is done. Mucolytic agents to loosen viscid mucus may be used. Acetylcysteine, used with a nebulizer attached to an oxygen or compressed air cylinder, is one of these.

The nursing equipment needed by the bedside is the same for children and adults. Nurses should, however, remember that they must be familiar with the type of tracheostomy tube in use. Most tubes have three parts: an outer tube, an inner tube and an introducer; the outer tube being the

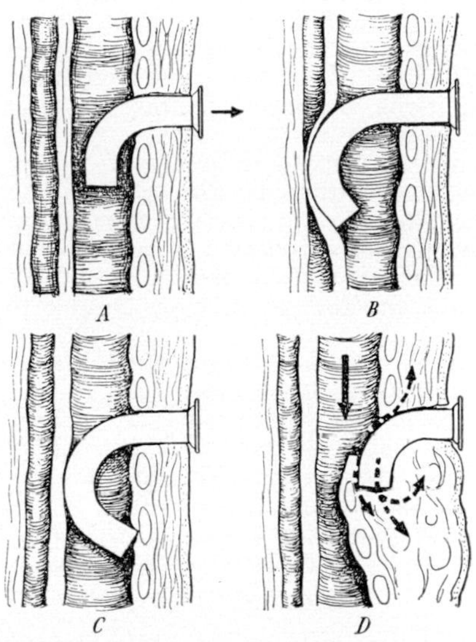

Fig. 30. DANGERS OF BADLY POSITIONED OR ACCIDENTALLY DISPLACED TRACHEOSTOMY TUBES.

A. Tube of correct dimension comfortably in place.
B. Too long a tube. The child will have dysphagia.
C. Too long and too curved a tube. Ulceration of the interior trocheal wall may occur from pressure. There will be a continual cough.
D. Disaster. Too short a tube has been inserted. It has been loosely tied in. The tube has slipped. Air enters through the narrowed larynx and the wound. The result may be asphyxia, surgical emphysema and possibly tension pneumothorax.

only one which has to be left in position the entire time. It is secured with tapes which are often wider at the back for added comfort. The outer tube is connected loosely with a plate which lies flush on the neck and is the part which is secured by the tapes. Some surgeons like to protect the skin by a key-hole dressing. Outer tube and plate must not be separated even though they appear to be only loosely connected. In the case of Durham's "lobster-tailed tube", the tube is connected to the plate by a movable collar and a long screw. The collar can be adjusted on the plate according to the distance of the trachea from the skin surface.

A tracheostomy does not interfere with feeding and the child should be given fluids and a light diet as soon as his condition permits, but extra care is needed to avoid any fluid from dribbling down the chin and into the tube. In paralytic conditions, however, feeding by naso-œsophageal tube may be necessary.

Tracheostomy performed in cases of acute illness, as in laryngotracheitis, can often be allowed to close after only a few days after plugging the tube for experimental periods. In cases of congenital abnormalities or neoplasm it may have to be permanent. Parents and children then have to learn how to manage the tube and the patient may be able to lead a fairly normal life.

After having had a tracheostomy for several days, children are rather apprehensive when the tube is to be removed. It is often helpful to give a sedative before attempting to do so. Occasionally the tube can be best removed while the child is drinking some favourite drink, as at this time normal rhythm between swallowing and breathing is easily established before the young patient is aware of what has been done.

Catarrhal Children

Children are very prone to upper respiratory tract infections, partly due to the close relationship of the organs concerned, partly because they have not acquired the necessary immunity against these infections. A great deal of schooling is missed in the first school years due to absence caused by coughs, colds, earache, throat infections and wheezy chests. Enlarged tonsils and adenoids are sometimes blamed for these periods of sickness, but it seems likely that they are not the cause but the effect and that they play a useful part in developing immunity.

Tonsillitis

Throat infections, most frequently caused by the hæmolytic streptococcus, are extremely common in children. The patient is often severely ill and this applies particularly to children under school age.

As children are not always capable of describing pain accurately, they may complain of abdominal pain. In addition, vomiting may be present and it is thus not easy to exclude acute appendicitis. As the neck is frequently held stiffly the condition may at first be mistaken for meningitis. Frequently mesenteric adenitis develops simultaneously causing general rigidity and confusing diagnosis still further.

The child is generally ill and fractious. The face is flushed, the temperature perhaps as high as 39·4° C. (103° F.) and headache may cause him to turn away from the light. Saliva may dribble from the mouth or alternatively the lips are parched and cracked.

When any other conditions have been excluded, a throat swab is taken to determine the causative organism and its sensitivity to drugs. Penicillin, given by injection, is the drug most commonly used.

Nursing Care. Patients suffering from tonsillitis should be barrier nursed for at least 24 hours after commencing treatment. If there is a high temperature the bed clothes should be light and supported by a bed cradle. An electric fan, well out of reach of the patient, may be used, and tepid sponging may be carried out with the doctor's permission. Mouth toilet, including mouth washes with a mild antiseptic such as glycothymoline or with saline, will help to keep the mouth clean.

Aspirin gargles may relieve the pain and are often given about 20 minutes before meals to make swallowing easier. As the child is likely to refuse solid foods in the early stages of the illness, he should be encouraged to take frequent drinks of cool, bland fluids. Ice cream is soothing and is often taken eagerly when other foods are refused. Later, extra nourishment in the form of milk and eggs should be given.

If the child is treated with modern drugs improvement is as a rule rapid and he may be ready for discharge in four or five days. On the other hand, the infection may spread to the middle ear and the cervical glands. Convulsions occur fairly frequently but are rarely of a serious nature, and the parents may be reassured about this.

Special Points. If nursed in an open ward, these children should never be placed next to others suffering from acute rheumatism, nephritis or congenital heart disease, as streptococcal infections are serious in patients suffering from these conditions.

Retropharyngeal Abscess

Retropharyngeal abscess occurs fairly frequently in young debilitated children. The abscess forms in a lymph gland in the pharynx and is situated underneath the mucous membrane between the post-pharyngeal wall and the cervical vertebræ. As it protrudes into the back of the throat it causes a swelling (which is always central), pain and difficulty in swallowing and breathing. The child is ill and toxic with a high temperature, flushed cheeks and sunken eyes. Fluids are obstinately refused and the child moves around restlessly in an attempt to find a position which allows for easier breathing. The head is held stiffly as every movement causes pain.

The illness is extremely acute and progresses with great rapidity. The obstruction to breathing soon becomes serious and the nurse should not leave her patient and, as emergency tracheostomy occasionally becomes necessary, a complete trolley for this operation should be at hand.

The abscess may burst spontaneously but although this may be followed by relief and general improvement there is a danger of inhalation of pus and subsequent lung infection. As a rule operation is therefore preferred. If time permits the child is prepared in the usual way in the ward and placed on the operating table with the head below the level of the body, or in the same position as for tonsillectomy. Occasionally the situation is a very urgent one and the opening has to be done without anæsthetic. In this case the child is wrapped in a blanket and restrained by an assistant. After inserting a mouth gag, a pair of closed sinus forceps or a guarded scalpel are used to puncture the abscess. Immediately this is done, the child is turned on his side with the head well below the level of the shoulders and the pus is removed by means of an electric sucker, and mouth and throat are thoroughly cleared with gauze swabs. A specimen of pus is sent to the laboratory for sensitivity tests.

Improvement is usually rapid and may be hastened by giving an appropriate antibiotic, abundant fluids, a light, high calorie diet, vitamins, iron and, eventually, a period of convalescence.

Quinsy or Peritonsillar Abscess

Quinsy is much more rare in childhood than retropharyngeal abscess. The abscess often follows tonsillitis and forms in one of the crypts of the tonsil. The swelling is therefore always a one-sided one. Pain is severe and prevents the patient from opening his mouth (trismus) and from swallowing. The illness may continue for a week or two and the difficulty of swallowing, taking nourishment and finding rest may seriously affect an already debilitated patient.

Treatment may be conservative or surgical. In the first instance hot gargles, warm compresses to the neck, Disprin-swallows, antibiotics and careful mouth toilet are given. Surgical treatment follows the same lines as those for retropharyngeal abscess. In either case removal of the diseased tonsils should be considered at a later date and treatment given for any dental caries and oral sepsis.

Tonsillectomy and Adenoidectomy

Operation for the removal of tonsils and adenoids is among the most common surgical procedures in a children's unit. Some nurses feel that they are here dealing with an undramatic and uninteresting routine job, but if they are made to realize how often the removal of diseased tonsils and hypertrophied adenoids improves the child's general health and how other illnesses such as recurrent tonsillitis, otitis media, sinusitis and even bronchiectasis and general development can be improved, they will realize the importance of this type of surgery and will find it of real interest.

Ideally patients for tonsillectomy should be admitted the day before operation in order to allow them to get used to the ward and the nurses. They should be told simply what is about to happen and expectations about parties, ice cream and the like which some parents still promise should be tactfully but firmly dispelled.

Temperature, pulse and respirations are taken and recorded four-hourly but as most of these children are mouth breathers, it is best to take the temperature in the axilla or rectum. Any fever and any other observations, such as coughs or purulent nasal discharge, are reported. Routine urine testing is carried out. A glucose drink is given 2 hours before the anæsthetic. The teeth should be cleaned as part of the immediate preoperative preparation. Premedication should include a sedative which will cause amnesia but at the same time is sufficiently light to allow for a rapid return of the cough reflex following operation. The hair of little girls should be kept out of the way with narrow ribbon and the operation gown should be left unbuttoned as the anæsthetist will want to slip it well off the shoulders when the patient is placed on the theatre table. In some units pyjama trousers only are worn by both girls and boys.

The operation differs in no way from that done in adults and on return to the ward the usual "tonsillectomy position" is adopted, i.e. the child lies on his side with the upper leg bent and the upper arm flexed in front of the head with the body leaning forward (Fig. 31). A pillow in the back will

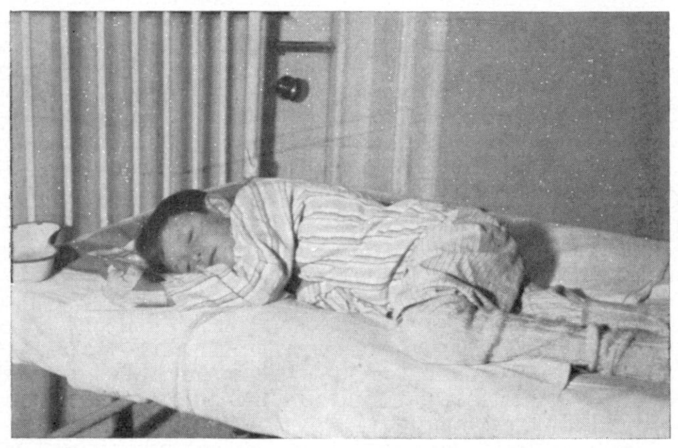

Fig. 31. POSITION AFTER TONSILLECTOMY.
Any blood or secretions can easily drain out of the mouth and inhalation is thus prevented.

assist in maintaining this position which will ensure that any blood trickles out of the mouth rather than down the throat. In that way the danger of inhaling blood is greatly reduced and any abnormal bleeding can easily be observed. The neck should remain exposed as regular swallowing movement of the neck muscles may be the first sign that there is some bleeding and that the child is swallowing blood. Some surgeons return the patient to the ward with tongue clips still holding the tongue safely forward, others ensure that the cough reflex is fully recovered before the patient leaves the theatre and that the level of consciousness is such that there is no danger of obstruction from the tongue falling back. Cold sponging of the face will hasten the return to consciousness and refresh the patient as he comes round from the anæsthetic. In some wards one prophylactic dose of procaine penicillin is given by intramuscular injection immediately after return from the theatre. The pulse is recorded very frequently for the first 24 hours, and some surgeons prefer the temperature not to be taken orally for the first three days.

Post-operative Bleeding. Restlessness and noisy, moist respirations are early indications of bleeding. If this goes unnoticed, the pulse rate may rise and the pulse volume become weaker. These signs and any vomit should be reported at once and vomit, if any, kept for inspection by an experienced nurse. Stale blood in the vomit is of little importance as it probably dates back to the time of operation, but any signs of fresh blood should be viewed with suspicion, and vigilance should be increased. If there is any bleeding, the mouth and nasopharynx are carefully swabbed and cleared of blood and the patient raised to the upright position, well supported by pillows and an injection of Nepenthe, previously ordered in case of any complication, given. In the majority of cases this is all that is needed. Sometimes however a clot on the tonsils or adenoid bed is the cause of the trouble and has to be removed with a sterile swab and forceps. Serious hæmorrhage necessitates a return to the theatre and ligaturing of the bleeding point. Blood loss can quickly prove serious and may have to be made good by blood transfusion or, in less serious cases, by iron therapy.

The younger the patient, the less severe are pain and general malaise. Fluids should be given as soon as the effect of the anæsthetic has worn off. Œdema and stiffness of the throat, associated with pain, can be greatly reduced by encouraging the child to swallow early. Cool drinks of fruit juice and ice cream are suitable but milk is inclined to coat the tonsil-bed and is best omitted for the first 24 hours. Children under the age of 8 years are usually ready for a light breakfast the morning after operation. Disprin 0·3 grammes (5 grains) crushed and dissolved in a little water can be given 20 minutes before meals and this reduces the pain and so encourages eating and drinking. A cheerful, matter of fact attitude by the nurses contributes considerably to an early recovery of these children.

Post-operatively these patients often complain of earache and of a stiff neck. In most cases neither of these conditions is serious and the referred pain causing the earache, and the stiff neck caused by the position on the theatre table, can be relieved by the application of warmth.

Breathing through the nose should be taught as soon as the post-operative œdema has subsided and the child told that the doctor would be looking forward to his efficiency in that respect on his return visit. Since modern antibiotics have become available the fear of infection and secondary hæmorrhage is much reduced and it is, therefore, unjustifiable to forbid visiting. The presence of the mother up to the time the premedication has taken effect and a short visit of mutual reassurance soon after the operation can be beneficial to both mother and child and may be the best means to ensure that there are no psychological after-effects.

Deafness

Deafness in childhood may be temporary or permanent. Permanent deafness may be congenital nerve deafness caused, e.g. by an attack of rubella in the mother, during the first 12 weeks of pregnancy. Cerebral palsy sufferers often also have an associated nerve deafness.

Among the acquired causes are repeated attacks of otitis media and perforation of the ear drum with subsequent scarring and adhesions or radical mastoidectomy. Transitory deafness may be caused by an accumulation of wax, a foreign body in the meatus, meatal boils and blocking of the Eustachian tube due to a cold, sinusitis or adenoids.

Children who are born deaf are usually dumb as well, as they have no perception of sound, but occasionally islands of hearing, or hearing at a certain pitch are present and can be developed by special education and the help of hearing aids. The problem of placing a child in an institution for the deaf at an early age is a very serious one, as separation from the family may add to the already heavy psychological burden these children have to bear. On the other hand, communication with the outside world can most easily be taught at an early age and schools for the deaf admit children from the age of 3 years. Each child will therefore have to be assessed as an individual before a decision can be made. Children who otherwise appear to be of normal intelligence but progress badly at school may be suffering from poor hearing and should be thoroughly investigated. Audiometry—exact measurement of hearing—is nowadays easily carried out at most large hospitals.

Otitis Media

In young children the structures of the ear, nose and throat are particularly closely related to one another, and their smallness easily accounts for frequent congestion and blocking and for the spread of infection from one to the other.

Otitis media is common as a secondary infection following a common cold, tonsillitis, infections of the mouth, infectious fevers and carious teeth. In babies the short, straight and rather wide Eustachian tube may even become blocked by vomitus, and special care should be taken with babies suffering from any kind of vomiting.

Signs and Symptoms. The onset of otitis media may be insidious and the first signs may be that the young child rolls his head on the pillow, pulls his ear and is abnormally irritable. Pain soon becomes severe, the temperature rises as high as 39·4° C. (103° F.) and the patient resents being touched. He looks toxic, and diarrhœa, vomiting and convulsions are common. On examination the blood vessels of the ear drum are found to be dilated and congested, the cone of light normally reflected from the handle of the malleus is absent, and the usual mobility of the drum is lost. The ear drum may be bulging and opaque owing to the pus which fills the cavity of the middle ear.

Treatment may be conservative, i.e. by means of drugs such as penicillin given systemically in fairly large dosage. The application of local heat may be soothing. At night several pillows should be used, as pain is more severe when the patient lies down flat. Disprin or some other analgesic should be given, as it is senseless to allow the child to suffer pain, and the loss of sleep which goes hand in hand with it can only prejudice the course of the illness. Sometimes sleep can be induced by such simple measures as a hot drink and a "cuddle" from a sympathetic nurse. One per cent. ephedrine nasal drops, which have the effect of shrinking the mucosa of the nose and Eustachian tube, are used to promote drainage, and older children can be given inhalations with the same purpose in mind.

Myringotomy

If there is no response to conservative treatment after 24 hours, myringotomy may be considered, as it is better to have a clean surgical incision which later heals by first intention than a spontaneous perforation with ragged edges which will result in scarring and adhesions of the ear drum. As soon as the tympanic membrane is perforated and pus released, pain subsides and the general condition of the patient improves.

Myringotomy is an exquisitely painful operation and for that reason should always be done under a light general anæsthetic, even though it takes only a matter of moments to perform.

Nursing Care following Myringotomy. On return from the theatre the patient is placed on the affected side to encourage drainage. The auditory meatus may have been loosely packed with a ribbon gauze wick to aid drainage of pus by capillary action and a light pad and bandage applied. These should be inspected and changed as soon as they have become saturated with discharge. Routine ear mopping (and in some cases syringing) is ordered, and started 12 hours after operation. The procedure is a strictly sterile one and is repeated as often as the need arises. The pain is as a rule relieved by the myringotomy, and analgesic drugs are rarely necessary. The patient may be allowed up the next day, as running around promotes drainage and means a happier patient. The course of penicillin will probably be continued. The diet should be a full, well-balanced one. Aural toilet is carried out as often as is necessary until the drainage has completely dried up and the ear drum has healed. In favourable cases there is little or no impairment of hearing.

Otorrhœa

Serous or purulent discharge from the ear may be either acute or chronic. In either case treatment will consist of three main factors:

Treatment by drugs such as sulphonamides, penicillin and other antibiotics.

Regular, thorough aural toilet by syringing or mopping.

Building up the patient's general health.

Ear Mopping

Ear mopping carried out by an efficient, experienced nurse should be painless. All the same the preparation involved may frighten the young patient, and it is well worth gaining the child's confidence before starting the actual procedure. Once he has learned that there is nothing to fear, even the youngest child will prove cooperative, and it is only the quiet patient, who needs little if any restraint, who makes thorough, gentle aural toilet possible.

Position. Infants and toddlers are best allowed to lie on their side either on their cot or on the nurse's knee. The nurse's one forearm can rest lightly on the child's head, the other on the body, thus giving light restraint and acting as an indication to the patient that he is required to keep still. Older children may be asked to stand between the nurse's legs as she sits, with the head on one of the mopper's knees (the left knee for the right ear and vice versa). Uncooperative patients and young babies may have to be restrained, as in Fig. 32.

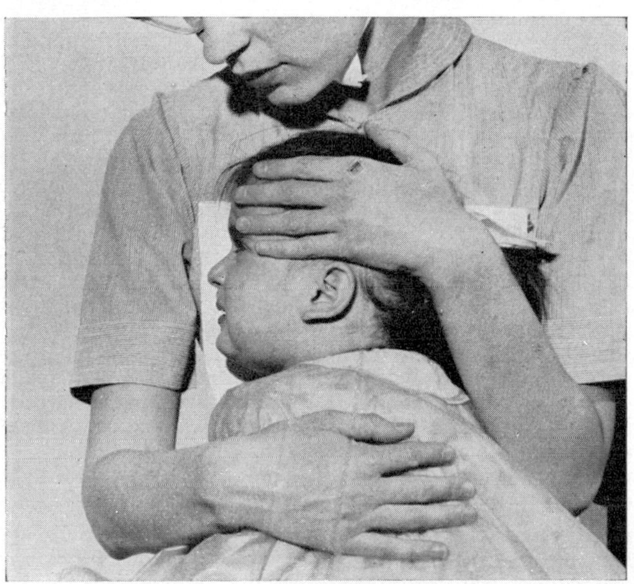

Fig. 32. SECURE COMFORTABLE RESTRAINT FOR EXAMINATION OR DRY MOPPING OF THE EAR.

Method. Whichever method is adopted the nurse should hold the wool carrier so lightly that she can easily let go as soon as the child moves his head. No harm is likely to come to the child who momentarily has a wool carrier sticking out of his ear, whereas a movement of the head with the operator clinging to the rigid stick may easily damage, and even perforate the ear drum, or at the best, is likely to cause pain. Alternatively the nurse can rest her hand on the patient's head so that they move together and so avoid trauma. Once the child has lost confidence the repeated aural toilet will also mean a repeated struggle.

Ear mopping is essentially the same in children as in adults. The auditory meatus in young children is, however, of different anatomical shape and in order to straighten it sufficiently to reach the bottom of the meatus when mopping, the pinna should be gently pulled in a backward direction up to the age of approximately 18 months, but in older patients in a backward and upward direction.

In some wards a graph record is kept of the number of mops used and the time intervals between treatments. The type of discharge, whether serous, purulent or blood-stained, its nature, whether ropy or watery and whether odourless or offensive, should all be reported.

The delicate skin of children easily becomes excoriated by aural discharge. The area around the ear should be gently washed with cotton wool and saline and zinc ointment or lanolin applied. As in the case of any open wound (and a discharging ear means a perforated drum, i.e. an open wound), it is important to keep all hair well out of the way. In little girls this can be achieved by wearing an Alice-band, hair grips or even a hair net. Any short, stray hair can be controlled by applying a little petroleum jelly to keep it away from the aural orifice. Babies and toddlers may have to have their arms restrained in order to prevent spread of infection. In all cases pillow slips should be changed whenever they become soiled.

Syringing Discharging Ears

In some units the doctor may order 4-hourly or twice daily syringing for a discharging ear. In young children this is best done with a sterilized rat-tail rubber bulb-syringe, in older children a sterilized Higginson's syringe with a special attachment is sometimes used. In either case the greatest care should be taken to use lotion at the correct temperature (37·8° C. (100° F.) in the jug) and to direct the stream on to the wall of the meatus and never on to the ear drum. The meatus should be straightened as described above. Careful drying of the meatus following the syringing is essential and the toilet is completed as described in the preceding paragraph. Note that ear syringing must never be undertaken except on doctor's orders.

Disease of the Mastoid Bone

Mastoiditis may be an immediate complication of otitis media or the sequel to long standing, badly drained infection of the middle ear. The organism is as a rule the streptococcus or staphylococcus but occasionally the mastoid infection is caused by the tubercle bacillus or *Escherichia* (*Bacterium*) *coli*. Chronic mastoiditis is associated with poor general health and aural discharge; at operation, granulations of the middle ear and necrosis of the mastoid bone are found. Neglected mastoid disease may lead to meningitis, brain abscess and lateral sinus thrombosis.

Acute Mastoiditis

Acute mastoiditis causes the child to be generally toxic, with a high temperature, vomiting and diarrhœa, acute misery and restlessness. He may refuse to lie down and holds his head stiffly, inclining it towards the affected side, in an instinctive attempt to relax the sternomastoid muscle which is attached to the mastoid bone. Œdema and swelling of the soft tissues behind the ear push the pinna forwards and downwards and the whole area may be red and shiny and very tender to touch. Although there is often a history of otitis media and aural discharge, discharge may be absent as the ear drum may never have perforated or the perforation may have closed up again causing the pus to trek backwards into the mastoid cells. Occasionally symptoms which resemble those of mastoiditis are caused by a meatal boil or an abscess of a superficial lymph gland behind the ear.

Treatment of mastoiditis may be conservative, that is to say by rest, warmth and chemotherapy. A well-balanced diet, rich in vitamins and abundant fluids is given at the same time. If the child is anæmic the anæmia should be treated and any septic foci which may be present should be eradicated.

Operations for the drainage of the mastoid antrum are similar to those performed on adults. There is also little that differs from the pre- and post-operative care.

Improvement in the child's condition usually follows operation rapidly and some children can be allowed up the day following operation.

Post-operative Care. In view of the painful nature of the first dressing an anæsthetic is given when this is done and a sedative may be necessary for the next and third dressings. The dressing is often left undisturbed for 8 to 10 days. By this time the post-auricular wound will probably have healed and some of the stitches can be removed. At the time of operation the auditory meatus will probably be packed tightly with ribbon gauze. When this is due for removal it can be softened by a solution of hydrogen peroxide 1 in 8. When the dressing is done, the pinna and the surrounding skin are thoroughly but gently cleaned with an antiseptic lotion and the meatus carefully mopped.

During the immediate post-operative period a mastoid bandage is usually necessary and young children may have to wear elbow splints to stop them from interfering with the dressing. On the second or third day older children are more comfortable if the mastoid dressing is kept in place by a mastoid cage in the day-time and a bandage worn at night only. As in the case of most head bandages, the bandage should be removed once daily and the child's hair given a brush. This is refreshing and prevents the hair from becoming tangled.

Myringoplasty (Tympanoplasty)

Occasionally a long-standing perforation of the ear drum is closed by skin graft. The necessary skin is taken from the upper arm, inner aspect of the thigh, a vein or from the ear. Working with the help of a microscope throughout the operation, the surgeon cleans the ear carefully and removes the upper skin of the tympanic membrane before applying the graft. The graft is kept in position by tiny plastic or nylon sponges, packed tightly into the auditory meatus and left undisturbed for at least 10 days. The operation is a very delicate one and only about half the cases are entirely successful. If the graft has taken discharge ceases and the danger that infection might enter the middle ear is eliminated. Hearing is not as a rule impaired. Tympanoplasty is a variant of this operation.

Cleft Lip and Cleft Palate

Approximately one baby in every thousand is born with a cleft lip or cleft palate so that most nurses are likely to meet this abnormality in the course of their pædiatric experience. Cleft lip and cleft palate are hereditary and are caused by a failure of development in the first three months of pregnancy. Many degrees of severity of this deformity occur and either condition can be present without the other. The cleft may be unilateral or bilateral, it may merely be a small notch in the upper lip, and it can be incomplete or extend deep into the nostrils. If the cleft is centrally placed the deformity is known as hare lip. Cleft palate may involve only the uvula or be a small hole in the soft or hard palate, but more often the cleft extends through both hard palate and soft palate. The cleft may be narrow or wide and may include the alveolar margin and if associated with a bad cleft lip causes an ugly protrusion of the premaxilla bone. In the majority of cases cleft lip is associated with an asymmetry and flattening of the nose (Fig. 33).

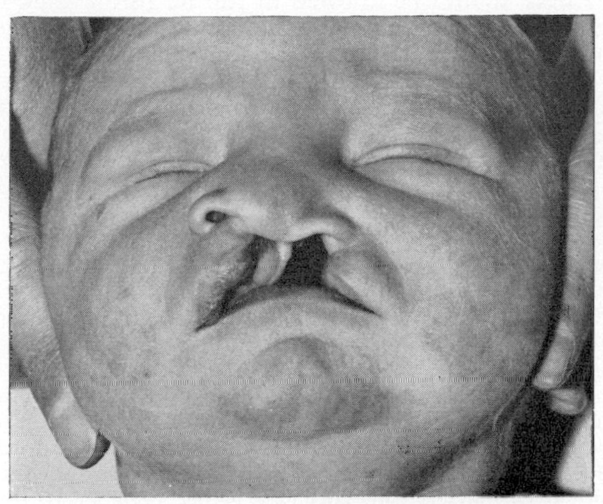

Fig. 33. Unilateral Cleft Lip and Cleft Palate.
Note the assymetry of the nose associated with the deformity.

Cleft Lip

General Points. As a mother who has a baby with a cleft lip is likely to be deeply distressed, repair is sometimes attempted in the first days after birth under local anæsthetic. The mother is thus saved the embarrassment of taking her baby home with an obvious and severe deformity. At the same time the closure of the cleft may help to push back the protruding premaxilla and later produce a better dental arch and a more regular development of the teeth. More usually, however, the operation is postponed until the baby is well established, that is to say when he is 3 months old and weighs about 12 pounds.

Cleft lip without cleft of the palate often does not interfere with sucking and in many cases breast feeding can be carried out successfully. Alternatively special nipple shields and teats are available and only severe cases of cleft lip and cleft palate need to be spoon-fed from birth. Even then the breasts should be expressed and the milk given to the infant as long as lactation can be maintained. When the cleft is complete feeding may be very difficult as regurgitation through the nose causes the baby to cough and sneeze. When spoon feeding, the milk should be allowed to run on to the back of the tongue or into the cheek, as this reduces regurgitation through the nose and checks irritation. Upper respiratory tract infections, inhalation pneumonia and otitis media are common.

Babies with cleft palates tend to swallow much air during feeding and special care must be taken when "bringing up the wind." A little boiled water is often given after feeds to clean the mouth and prevent crusts of milk from forming around the cleft edges.

Repair of Cleft Lip. The baby is usually admitted to a cubicle several days before the operation. The surgeon may wish to have a photograph taken for record purposes and nose and throat swabs are sent for culture as it is important that the baby should be free from infection. The hæmoglobin level should be 80 per cent. or higher. Spoon feeding is started and the baby should be nursed by as few nurses as possible, so that both baby and nurse can get used to each other. Ideally the mother is admitted with her baby and can be allowed to look after him herself most of the time. For spoon-feeding, a special spoon with the sides bent in to form a trough is often useful and great care must be taken not to injure the mucous membrane of the mouth. After feeds the chin should be well dried to avoid the skin getting sore from dribbling while being fed. Systemic penicillin is sometimes ordered to help reduce the risk of infection. In the newly-born infant the operation may be done under a local anæsthetic. A sedative such as chloral hydrate 60 to 300 milligrammes (1 to 5 grams) is given and the baby is placed on a T-shaped splint. If a general anæsthetic is to be given, splinting is not necessary but atropine 0·3 milligramme (gr. $\frac{1}{200}$) by hypodermic injection is ordered. Feeds are discontinued 4 to 6 hours before operation but a drink of 3 ounces of dextrose 5 per cent. is given 2 hours before the child goes to the theatre.

Post-operatively the baby is received into a warmed cot protected from draughts. While unconscious he is nursed on his side and the foot-end of the bed may be raised to help with the drainage of any saliva and blood, although bleeding is not likely to occur. A stimulant tray, oxygen and an electric sucker with small sterilized ends should be by the cot side. The sucker is used only if other means of evacuating secretions or blood prove ineffective, as the suture line can easily be damaged. It is of particular importance to watch the infant's colour and to ensure an adequate air-way as the closure of the cleft and the œdema arising from the local anæsthetic and surgical manœuvre may obstruct much of the airway to which the infant has been accustomed. If a general anæsthetic has been given, via an endotracheal tube, laryngotracheal œdema is a common complication which may require treatment by steam therapy.

A covered sterile tray, ready for use for the toilet of the suture line and nostrils, is kept by the bedside and its contents boiled at least once a day. It should contain fine dressing forceps, swabs, sterile saline and, if desired by the surgeon, some antiseptic lotion such as an aqueous solution of acriflavine 1 in 1,000, or Roccal 1 in 160. Sometimes liquid paraffin or Polyfax ointment, a mild antiseptic, which keeps the scar soft, may be applied. While the infant is still unconscious elbow splints are applied and in addition it may later be necessary to secure the splinted arms to the cot frame. The splints are removed at least twice daily and the child allowed to exercise his arms. As soon as the baby has regained consciousness, he is sat up well supported by pillows to facilitate breathing and avoid chest complications. As it is vital that all tension on the stitches should be reduced to a minimum everything possible should be done to stop the baby from crying. Picking him up and nursing him will not spoil the infant but is mere common sense at such a time. Occasionally a Logan's bow is applied to relieve tension (Fig. 34). Feeding can usually be resumed about two hours after return to the ward. As the infant has had atropine he is as a rule particularly thirsty and liable to cry for that reason. The first feed given is plain boiled water or sterile dextrose 5 per cent. If this is well tolerated, the next feed can be half strength milk and this can be rapidly increased to the feed the baby had been used to before operation.

Local care includes careful mouth toilet. If a nasal plug is in position, this is changed as soon and as often as it becomes soaked until it can be omitted according to the surgeon's instructions, probably after 48 hours. The lip is cleaned and any crusts gently removed. Hydrogen peroxide in a 1 in 8 solution may help to loosen any crusts of blood. If a Logan's bow is used, the skin should be watched for reaction to the strapping.

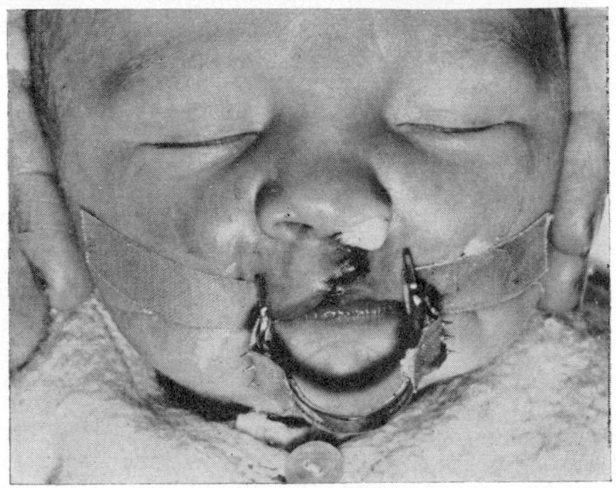

Fig. 34. LOGAN'S BOW.

After operation for repair of cleft lip, tension on the suture line may be reduced by using a Logan's bow. Note the pledget of cotton wool in the nostril to help absorb any nasal discharge and keep the stitches dry.

The catgut sutures used on the mucosa of the lip are not removed, as they gradually become absorbed, but the fine silk sutures should be removed on the 6th and 7th days respectively. Skilled restraint of the baby during this procedure is essential if scarring is to be prevented. Special care should be taken not to overlook the fine stitches which often continue well up into the floor of the nose.

In uncomplicated cases the infant may be ready for discharge once the sutures have been removed, although he may go home still wearing the Logan's bow, and the arm splints are not left off until this has been removed. Breast feeding and sucking from a teat can be started again as soon as stitches and bow have been removed, provided that an associated cleft palate does not make this impossible.

Cleft Palate

Repair of Cleft Palate. The usual age for repair of cleft palate is 18 to 24 months, that is to say before the child begins to talk, so that any bad habits of speech may be prevented from developing. Children with cleft palates are often late in commencing to talk.

As in the case of babies admitted for repair of cleft lip, these children are brought to hospital a few days prior to operation for thorough assessment and to allow them to get used to the unfamiliar people and surroundings. Elbow splints are applied for short periods so that the child may gradually become used to them. Nose and throat swabs are sent for culture and sensitivity tests and blood is taken to ensure that the hæmoglobin is no lower than 80 per cent. As post-operative blood transfusion is occasionally necessary the blood is also grouped.

Feeding and pre-operative care differ little from that for any other operation, and the immediate post-operative care is similar to that described under the heading of hare lip. The danger of an obstructed airway is, however, even greater. Careful watch has to be kept for excessive oozing of blood from the suture line. If vomiting occurs, stale blood may be seen. The immediate post-operative considerations and nursing observations are, for obvious reasons, very similar to those necessary for patients who have had a tonsillectomy (see page 134). Sometimes ribbon gauze packs soaked in Whitehead's varnish are used to relieve tension either side of the suture line. Although they are as a rule kept in position by the normal pressure of the tongue, the mouth should be inspected from time to time to see if they are still in position, as the child may try to dislodge them with his tongue. In this case his attention should be distracted and a sedative given. Elbow splints are used continuously until healing has taken place.

For the first 10 days all food should be liquid or semi-solid and meals should be followed by a drink of plain water to wash down any remains of food. The diet should be rich in vitamins, protein and iron.

Drugs. Sedatives should not be withheld for the first 2 or 3 days, as crying and fretfulness may prejudice the good result of the operation. Iron in the form of Colliron is often given and vitamin C in the form of ascorbic acid or fresh fruit juices will enhance healing. Government concentrated orange juice is inclined to sting on the raw wound edges and for that reason is best discontinued for the time being. Catgut is used for suturing and as this dissolves, removal is not necessary. Some surgeons favour silk sutures. These can be "sucked out" by the patient and will disappear within about ten days. Even though the child's arms are effectively splinted, the toys chosen to occupy and amuse him should be of a kind which cannot be put into the mouth, as this would easily cause damage to the suture lines and might introduce infection. It is also important that neither boiled, hard sweets, nor toffees should be given and in wards where unrestricted visiting is the custom, this should be explained to the mother.

Speech therapy is of great importance in promoting early, normal speech. As soon as the post-operative œdema has subsided the nurse can start to play games, such as blowing bubbles and practising the consonants K and T in order to encourage normal articulation. On discharge the child is referred to an expert speech therapist for assessment and in some cases the mother can be taught exercises which can be practised at home until such time as the child is old enough to benefit from organized speech therapy. The best results are obtained where there is good team work between surgeon, nurse, speech therapist and orthodontic surgeon.

Points of Interest

1 in 1,000 babies have a cleft lip or palate.

Mental subnormality is ten times more frequent in children with cleft lip or palate than in others.

Grades of deformity:

Lip only: 25 per cent. Palate only: 25 per cent.
Complete: 50 per cent.

Two males are affected to every female, and the deformity occurs in a proportion of two left clefts to every right.

10

THE CARDIOVASCULAR SYSTEM

The relationship between temperature, pulse and respirations in children is of great importance and should therefore always be reported together.

The Pulse

Owing to the small size of the structures involved, even simple procedures such as taking the pulse or the blood pressure and obtaining a sample of venous blood may present special difficulties in children; the younger the child, the more difficult it may be to feel and count the pulse beat over the radial artery at the wrist as he may resent being touched and may struggle or cry, overlying fat may make it hard to feel the pulse and may alter the volume and make assessment difficult. It is often a good plan to try to take the pulse while the patient is sleeping and this is often best done over the temporal artery immediately in front of the ear or in the case of infants over the fontanelle. The pulse should be taken and counted for one minute. Changes in the rate, volume or rhythm should be reported at once. In certain diseases, for instance in some types of congenital heart disease, the pulse beat can be plainly seen at the side of the neck, in others it is not palpable in the groin, as it is in normal children. The pulse rate alters as the child grows older and during exercise, excitement or disease. Infection and febrile conditions in infancy are not, however, necessarily accompanied by a rapid pulse as with adults, a fact which must be borne in mind when assessing a child's condition.

The Sleeping Pulse. When metabolism is at its lowest during sleep the pulse rate normally drops to approximately 10 beats below the waking pulse rate. Overaction of the heart, as it occurs in certain diseases, may cause both sleeping and waking pulse rates to be raised and at the same time the beat may be irregular. In certain diseases such as rheumatic carditis, there may be little or no difference between the sleeping and waking pulse and both may be significantly raised. A special record of the sleeping pulse is usually kept in these cases. It is of course important to avoid rousing the child when the pulse is taken. The temporal pulse is often the site of choice.

The Apical Beat (Apex Beat). In some diseases not every beat of the heart is transmitted to the radial pulse and it is important to record the difference by counting not only the peripheral pulse but also the apex beat. In children the apex beat is usually found just below the left nipple and can be heard with the help of a stethoscope. A difference between the apex beat and the radial pulse is known as pulse deficit.

Sinus arrhythmia is often noticed in children and, when present, does not necessarily imply disease. The pulse rate is accelerated during inspiration and slowed during expiration.

Extra-systole or premature contractions may be present in the healthy child but occurs more commonly when the heart is diseased. The extra-systole can be heard with a stethoscope or may be felt in a peripheral pulse. It is rhythmic and is sometimes likened to an "echo" of the real beat. This "echo" may take the place of the next beat and so cause a beat to be missed. Another abnormal pulse is known as *Heart Block.* In this condition there is failure in the conduction of nerve impulses from the atrium to the ventricle through the atrio-ventricular node. In consequence, although the heart may be beating rapidly, the pulse rate may be slowed to below 50 beats per minute or with partial heart block be irregular in rhythm. It is rare to find this abnormality in children.

Taking the Blood Pressure

In infants and young children it is difficult to estimate the blood pressure with accuracy. Special narrow cuffs may have to be used but they should not be wider than two-thirds of the length of the child's upper arm. Variations may be considerable even in healthy children, but average systolic readings are likely to be 60 to 80 millimetres of mercury and the diastolic pressure 50 to 60 millimetres of mercury in the first year and 100–110/80 (systolic/diastolic) at 10 years of age, while at rest.

Daily blood pressure readings may be required in certain heart diseases, diseases of the kidney, when increased intra-cranial pressure is suspected and in the case of patients on steroid therapy. A nurse who experiences difficulties should always seek help and advice, as the pædiatrician will rely on the accuracy of the charting notwithstanding the difficult nature of the procedure. Children are sometimes frightened by the apparatus, and it may be wise to "reassure" them by taking the teddy bear's blood pressure first and letting them handle the rubber bulb, making the mercury rise and fall themselves.

Lack of oxygen in the circulation causes cyanosis more readily in young children than in adults. Cyanosis is always a serious sign. It should be relieved without delay by the administration of oxygen. It may be particularly marked in respiratory abnormalities of the newly born, congenital heart lesions and in obstructed breathing. Occasionally young children have breath-holding attacks which cause cyanosis. These attacks are often due to behaviour disturbances and are of little pathological significance.

Types of Heart Disease in Childhood

There are two main types of heart diseases in childhood:

1. Inflammatory lesions in the heart, causing carditis.
2. Congenital malformations of the heart or blood vessels (Fig. 35).

Both these may interfere with the action of the heart and can, in their turn, cause chronic heart disease, due to failure of the heart to compensate for the extra strain placed on it by the cardiac abnormality. Chronic heart failure develops gradually and is therefore rarely seen before the patient has reached adolescence.

Inflammatory Heart Disease

Although endocarditis, myocarditis and pericarditis are separate entities, any one of them is bound to affect all parts of the heart as the various structures are so intimately connected.

Inflammation may be caused by toxins reaching the heart as in pneumonia, influenza, general septicæmia and especially diphtheria and the result may be heart failure. Alternatively the heart may be affected by bacterial invasion as for example in bacterial endocarditis. Inflammatory heart disease is one of the possible complications of rheumatic fever and chorea, and it is the possibility of permanent cardiac damage which gives these conditions their serious character.

Bacterial Endocarditis

Bacterial endocarditis is an acute, or more commonly a subacute infection of the endocardium and the condition often follows throat, dental or middle ear infections caused by the *Streptococcus viridans*. Bacterial endocarditis usually arises as a complication of congenital or rheumatic heart disease. It is rare in childhood.

The *symptoms* are similar to those of rheumatic carditis but the child is extremely toxic. He looks seriously ill, the eyes are sunken and surrounded by deep shadows and though he seems weary he tosses about restlessly. Pulse and respiration rates are increased and the temperature may rise to 40° C. (104° F.) or more. The skin becomes dry, the urinary output is low, the tongue is furred and the lips dry and inclined to crack. Petechial spots may appear on the skin.

Nursing Care. The child will be nursed in a similar manner to that described for other acute cardiac conditions. Abundant fluids are given to help reduce the toxæmia by assisting with the elimination of toxins via the kidney. The diet should be nutritious and well balanced but light and easily digested. It should be attractively served and contain an adequate vitamin intake to help raise the child's resistance to further infection.

Drug therapy is directed towards overcoming the infection by giving suitable antibiotics. Frequently very large doses of penicillin are ordered.

Complications. The most dreaded complication is embolism caused by a breakdown of septic particles from the diseased endocardium and the cardiac valves. The chance of permanent damage is great and what has been said about the nursing care and preventive measures in other acute heart conditions applies here in every detail. Recovery may be complete but the illness and period of convalescence may extend over some months and a careful follow up is usually arranged.

Pericarditis

Pericarditis may occur either as a result of rheumatic inflammation or bacterial infection. In the early stages the two inflamed surfaces moving upon each other cause friction and pain, but after some time the exudate of serous fluid which forms, separates the two surfaces and this relieves the pain. The pain is felt behind the sternum and, as it is increased by breathing, the child restricts respirations so that they become shallow and rapid. Dyspnœa and cyanosis may become apparent. The effusion is either absorbed or becomes fibrinous causing permanent adhesions. If the effusion is considerable, an aspiration of the pericardial sac may be undertaken. The procedure is similar to that of an ordinary chest aspiration as described on page 106.

The *nursing care* is like that of the other acute cardiac conditions but it should be realized that the pain, coupled with shortness of breath, may make the child very anxious and even severely frightened. At night it may be necessary to have a nurse near the child all the time and an adequate light should be left burning to comfort him. Fear of impending death is not uncommon.

Chronic Heart Disease

Chronic heart disease is a term given to illnesses which cause progressive or permanent damage to the heart and eventually lead to heart failure. It is uncommon in childhood as it rarely develops before the age of adolescence. Among the lesions causing chronic heart disease are mitral stenosis and mitral valve incompetence which leads to hypertrophy of the left ventricle.

At times the heart is able to overcome the defect by hypertrophy or increased effort although this puts an extra strain on the organ. Symptoms may at first be absent, though the heart is all the time subjected to additional strain when such compensation is no longer possible. Chronic cardiac failure then arises and symptoms due to failure in the circulation of the blood to the organs becomes apparent.

Signs and symptoms of chronic heart disease include cyanosis, breathlessness and a dry cough. The pulse becomes irregular, the rate varying considerably throughout the day and heart block may occur. The failing circulation causes retention of fluid in the tissues with symptoms of ascites, pleural effusion and pitting œdema in the pendent parts. The urinary output is low and the urine may be concentrated and contain albumen. The child is prone to develop pressure sores and this tendency is aggravated by restlessness and the need for sitting upright to relieve dyspnœa. The hands and feet tend to be cold and clammy.

Nursing care differs little from that for adults. The nurse will have to consider the patient's position and arrange adequate support for him. Whether in bed or in a comfortable armchair, she will have to treat the pressure areas and supply nursing aids such as a bed table to lean on and an air ring, sorbo cushion or water bed. Warm pyjamas and a chest blanket and bed socks are needed to help keep the patient warm. The weight of the bedclothes can be taken by a bed cradle.

Intake and output balance needs to be watched carefully and any change in this and in the pulse volume and rate reported immediately. Restful sleep should be secured by quiet, warm drinks and general comforting though a sedative such as choral hydrate or phenobarbitone may have to be prescribed. Oxygen is given by whichever method seems most suitable and comfortable to the individual patient. If œdema is present a low-salt diet may be ordered but it should contain the essential nutrients and adequate amounts of fruit and roughage to ensure easy bowel actions. Constipation may be obstinate and glycerin suppositories and mild laxatives may have to be used. Salt-free diets can be tiresome and variety and attractive appearance can do much to stimulate appetite. The food should be colourful whenever possible and attractive crockery may be used as a special treat. A low-sodium milk powder available under the name of Edosol can be used in the place of cow's milk both as a drink and for cooking purposes.

Prognosis

Many of these children recover a limited degree of normal health but the majority will have to attend special schools for the physically handicapped or residential homes for cardiac cripples. Here they not only receive ordinary education but are trained for occupations which may eventually enable them to earn their own living.

Congenital Heart Disease or Congenital Morbus Cordis

Errors in the structural development of the heart before birth may take a variety of forms and according to the type of defect may be incompatible with life or affect the patient in a greater or lesser degree. Some congenital defects are so minor, or so well compensated, that the child is able to lead a normal life. Cyanosis does not necessarily occur as long as the pulmonary circulation remains normal and this depends on the type of malformation affecting the child.

Shunts

When there is a communication between the left and right chambers of the heart through a defect in the septum, blood from the side of the heart where the pressure is greater will be forced into the opposite side of the heart where pressure is lower. A *left to right shunt* may thus occur. Blood from the left ventricle where it is under pressure is forced into the right ventricle through the abnormal opening in the septum between them, short-circuiting the lungs.

A right to left shunt occurs when blood is forced from the right ventricle or atrium when it is under greater pressure than the blood in the left ventricle or atrium. A typical example is high right ventricular pressure due to stenosis of the pulmonary artery. A typical example of a left to right shunt on the other hand, is the condition of atrial septal defect (Fig. 35).

The following is a short summary of abnormalities of the heart and its vessels.

Acyanotic Types of Congenital Heart Disease

Hypertrophy of the heart (very rare).
Dextrocardia.
Aortic stenosis.
Pulmonary stenosis.
Coarctation of the aorta.
Patent ductus arteriosus.
Atrial septal defect.
Interventricular septal defect.

Cyanotic Type of Congenital Heart Disease

Pulmonary stenosis with septal defect.
Dextraposition of the aorta.
Fallot's tetralogy.

Many of these abnormalities can now be relieved by operation but frequently these patients are admitted to medical pædiatric units for preliminary investigations and assessment. Certain terms used in the discussion of the child's symptoms and their nursing care should be understood by the nurse caring for these children.

It is not always easy to diagnose children with congenital heart disease in the neonatal period as signs and symptoms may be somewhat indefinite. Many infants go into heart failure at an early age, and it is important to be conversant with these signs and symptoms.

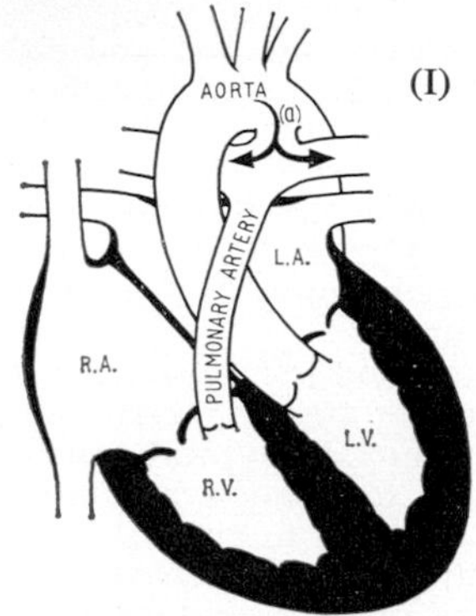

I. (a) indicates
Patent ductus arteriosus

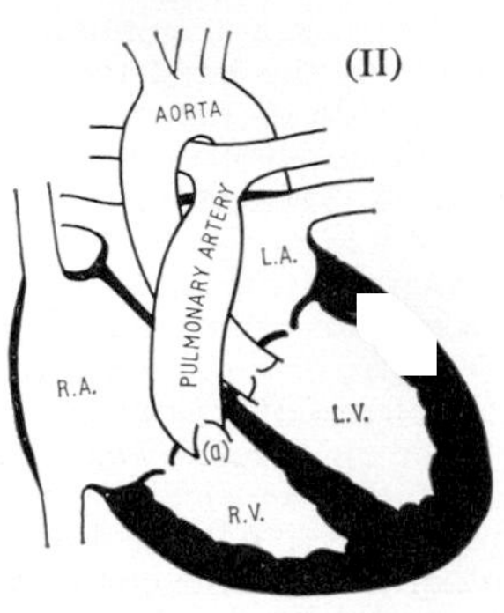

II. (a) indicates
Pulmonary valvular stenosis

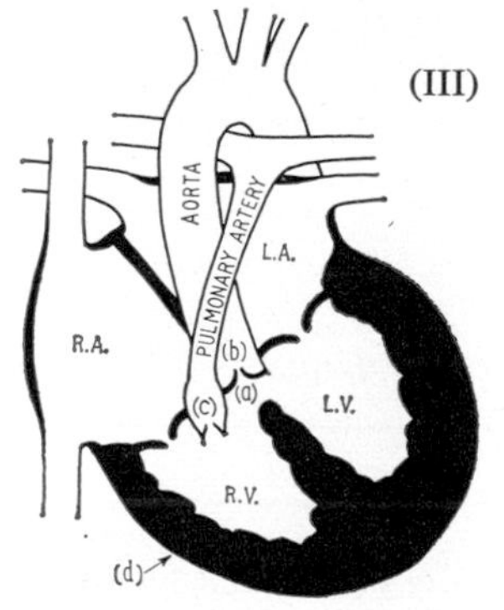

III. *Fallot's tetralogy*
(a) Ventricular septal defect
(b) Dextro position of aorta
(c) Pulmonary valvular stenosis
(d) Thickened wall of right ventricle

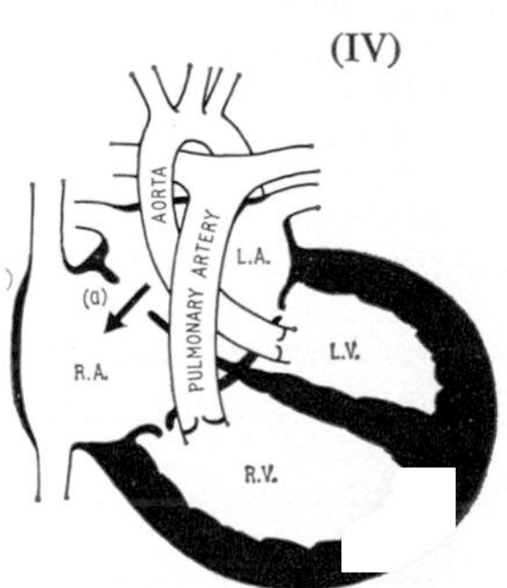

IV. (a) indicates
Atrial septal defect

Fig. 35. Congenital Malformations of the Heart and Great Vessels.

Babies with heart failure show a tendency to cold extremities, are puny in appearance and fail to thrive although œdema sometimes masks the fact by causing a false gain in weight and giving nicely rounded contours. The heart soon hypertrophies and causes the sternum and ribs to bulge forward. There is subcostal retraction and the apex beat is displaced. Respirations are rapid and the airway easily becomes blocked by thick, viscid secretions. Because of the difficulty in breathing the infant is often restless and irritable and throws his head back in an attempt to improve the air intake. Heart and liver are both enlarged and the lungs are congested. A persistent cough is common and leaves the infant exhausted. Pallor is more frequently present than cyanosis. Feeds are taken slowly and rarely finished, and vomiting is a fairly consistent feature. Clubbing of fingers and toes develops at an early stage.

Babies in heart failure need rest above all. They are best nursed in an oxygen tent (40 per cent. concentration) and in

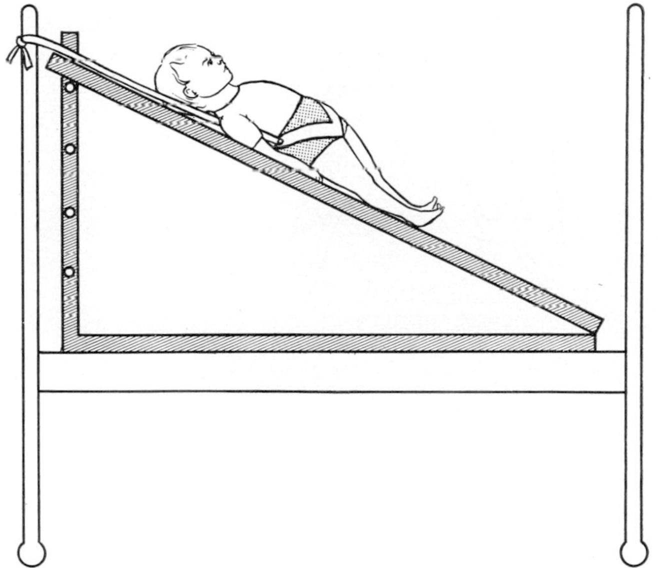

Fig. 36. Inclined Bed for Infants in Cardiac Failure.

high humidity. Sometimes a special frame is used which helps to keep the baby in an almost upright position (Figs. 36–7). Heat is easily lost and a rectal temperature of 36° to 36·6° C. (97° to 98° F.) should be maintained. The clothing, if any, should be light enough not to restrict breathing by its weight.

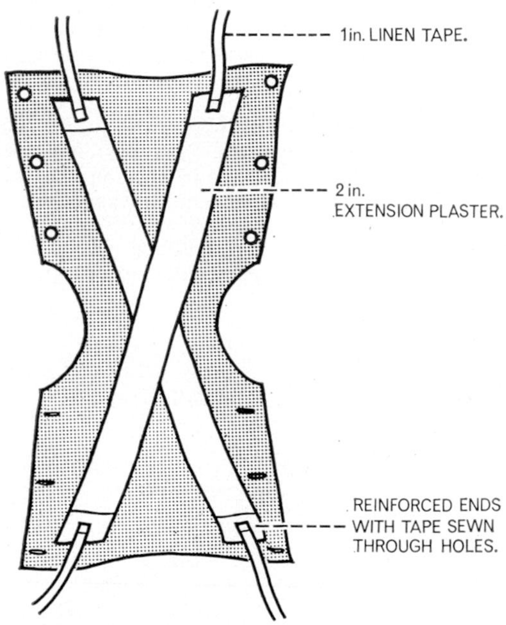

Fig. 37. A Good and Simple Method of Supporting Babies in the Upright Position.

This design, making use of ordinary plastic pants, was thought out by a staff nurse in her first post-registration year.

Tracheostomy often relieves the respiratory difficulties and makes it easier to suck out the viscid secretions. It also serves to reduce the "dead space" in the trachea. Secretions may at times be loosened by dropping 3 or 4 millilitres of a saturated solution of sodium bicarbonate into the tube immediately before turning on the suction and passing a fine catheter (no. 3 to 5 Jaques) well down into the tube.

Drugs given usually include diuretics such as chlorothiazide or Neptal; digoxin in large dosage; antibiotics; antispasmodic drugs to aid breathing and morphine as a sedative.

Children with congenital heart disease are prone to a variety of complications, many due to poor circulation of badly oxygenated blood. Bronchitis, pneumonia, sepsis, bacterial endocarditis and brain abscess are all seen with far greater frequency than in other children. Poor appetite, digestive difficulties and restricted exercise contribute to retardation of growth. Reduced peripheral circulation coupled with comparative immobility make these children very prone to pressure sores which are difficult to heal once they have occurred. Chronic heart failure may gradually develop and cause signs of peripheral œdema, ascites, nervous symptoms and distressed breathing. In those cases in which there is œdema, every effort should be made to allow the fluid to gravitate to the lower extremities and abdomen in order to prevent pulmonary œdema and embarrassment of breathing. The feeds of babies and the general diet may have to be salt free and a strict fluid balance chart kept. If the patient is having digoxin the dose may be increased to encourage diuresis and a diuretic such as hydrochlorothiazide given by mouth may be prescribed. Mercurial diuretics are not suitable for these patients on account of impaired renal function due to the poor renal circulation. A careful weight chart is the best means of spotting incipient œdema. The prognosis depends on the anatomy and the severity of the abnormality and several abnormalities occurring together obviously carry a greater risk than those occurring singly. Congenital disease of the heart and its vessels can now often be cured or alleviated by surgical intervention. In many cases, children who have never walked before can carry on with a normal life after successful operation, and others improve sufficiently to lead a useful, if restricted existence.

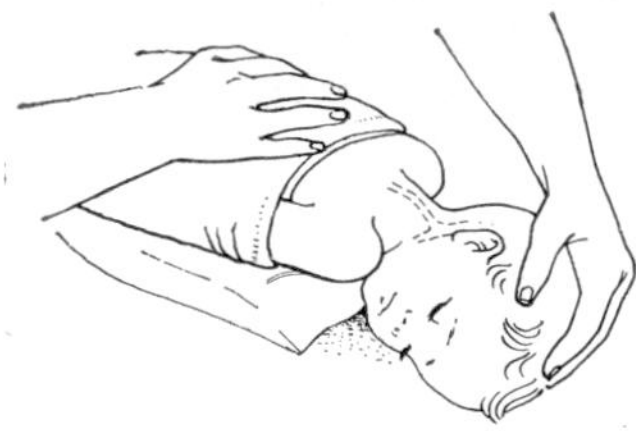

Fig. 38. METHOD OF RESTRAINING AND POSITIONING AN INFANT FOR VENEPUNCTURE.

Owing to the small size of the veins, either the external or the internal jugular vein is often used when a sample of blood is required.

Until such time as the child is old enough for surgical treatment or even if his condition is unsuitable for this, he is kept under careful supervision by a "cardiac team" as an out-patient.

Careful records are kept on the rate of growth and general exercise tolerance and the degree of disability. If admitted to the ward, special care is taken to reduce the risk of cross-infection to a minimum. The child is best placed in a bed where he can be easily watched and protected from colds and draughts. As breathing usually improves if the child is sitting up, he should be well supported with an adequate number of pillows and a back rest. Bed socks and mittens may help to keep the extremities warm and an air ring is useful in the prevention of pressure sores. The daily toilet includes a bed bath, as baths in the bathroom would prove too much of a strain in the majority of cases.

The diet should be light but nutritious and high in protein value. Small meals given frequently will prevent distension of the stomach and further embarrassment of breathing from pressure on the diaphragm. As the patient's appetite is likely to be capricious special care should be taken in serving the food attractively and it may be possible to allow him to take his meals in the company of and in competition with other children. Adequate amounts of fruit and vegetables and wholemeal bread and cereals in the diet, help to prevent constipation, an important point as the straining at defæcation may seriously tax the heart and cause cyanotic attacks. Infants may have to be fed by gastric tube which is often best left *in situ* for several days without changing. Very fine polythene tubing is used, for it is essential that the nostril should not be blocked by the tube as these babies already have difficulty in breathing, and even the slightest additional obstruction may prove too much for them. (Allen and Hanbury polythene tubing No. 2 connected to the rubber tubing by a 25 millimetre or 1 inch hypodermic needle is suitable.)

Like all chronically sick people, these children may have become spoilt and over-protected at home in an attempt at avoiding cyanotic attacks and exhaustion. They are often highly intelligent but inclined to be irritable, to tire easily and to show emotional instability but many are educationally backward. While doing everything necessary for the patient, the nurse should encourage him to make any small efforts his condition may allow such as cleaning his teeth, dressing and feeding himself, but at the same time she should watch to see how each small effort affects her young patient. Greater self-reliance and activity make the life of these children happier and their care at home easier.

Walking is often delayed, but with the permission of the specialist these children should be allowed to get up and play with the other children and take part in schooling and other activities. This enables the medical and nursing staffs to assess their exercise tolerance and also teaches children to adapt themselves to other children and to a more active existence than they often are allowed at home.

The nurse should learn to choose suitable toys and educational games which do not require too much energy. Free visiting and every other possible means of keeping in touch with the outside world are essential for these patients who are often in hospital for a considerable time.

Cyanotic Attacks. Some children with certain heart defects have frequent cyanotic attacks which may be so severe as to cause loss of consciousness. Oxygen is given by means of a light plastic mask or by oxygen tent, and care must be taken to protect these children from general injury. If the cyanosis is due to a right to left shunt, however, it cannot be relieved by giving oxygen as the blood does not circulate through the lungs. Many children obtain relief when placed on their right side; others when they are placed in the squatting position and their thighs doubled up on to the abdomen. The mother can often give valuable information about this and the intelligent nurse can find out the best means of relief by experiment and keen observation.

Charts kept include intake and output charts to detect incipient œdema at an early stage. The urine is tested weekly for the presence of albumin. The pulse rate and volume, the respiratory rate and depth, its character and the degree of cyanosis must all be carefully observed and changes reported at once. Reaction to exertion, time of administration of oxygen, response to drugs, cyanotic attacks, variations in weight are all charted regularly and help greatly in the assessment of the severity of the illness.

Drugs in common use include digoxin, which is employed particularly in cases in which the pulse is irregular. The dose will vary with the age of the child. A large, initial dose, e.g. 0·1–0·5 milligram may be followed by 0·0125–0·05 milligram at 4- or 8-hourly intervals. Some physicians give antibiotics prophylactically and vitamins and iron preparations may also be prescribed. When constipation is present a mild aperient such as milk of magnesia or Senokot may be given. Glycerin suppositories are often helpful.

Special Investigations. Electrocardiography, hæmatocrit estimation,* straight X-ray, barium swallow and X-ray screening, full blood picture, cardiac catheterization and angiocardiography are among the highly specialized tests carried out to help with diagnosis and to assess the child's suitability for surgical intervention.

Malformations of the Heart and its Vessels which do not cause Cyanosis

Dextrocardia (with situs inversus)

As the word implies in this condition the heart lies on the right side of the thoracic cavity and this phenomenon may also be accompanied by a complete reversal of the organs of the abdominal cavity. Thus for instance the liver is on the left, the spleen on the right, the appendix on the left and the flexures of the colon are reversed. The condition, if uncomplicated, does not interfere in any way with normal life.

Aortic Stenosis

When a thickening of the aortic semilunar valves occurs it is spoken of as aortic stenosis. The narrowing restricts circulation and causes a lowering of blood pressure in the peripheral arteries, and hypertrophy of the left ventricle develops as the heart attempts to overcome the obstruction. Valvotomy is carried out by opening the heart and operating under direct vision. A heart-lung machine is used.

Coarctation of the Aorta

Coarctation means narrowing and in this case narrowing occurs along the course of the aortic arch. The blood supply to the distal part of the aorta is thus reduced, while pressure is high in that part of the aorta and the arteries supplied by it which lie between the left ventricle of the heart and the narrowing, that is to say the proximal part. The systolic blood pressure in the arm is high, the heart muscle hypertrophies in an attempt at increasing its pumping action and subsidiary vessels develop. Pulsation in these vessels can be felt on the chest and back, while the femoral pulse is feeble or impalpable. Excision of the coarctation and if necessary

* The hæmatocrit value or packed cell value (P.C.V.) is a very accurate test for anæmia. The normal range is: at 1 year (mean) 35 per cent.; at 10 years (mean) 37·5 per cent. In full term cord blood: 44–62 per cent.

arterial grafting can be undertaken to relieve the condition in a high proportion of cases. The operation is ideally done at the age of about 10 years while the vessels are still highly elastic but already of reasonable size.

In successful cases the prognosis is good. The circulation becomes normal, the blood pressure falls to ordinary levels and the patient is able to live an active, unrestricted life.

Atrial Septal Defect

Atrial septal defect as a form of congenital heart disease is due to the persistence of an opening in the septum necessary in fœtal life but closing at birth in the normal child. The hole can be closed surgically and depending on the type of defect this is done either under controlled hypothermia or with the help of a heart-lung machine (cooling plus extra-corporeal circulation).

Patent Ductus Arteriosus

The ductus arteriosus is another anatomical feature necessary to the fœtal circulation, but failure to close after birth causes oxygenated blood from the aorta, which is under high pressure as it leaves the ventricle, to be pumped back into the pulmonary artery where the blood is under low pressure. The left ventricle has to do extra work to send blood to the pulmonary artery as well as supplying the systemic circulation. It hypertrophies and in infancy may fail. Owing to the leak from the aorta, continuing after the aortic valves have closed the diastolic blood pressure is low, thus producing the characteristic collapsing pulse.

Growth is often stunted on account of the restricted blood supply although otherwise there may be no symptoms. Diagnosis may not be made until the child is 3 or 4 years old as there are no early symptoms. The operation performed for this condition is best carried out during infancy or as soon as the diagnosis has been made. It consists of tying the ductus in two places and dividing it. Failure to operate may cause bacterial endocarditis or cardiac failure, while operation usually restores the patient to complete health.

Malformations of the Heart which cause Cyanosis

Any cardiac malformation which leads to heart failure may cause cyanosis but cyanosis occurring without heart failure is produced by blood from the right (venous) side of the neart getting into the systemic circulation. This produces the "blue baby". There are two main causes.

Transposition of the great vessels in which the aorta arises from the right instead of the left ventricle and the pulmonary artery arises from the left ventricle. There is as yet no satisfactory surgical treatment and death usually takes place within a few weeks, although, owing to other factors (an atrial septal defect and circulation through the brachial arteries) occasionally life continues for years.

Fallot's tetralogy is the other main type. Tetra signifies four but there are really two primary abnormalities with two others produced by them. The first is *ventricular septal defect*, which as we have seen causes by itself a shunt of blood from left to right; in this case there is yet another abnormality: *pulmonary stenosis*, which causes the right ventricle to work harder, raising its blood pressure so that blood flows from right to left through the ventricular septal defect. This right ventricular blood has not been through the lungs and therefore remains deoxygenated; as it is sent out with the left ventricular blood into the systemic circulation it produces cyanosis. The secondary abnormalities of the tetralogy are *hypertrophy of the right ventricle* which is produced by its struggle to push blood through the narrow pulmonary valve while at the same time satisfying the leak through the septal defect. As part of the dilatation and hypertrophy, *displacement of the septum between the ventricles* to the left occurs so that the septum lies underneath the opening of the aorta, which can thus easily receive blood from both ventricles. The septal defect is at the top of the septum just below the aorta.

The tetralogy thus consists of:

(1) ventricular septal defect;
(2) pulmonary stenosis;
(3) right ventricular hypertrophy, and
(4) transposition of the aorta, which is really transposition to the left of the ventricular septum.

Treatment

Treatment demands cure of the two primary defects, opening of the pulmonary stenosis by performing pulmonary valvotomy and closure of the septal defect.

Surgery of the Heart and Great Vessels

In the course of the last 15 years many abnormalities of the heart and great vessels have become amenable to surgery, assisted by new methods of anæsthesia, hypothermia, extra-corporeal circulation pace-makers and other modern advances. Under ideal conditions cardiac surgery can now be accepted in the same way as other types of surgery. Heart and great vessels can be regarded as specialized muscular tubes rather than inaccessible structures and much of the usual alarm about cardiac surgery is now no longer justified.

Pre-operative Care and Investigations

Ideally children are admitted about a week prior to the date of operation to allow them to get used to their surroundings and make friends with the staff. Breathing exercises are started so that the patient can do these effectively after operation. An antibiotic may be given in large dosage, any iron deficiency is treated, and the patient's likes and dislikes with regard to food are observed. It is important to know the patient well as this makes it easier to assess his condition accurately after operation. Pulse rate and rhythm should be known and the blood pressure readings in arms and legs are recorded as this enables doctors and nurses to recognize significant changes postoperatively. The width of the cuff used is important and all readings should be taken with the same cuff. If cyanosis is present the degree must be noted and a note made of the child's exercise tolerance and general activities. Height and weight are recorded and the sleeping pulse rate charted.

Laboratory tests include a full blood picture, blood grouping, and urine testing. Any other more elaborate tests such as angiocardiography, electrocardiography, cardiac catheterization, X-ray screening and barium swallow, auricular or ventricular puncture and arterial blood saturation tests will have been carried out previously. These tests are very specialized and cannot be described within the scope of this book. Decayed teeth and septic tonsils are treated before admission. The child should be free from coughs and colds but if old enough he should be taught to blow his nose and to cough effectively. Many of these children are mouth breathers and for that reason may have cracked lips which should be treated by the application of a greasy cream or petroleum jelly morning and evening and after meals. As there is a tendency to thrombosis a liberal fluid intake is essential unless œdema is present. The child's nurse will have an opportunity to get to know his likes and dislikes in this respect during the pre-operative period, and he can often be made to take an interest in his fluid chart. If the child is at all apprehensive he is allowed to spend a short time in an oxygen tent.

Cardiac surgery still holds special terror for many people and children undergoing this kind of surgery are often only children and particularly precious to their parents; these should be treated with great sympathy. It is important for all members of the cardiac team to gain their confidence and to help them through this period of great anxiety. At the same time it may be necessary to temper their hopes for the future, as these are often greater than is justified.

Immediate preparation differs little from that for any other major operation. If his condition permits, the child is given a bath the morning before operation and special attention is paid to axillæ, chest and back. Enemata are avoided as they cause extra strain on the patient and daily bowel movements will have been ensured by giving suitable diet, abundant fluids and, if necessary, a mild laxative. A sleeping draught such as chloral hydrate or Nembutal is given the night before operation to ensure a good rest. Rectal Pentothal, Omnopon and atropine are the usual pre-operative drugs.

Cardiac Surgery

The detail of technique in cardiac surgery varies from one hospital to another and sometimes unexpected decisions have to be made at time of operation. In all cases, however, thoracotomy is performed and in some cases this may have to be bilateral and include division of the sternum and resection of one or more ribs.

Occasionally intrapericardial procaine is injected during operation to reduce the irritating effect of the handling of the heart to a minimum and an injection of potassium citrate enables the surgeon to stop the heart temporarily at will. Other drugs may be used to lower blood pressure sufficiently to make the control of bleeding from the enlarged collateral vessels in the chest wall easier. During recent years special techniques have been evolved which make it possible to interrupt circulation temporarily. When the surgeon opens the heart to carry out surgery inside it under direct vision, a heart-lung machine may be used which takes over circulation for a short time.

One or more lobes of the lung are allowed to collapse in order to reach the heart and special anæsthetic techniques make it possible to inflate and deflate the lungs as required. Blood loss is carefully measured (all sponges or swabs are weighed before and after use) and replaced by blood transfusion, while the patient is still in the theatre. The vein is kept open in case of an emergency by giving intravenous fluids slowly, for about 12 hours after operation. (For details on hypothermia see page 170.)

Post-operative Care

On return from the theatre the child is nursed flat and as a rule an oxygen tent is needed. Until the lungs have fully re-expanded, intercostal drainage is carried out. The intercostal tube is connected to an under-water seal on return from the theatre and the rise and fall of the fluid level is carefully watched (for details of intercostal drainage, see page 171).

A sphygmomanometer cuff is left on the arm and the blood pressure taken and recorded half-hourly together with pulse and respiration. As soon as the patient has regained consciousness and the blood pressure has returned to normal he is given several pillows, his face and hands are sponged and he is made as comfortable as possible. When intercardiac surgery has been done, shock is usually severe and sitting the patient up is best delayed. Bed blocks may be used at first to raise the foot end of the bed to counteract shock, and later to help the patient from slipping down in the bed. The pillows should be so arranged as to make a hollow for the drainage tube to prevent it from kinking or from being compressed by the weight of the body. A blood transfusion is often started in the theatre and when this is discontinued the vein is kept open by a slowly dripping infusion so as to have a vein readily available should a further transfusion be necessary.

Before moving the patient an injection of morphine is usually given as it is important to relieve pain which may cause the child to restrict his chest movements and cause unnecessary fear and discomfort. Morphine by injection, Disprin and chloral hydrate are given freely during the first 24 hours but after that time pain is rarely severe. If hypothermia has been used, the excretion rate is slowed down and long acting drugs such as morphine or digoxin may have to be given in reduced amounts, or even withheld altogether until the temperature has returned to normal. In young children the dosage of morphine sulphate is usually calculated on the basis of 0·1 milligramme per pound of body weight.

In order to encourage the patient to move freely, a piece of webbing may be attached to the foot end of the bed and the child can use this in the manner of a pair of reins to pull himself forward. Physiotherapy is started after approximately 4 hours. In this connection it is very important to remember that the child must first of all be made to breathe out fully in order to prevent him from moving any mucus further down the bronchial tree instead of coughing it up. Only after full expiration should deep breathing be started. He will then probably be laid flat on "the good side" and the back and chest vibrated and percussed to move secretions. Older children are encouraged to expectorate but sometimes the electric sucker may have to be used and very occasionally post-operative bronchoscopy is necessary. Mucus obstructing the bronchial tree may lead to fever, raised pulse and respirations, dyspnœa and cyanosis and failure to make general progress. Since the physiotherapist cannot be available all the time nurses should know how to carry out modified exercises and they should use every opportunity for encouraging deep breathing, coughing and chest expansion. They should also watch posture and prevent scoliosis from developing. Movement of the lower limbs is important to prevent thrombosis and during bedmaking the patient should be rolled from side to side as this helps to move mucus and secretions. Pressure sores develop quickly particularly in the first hours after operation as these patients have lain on the operating table in the same position for several hours. Furthermore the skin is devitalized by poor circulation and sometimes by the use of hypothermia. Nurses need not be afraid of moving their patients adequately to treat the pressure areas even in the first post-operative hours.

Lung expansion can be watched by observing the degree of fluctuation in the tube and the amount of drainage. If there is no drainage tube, early X-ray with the portable machine is taken and occasionally air or blood have to be aspirated with syringe and needle from the pleural space.

During the first 24 hours special nursing care will absorb much of the nurse's time. Complications are most likely to occur during that time and the nurse should be observant and must understand the significance of any changes and report promptly and accurately. Speed in taking action may be very important.

Complications include spontaneous filling of the pleural space with air: pneumothorax, or with blood from a bleeding point in the heart itself or from one of the great vessels: hæmothorax; signs include accelerated and distressed breathing and general collapse. Frank blood may appear in the drainage tube, but the possibility of a concealed intrathoracic hæmorrhage must always be kept in mind. Morphine and a blood transfusion are given at once and the patient returned to the theatre for ligation of the bleeding point and evacuation of the free blood from the hæmothorax.

The long intratracheal anæsthetic may cause œdema of the larynx which usually responds to steam therapy but very occasionally tracheostomy becomes necessary. Damage to the cervical sympathetic chain and the recurrent laryngeal nerve may cause paralysis of the vocal cords which may take a long time to recover or may even be irreversible; this is known as Horner's syndrome. Cardiac irregularities may occur. Other complications include cerebral thrombosis, and cerebral abscess. The reason for these last two complications is probably not yet fully understood. A warning sign of cerebral thrombosis is delayed return to consciousness and hemiplegia. Cerebral abscess develops gradually. The patient may have an unexplained fever, he is irritable and drowsy and may have convulsions and develop slow mental changes. Neurosurgery may be necessary to drain the abscess.

Once the immediate post-operative period is over, it is often difficult to restrain these children who are eager to try out their newly found strength. Following the simple types of thoracic operations they are often able to sit in a chair during bedmaking on the day after operation and allowed to walk a few steps on the third day. When intracardiac surgery has been performed shock is more severe and greater care has to be taken. The child may be allowed to dress in day clothes and sit on top of his bed and move around freely on the third day, but too early ambulation may lead to unexplained thoracic pain and malaise towards the tenth day. As soon as the patient is up and about he should be encouraged to watch his posture in front of a mirror. The child should wear his own, well fitting shoes and not be allowed to walk around in slippers. Muscular pains in the back and legs are usual at first but they can easily be relieved by giving Disprin. They disappear as the patient gets used to exercise and as the muscles grow stronger. The diet should be built up from a very light, easily digested one to one rich in protein, minerals and vitamins and fluids should be given in adequate amounts. The child is usually hungry as a result of his increased exercise tolerance. Babies may have to have ½-strength feeds at first and it should be remembered that after hypothermia the calorie requirements are low until normal temperature has been regained.

After relief of a serious cardiac disability babies often find themselves enjoying their feeds for the first time in their lives. They are inclined to take them greedily and often demand more than is offered. Temptation to give in to their newly found appetite must be resisted as there is great danger of collapse if the stomach is allowed to become distended with feed and expansion of the lungs may be delayed by pressure on the diaphragm. The baby may have to be pacified by giving a sedative, rather than by extra feeding.

The nursing care outlined briefly in the last paragraph is one that may be used as a general guide in the nursing care of any child who has undergone thoracic surgery. Each hospital will, however, have its own special way of managing these children and each type of operation presents special problems. A description of the various types of operation and their management should be sought in a more detailed text book.

Hypothermia

The ability of certain organs of the human body to remain undamaged if deprived of oxygen at normal temperature is known to vary and it is known that the brain tissues are the first to suffer and that the maximum period of deprivation is 12 minutes without causing irreparable damage. By cooling the body to temperatures as low as 12° to 15° C. (53° to 60° F.) the chemical processes of the body are slowed down and the oxygen requirements reduced. Operations involving a temporary interruption of circulation can therefore be undertaken while the patient is in a state comparable to that of a hibernating animal.

Cooling the body can be achieved by the use of ice packs, by immersion into cooled water or by allowing the blood to flow through a cannula and tubing from the superior vena cava through a refrigerating circuit and pumping it back into the circulation via the inferior vena cava. At this low body temperature large vessels can be clamped off, the heart opened and operations performed under direct vision. When the operation is complete, normal circulation is restarted and the patient is allowed to warm up gradually. This may be done by warming up the operating theatre, by using electric blankets, by placing the patient on blankets perfused with water at a temperature of 40° C. (104° F.) or by extracorporeal warming of the blood. The warming-up process may either be carried out entirely in the theatre or started there and completed in the ward. It should be done very gradually. During this time the temperature is taken rectally every quarter of an hour. A special device called a Thermocouple may be used, the lead of which is inserted into the rectum and frequent, accurate recordings are made without disturbing the patient. A rise of more than half a degree in a quarter of an hour is the signal for discontinuing active warming-up procedures. Reactionary hyperpyrexia develops occasionally and tepid sponging, cooling the room or the oxygen tent and using an electric fan is as a rule all that is needed, but occasionally it may be necessary to cover the wound with a plastic seal and lower the patient into a bath of water at 32° C. (90° F.). Whenever heat is applied great care must be taken as the skin is devitalized by hypothermia and low blood pressure during operation. Even after the body temperature has returned to normal, hands and feet may remain cold and the child may need mittens and bootees even though he may be nursed otherwise naked with only a light cotton cover. Overheating and dehydration must both be avoided by good nursing care.

Intercostal Drainage

Following extensive intrathoracic surgery one or two tubes are stitched into position to allow fluid and air to escape from the pleural cavity, until the lungs have completely re-expanded. The drainage tube which forms an air-tight seal into the pleural cavity is connected to a graduated bottle and an under-water seal, thus every expansion of the chest on inspiration increases the intrapleural vacuum and water is drawn up in the tube. The weight of the column of water prevents it from rising more than a few centimetres within the tube so that the intrapleural vacuum is preserved all the time. The fluctuations of the water column are a useful guide as to the degree of chest movement and at the same time show that the tube is remaining patent and that there is no escape of air from the lungs. The swing is usually best seen in the glass tube which goes through the rubber bung, but, in infants, drainage may be infinitesimal and semi-transparent latex tubes make it possible to watch drainage of serum and blood and fluctuations at the proximal end of the tube. When the lungs are once again fully expanded, drainage ceases and after confirming this by X-ray, the tube is removed. In children an extra length of tubing is used to allow for free movement. The tube must be clipped off securely when changing the bottle and the latter must never be raised above the level of the patient, or air and fluid may be sucked into the pleural cavity. The type and amount of drainage are carefully noted at regular intervals and at night a good light is needed to enable the nurse to read the markings on the graduated bottle accurately.

11

RHEUMATIC AND COLLAGEN DISEASES

All the diseases described in this chapter are thought to be due to a hypersensitivity or auto-immunity reaction. In persons affected by any of these conditions, the normal immune reaction is replaced by an abnormal sensitivity to infection or a definite destructive reaction within the body. In addition to the conditions described in this chapter, the following diseases are sometimes included in this broad group:

Anaphylactoid purpura (see page 194).

Idiopathic and symptomatic thrombocytopenic purpura (see pages 193 and 194).

Nephritis, nephrosis (see page 274).

Ulcerative colitis.

Subacute Rheumatism

In the outpatient department children are often said to be listless, "off colour", disinterested in food, pale and failing to gain weight. They complain of indefinite aches and pains and frequently the tonsils may show signs of recent inflammation or sepsis. These children are sometimes said to be suffering merely from growing pains and at times little note is taken of what appears to be a phase in the normal development of the child. This however, is an outdated and dangerous idea. Subacute rheumatism is a most serious condition and any child complaining of the symptoms described should be seen by a doctor without delay. Normal growth does not cause pain and neglect of subacute rheumatism may cause carditis and permanent damage to the heart. The diagnosis can easily be confirmed: the erythrocyte sedimentation rate will be significantly raised and as a rule the case history will be typical.

Treatment consists of resting the child in bed and of careful observation of pulse rate and rhythm and of changes in the sedimentation rate. Return to normal activities and schooling should be very gradual and carefully supervised. Many physicians prescribe a prolonged course of sulphonamides or penicillin as a prophylaxis against recurrence of the streptococcal infection which usually precedes a relapse. Treatment for diseased tonsils and dental decay should be considered and the child's health should be built up generally. He needs a well balanced diet, an adequate vitamin intake and possibly an iron mixture. Clothing should be warm and if rehousing is possible this may have to be considered where living conditions are poor.

Acute Rheumatic Fever and Rheumatic Carditis

In acute rheumatic fever there is commonly a history of a sore throat or tonsillitis two or three weeks before the onset of symptoms.

Streptococcus pyogenes is usually the causative organism, but this is not always present on culture when a throat swab is taken. The infection may have been overcome although the streptococcal toxin has set up an auto-immune reaction in the body.

The child suffering from acute rheumatism often has a moderate pyrexia of about 37·2° to 37·8° C. (99° to 100° F.), but it may be much higher. The pulse rate is raised and toxic signs such as headache, vomiting, furred tongue, sweating and constipation are likely to be present. The child may complain of severe pain in the knee, elbow, ankle and wrist joints. These severe pains may affect one joint one day and others the next and although there may be redness, heat and swelling there is no permanent damage to the joints. In long standing cases anæmia may develop and there is danger of permanent cardiac damage. The latter fact makes good medical care and careful nursing all-important. A constant watch has to be kept for early signs of carditis (see page 175).

Occasionally a faint, slightly raised pink rash appears on the trunk and this may recur intermittently for several months (erythema marginatum). On examination rheumatic nodules are sometimes found over the elbows, shins, knuckles, knees, occiput and spine (erythema nodosum). These nodules are better felt than seen, but when the skin over them is stretched they show up clearly as raised, white areas. They may appear in crops for many weeks and may go only after some considerable time. These nodules are usually a sign that the illness is taking a serious course and they are rarely found unless the heart has become affected.

Treatment of Rheumatic Fever and Rheumatic Carditis

Little treatment can be given apart from adequate drug therapy and careful nursing care and rest.

Drug Therapy. Salicylates are the specific drugs for the treatment of acute rheumatic conditions. Usually at least 0·6 grammes four times a day are given in the form of aspirin or, preferably, Disprin or Solprin, since the two latter are less irritant to the gastric mucosa. Relief from pain may be very rapid. Signs of intolerance or overdose, which used to be very common when sodium salicylate was used, are now unusual but if they occur they should be reported at once. They include nausea, tinnitus, vomiting, deafness, albuminuria, a discreet erythematous rash, sighing respirations and purpura. Prophylactic drug therapy against recurrent streptococcal infections is sometimes prescribed and usually carried on for a period of at least five years or until the child leaves school, whichever is the longer. During that time the patient may be ordered penicillin by mouth or one of the sulphonamide group of drugs. Steroids are valuable in severe cases or where there are signs of cardiac involvement, since the early use of these drugs has been found to prevent or minimize permanent cardiac damage. If there is any cardiac incompetence due to carditis, digoxin may be ordered.

Nursing Care. Children suffering from acute rheumatism should be nursed in a warm, well-ventilated, pleasant room. If admitted to a ward they should be given a bed in a quiet corner where there is little danger of other children or passers-by knocking into their beds, as at first pain is severe and even slight vibration, caused by someone passing or holding on to the bed while talking to the patient, may cause the child to cry out in agony. Complete rest is enforced, that is to say he is not allowed to do anything for himself. The nurse will have to explain this if the child is old enough and capable of cooperation. He will be washed and, unless a very light patient, two nurses will be required for giving a bed pan which he is asked to use in a lying down position. In many cases the child will have to be fed, but some pædiatricians feel that, provided the patient is well supported by pillows, he may be allowed to feed himself as this may improve the appetite and is often less strain than being fed. When pain is present the use of small pillows or pads of cotton wool to support the affected limb may give comfort. A soft, firm mattress should be used and the weight of the bedclothes taken by a bed cradle. But no definite rule can be laid down and the nursing routine will largely depend on the history, the severity of the illness, whether the heart is involved and the patient's response to treatment. It is, however, always best to be too careful in view of the serious consequences a neglect of the illness may have.

The *diet* should be light and nutritious as the illness is a long and debilitating one and no trouble should be spared in tempting the child with dishes he enjoys.

Drinking in the recumbent position can be a serious problem. A feeding cup may be used and the nurse can play a suitable game with her patient while teaching him how to drink from it. Polythene tubing is more suitable than a straw to assist with drinking, as it bends easily. Owing to its transparency the fluid can be seen going up and down the tube, a fact which amuses children and makes drinking a pleasure. Nowadays coloured straws which can be bent and moulded have become available. A story told or read while feeding a child is permissible if this means a contented patient who takes his food willingly.

As exertion should be reduced to a minimum, it is useful to let the child wear an open back gown in the acute stages as this makes dressing and undressing easy and also prevents him from lying on wrinkles and creases. The nurse can use her nursing skill and imagination in many ways to relieve pain and boredom and to make the irksome rest and the difficulties of taking food in the recumbent position as bearable as possible. Some ways of relieving pain and preventing painful movement are mentioned above. In the relief of boredom a good pædiatric staff will cooperate in setting some time aside during which the nurse can read to the child or sit down beside him to talk to him or draw for him. A book-rest may be supplied to make reading possible without exertion or light toys or comics may be provided. It may be possible to move the bed near a window and let the child watch the happenings in the street by means of a spy mirror fixed to the bed. Extra visiting helps to allay boredom and a wireless set by the bedside is often greatly appreciated and may give hours of restful entertainment.

Rheumatic carditis most commonly follows an attack of acute rheumatism often preceded by a sore throat, but may occasionally arise without any evidence of previous infection. Endocarditis with some involvement of the myocardium is the most common manifestation and the pathology is similar to that of endocarditis in the adult. The lesions resulting from the inflammatory process are scarring and growth of vegetations around the cardiac valves; the most commonly affected one being the mitral valve. Over a period of years, mitral stenosis accompanied by aortic regurgitation and enlargement of the left ventricle develops. In the young adult this damage leads to dyspnœa, congestion of the lungs, œdema and generalized cardiac crippling.

The child who has an attack of acute rheumatism fails to improve and remains tired, irritable and unhappy. His appetite is poor, his sleep restless, his colour grey or dusky, his skin feels clammy and the face looks pinched and the nose pointed. The pulse rate is rapid and the sleeping pulse rate may rise to approximate the waking pulse. Irregularities of volume and rhythm may occur. A mild pyrexia of 37·2° to 37·8° C. (99° to 100° F.) is common. The child frequently suffers from dyspnœa.

On examination heart murmurs can be heard and the erythrocyte sedimentation rate may be raised from 10 millimetres to 60 or 80 millimetres per hour. The urinary output is often diminished and œdema may develop due to heart failure.

Complications arising from rheumatic carditis may become apparent during the attack or occur later, and are due to permanent damage to the heart and its valves. They include heart failure, mitral stenosis, aortic valve incompetence and pericarditis. All these are likely to make the patient into a permanent invalid and to shorten life. No trouble or expenditure of time is therefore too much to give when nursing those children and a very great responsibility rests upon the nurse in this respect.

A child with rheumatic carditis will be in bed for a number of weeks or months and passive exercises, particularly to the limbs, are sometimes given to help to maintain muscle tone and prevent foot drop, without causing the patient any exertion. The position in the bed will depend on the wishes of the physician and on the degree of dyspnœa present. A semi-recumbent position with two or three pillows giving adequate support to the trunk, neck and head, is often considered more satisfactory than the recumbent position with only a small pillow for the head, as it may be difficult to keep a child quiet and content with most of his outlook confined to watching the ceiling. If one pillow only is allowed, raising the head end of the bed on blocks overcomes some of the difficulty. It is sometimes considered wise to nurse these children in a cubicle or side ward to ensure better rest and quiet. This needs to be considered carefully, however, as many children will lie still more readily when they can watch what is going on around them, provided a long night's rest and a good sleep at midday can be guaranteed. The blanket bed, so commonly used at one time, is now not considered necessary but a small flannelette blanket next to the patient may give comfort and extra warmth. A daily blanket bath should be given, particularly if perspiration is profuse. Oral toilet and regular attention to all pressure areas are important in a patient who will be ill for some time and who as a rule has to lie still, is on a very light diet and is probably thin and in indifferent general health.

Charts and Observations. Four-hourly recordings of temperature, pulse and respirations will be made and the sleeping pulse taken and recorded four-hourly throughout the night. The nurse should note particularly the quality and rhythm of the pulse rate and report any irregularities without delay, as they may be the earliest signs of cardiac involvement. The nurse's intelligent observations and careful recording can be of great value to the doctor in charge. A fluid balance chart is kept up and the urinary output watched conscientiously. An imbalance in the intake and output may be an early sign of cardiac failure. The child's weight is checked weekly, provided special scales which enable even older children to be weighed lying down, are available for the purpose.

The *erythrocyte sedimentation rate* is taken weekly and together with the sleeping pulse recordings will give a good indication as to the patient's progress. Guided by these and a lessening in the abnormal heart sounds, a gradual increase in exercise is allowed, though the child may need to remain at rest for several weeks or even months. If symptoms persist and the heart lesion fails to improve, transfer to a long-stay Hospital and special schooling may have to be arranged.

Chorea (Sydenham's Chorea, "St. Vitus's Dance")

Chorea is sometimes described as rheumatism of the brain. Attacks may be so mild as almost to escape notice or of extreme severity. In its severest form chorea is now rarely seen, but the seriousness of the attack cannot be overestimated even if it is a mild one. In this chapter a severe case and its nursing care is described and the intelligent nurse will modify the nursing treatment according to her patient. The characteristic features of the disease are the involuntary, uncoordinated and purposeless movements.

Signs and Symptoms. The onset is often insidious but emotional factors do appear to play a part in starting the disease. Anxieties over schoolwork, sudden frights or bereavement are among these emotional causes. Parents and teachers may merely complain that the child has become fidgety, that he is dropping things at school and that his handwriting is deteriorating. The usually bright pupil becomes inattentive and giggles and grimaces during lessons. As time goes on the movements become more marked and emotional disturbances develop. The child laughs and cries without any apparent reason. Examination of the patient includes some simple, but almost diagnostic tests. The child who is asked to put out his tongue does so, but moves it in and out, unable to keep it still. Asked to unbutton his coat he is unable to do so on

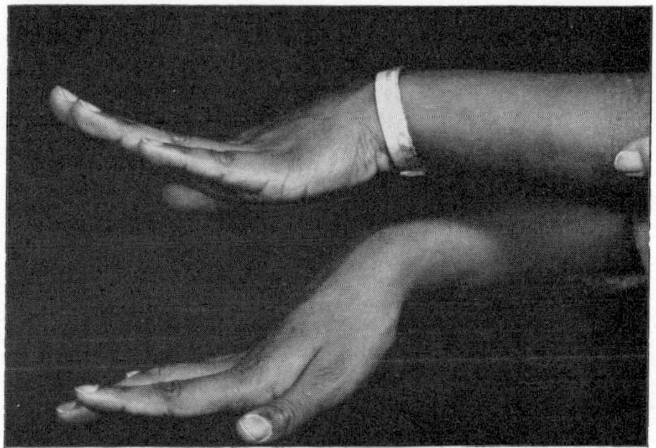

Fig. 39. CHOREA.
Typical position of the hand, known as spooning.

account of irregular, unco-ordinated movements and when asked to hold out his hands in front of him he shoots them forward like a gun. Hyperflexion of the wrist and hyperextension of the metacarpophalangeal joints causes a "dinner fork" deformity of the hands. Speech is jerky and difficult to understand and in the severest form may be altogether impossible. During the medical examination the child is sometimes asked to count rapidly, a task he finds himself unable to perform. He finds writing and drawing extremely difficult and it is often interesting to give the patient a weekly drawing task in which improvement in the co-ordinated movements can be seen when the successive drawings are compared. The child has a friendly smile which may seem very attractive, but it is exaggerated in relation to the circumstances and to his emotional state. He easily bursts into tears and has emotional upsets and temper tantrums.

Eating and drinking are difficult as the patient is constantly moving and throwing himself about. The difficulty of getting the child to take sufficient nourishment, together with the constant movements, leads to wasting and this coupled with the rubbing of occiput, elbows and heels on the bedclothes presents a serious nursing problem, if bedsores are to be prevented. An interesting feature is the fact that movements cease during sleep.

Nursing Care. The child is best nursed in a quiet part of the ward. Cot sides should be used to prevent him falling out of bed and in severe cases these need to be padded to prevent injury. The head bars of the bed should be protected by tying a pillow in position. As movements are so uncoordinated, there is a real danger of suffocation and loose, soft pillows must never be used. Sudden noises or lights should be avoided and all excitement kept from the patient. All sources of danger such as buttons, pins, long fingernails and sharp or even hard eating utensils must be eliminated. The mouth should be given special attention as the child frequently bites his tongue, lips or cheeks and ulceration easily occurs. The corners of the mouth should be protected against the constant dribble of saliva by lanolin or petroleum jelly. Feeding presents many difficulties. The child will move his head around continuously and it is often almost impossible to "aim" at the mouth. Inhalation of food, drink and saliva is a real danger and not easy to prevent. Plastic spoons and polythene tubing are useful but at times it becomes necessary to resort to tube feeding. The diet should have a high calorie value and should require little mastication.

The giving of bed pans may also present difficulties. As the patient cannot keep still on the bed pan, abrasions must be prevented from the start by padding the hard edges or by using rubber bed pans. The temperature must be taken in the groin or axilla to prevent accidents.

Every attempt should be made to ensure as much rest and sleep as possible by good nursing attention. Warm sponging may not only keep the skin healthy but may help to induce sleep. Toys should be of a simple, soft type and should have no hard bits or parts which could come off and be swallowed. Hairslides should be replaced by ribbon.

The temperature, pulse and respirations are recorded every

four hours and observations on the pulse and the recording of the sleeping pulse are of particular importance. Whenever possible a weekly weight chart is kept, as well as a note on the patient's emotional behaviour, movements and general

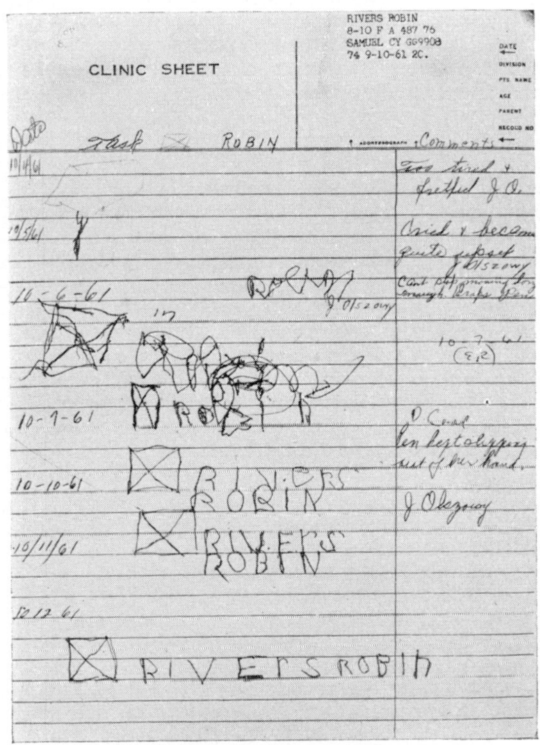
RIVERS ROBIN
8-10 F A 487 76
SAMUEL CY G69908
74 9-10-61 2C.
CLINIC SHEET
DATE
DIVISION
PTS. NAME
AGE
PARENT
RECORD NO
Date
Task
ROBIN
Comments
10/4/61
10/5/61
10-6-61
10-7-61
10-10-61
RIVERS ROBIN
10/11/61
RIVERS ROBIN
10-12-61
RIVERS ROBIN

Fig. 40. Chorea.
Samples of the patient's hand-writing, illustrating clearly the initial difficulties and the steady increase in legibility as the clinical condition improves.

condition. A weekly sample of his writing or drawing performance can be filed for comparison.

Treatment. Apart from careful nursing, every effort should be made to reduce exertion and excitement to a minimum. The nurse should spare the time to sit by the child and read and talk to him and extra visiting by the mother will help to keep him happy and occupied. There is little medical treatment apart from sedatives. Some physicians prescribe a course of penicillin or sulphonamides prophylactically over a period of years. Erythrocyte sedimentation rate and cardiography give a useful guide to progress.

Complete recovery may be expected after several weeks but there is a strong tendency to recurrence and the danger of cardiac involvement is considerable.

Still's Disease (Rheumatoid Arthritis)

Although Still's disease is not common in childhood, characteristic manifestations and the careful nursing required make it a condition of some interest to the general-trained nurse, who will already have met a similar condition in the adult wards.

Still's disease most commonly starts at the age of 3 to 6 years and the earlier the onset the less favourable the prognosis. The cause remains unknown.

Signs and Symptoms. Occasionally the onset is acute and may easily be mistaken for acute rheumatic fever. The child is feverish and complains of general malaise. Pain and swelling of the joints may be both acute and severe. More often, however, the disease develops gradually. The usually bright child becomes listless, miserable and pale. Loss of appetite soon causes him to lose weight and he fails to make general progress. He has a low grade fever, the skin is moist and clammy and the blood sedimentation rate is raised (50 to 100 millimetres) and the Rose Waaler test is positive. The hæmoglobin level falls and there may be a mild degree of tachycardia. On examination, subcutaneous nodules may be found although more rarely than in rheumatic fever. As the illness progresses the joints become painful and swollen and the overlying skin looks white and shiny, though at the same time it may be hot to the touch. Periarticular swelling and wasting gradually cause the fingers to take on a spindle-shaped appearance.

As a rule the fingers, wrists, elbows and knees are affected most and the swelling and deformity occur symmetrically. Despite marked swelling in the acute stages, the joints are not always permanently damaged, though fibrous ankylosis is very often the cause of extensive crippling and may necessitate corrective orthopædic surgery. Osteoporosis may be considerable and may be the cause of pathological fractures.

Occasionally a fine erythematous rash appears and may not fade for many weeks. Both the peripheral lymphatic glands and the spleen may be enlarged. Pericarditis is an occasional complication.

Treatment. In the acute stage this aims at resting both the patient and the affected part and splints are applied to avoid deformity. The child should be nursed in a well ventilated room and the bed should be protected from any jarring movement. Whenever possible he should be carried on to a balcony or into the garden but draughts and cold should be avoided. The bedclothes should be light and bed cradles should be used. Sand bags, small pillows and foot rests and light plaster of Paris splints help to make the patient more comfortable and may prevent deformities. Even in the acute stages physiotherapy should ensure movement throughout the whole range at least once daily. Movement may be made easier by heat therapy prior to physiotherapy and this can be achieved by the use of radiant heat, wax baths or infra-red ray treatment, but it should be remembered that the child must not be left even for a short while during such treatment.

The diet should be light and nutritious and should contain adequate amounts of vitamins. Fresh fruit is wholesome and may help to prevent constipation. Poor general health and immobility make careful attention to all pressure areas important. Children with Still's disease are inclined to become over-anxious and introspective, and schooling and adequate occupation should be provided to keep up the child's morale and interest. At the same time occupational therapy will help to keep the affected joints moving.

Drug Therapy. Salicylates which abolish pain and fever in acute rheumatism have little effect in Still's disease (a point which may help in making the initial diagnosis), but Disprin and other analgesic drugs may relieve pain. Iron is given to combat anæmia and occasionally a small blood transfusion may help to build up the child's health generally, as well as raising the hæmoglobin level. Steroids are used with some success, but the side effects which occur, and the need to keep up the steroid therapy, limit their usefulness.

Collagen Diseases

Sometimes a hypersensitivity or auto-immune reaction affects the connective tissue, and in that case one of four rare diseases, grouped together as collagen diseases, may occur. These diseases are briefly described below. All may have a poor prognosis in spite of treatment with steroids and death is often caused by renal failure. The serum proteins are abnormal in all four conditions and the erythrocyte sedimentation rate is raised.

Polyarteritis Nodosa (Periarteritis Nodosa)

Polyarteritis nodosa is an acute inflammation of the small arterioles, with aneurysm formation which can sometimes be quite easily felt as nodules under the skin. The damage to the arterioles may lead to thrombosis and to hæmorrhage. The main signs and symptoms are fever, tachycardia, joint and muscle pains and proteinuria which may progress to renal failure. There is hypertension and a polymorphonuclear leucocytosis, and anæmia is common. Temporal arteritis may cause severe headaches and possibly cerebral hæmorrhage. Renal and muscle biopsy will confirm the diagnosis.

Scleroderma

Scleroderma is very rare in childhood. It is a condition in which the affected skin becomes fibrosed to the subcutaneous tissues, causing stiffness which in turn leads to joint fixation and bone and joint destruction. The skin appears shiny, often pigmented, and the loss of mobility of the face leads to difficulty in opening the mouth. Later there may be dysphagia, dyspnœa, cardiac failure and uræmia. Although spontaneous remissions may occur, the disease, in spite of steroid therapy, often runs a rapidly downhill course.

Dermatomyositis

Dermatomyositis has an insidious onset. Muscle, skin and subcutaneous tissues become inflamed. The muscles are stiff, tender and swollen and become weak with atrophy, contractions and fibrosis. The heart muscle may be affected, causing myocarditis and tachycardia. There is a typical, violet-coloured rash on cheeks and eyelids, circumoral pallor, and an erythematous and sometimes urticarial rash on trunk, limbs and knuckles. The subcutaneous tissues become inelastic and there is a low grade pyrexia and progressive disability which may include muscles of respiration, speech and swallowing. The urinary creatinine levels are greatly elevated in the acute phase, and muscle biopsy and electromyogram confirm the diagnosis. The condition may become chronic with signs similar to scleroderma, but in spite of steroid therapy acute cases may die of cardiac or renal failure or intercurrent infections.

Lupus Erythematosus

The disseminated form of lupus erythematosus is rare in childhood, and has an even worse prognosis than in later life. The most characteristic lesion is a purplish-red, raised and indurated "butterfly" rash over the cheeks and nose. All the mesenchymal tissues are affected, leading to hypertension, anæmia, pyrexia, painful swelling of joints, enlargement of liver and spleen, pleurisy, endocarditis, proteinuria and renal lesions. The bone marrow is depressed, causing leucopenia, and the blood sedimentation rate is very high. Atypical antibodies from the auto-immune reaction—lupus erythematosus (L.E.) cells—can be seen in blood tests and are specifically diagnostic. Although steroid therapy may relieve symptoms, it does not appear to affect an eventual poor prognosis.

12

DISEASES OF THE BLOOD

The Blood

Some typical figures connected with the blood are the following:

Red Cell Count. The number of red cells normally present at birth is 6 to 7 millions per cubic millilitre; these rapidly decrease to 4½ to 5½ millions, the adult level.

Hæmoglobin. The hæmoglobin level is 14·0 to 19·2 grammes per 100 millilitres (95 to 130 per cent) at birth. After an initial fall the level rises again gradually during childhood to 13·3 or 14·8 grammes per 100 millilitres (90 to 100 per cent.).

White Cell Counts. The number of white cells present at birth is 10,000 to 25,000 per cubic millimetre, with a high number of lymphocytes. During the first 3 or 4 years of life it drops to between 6,000 and 13,000, of which about half are lymphocytes.

Blood Volume. The average baby [3·2 kilogrammes (7 pounds) birth weight] has a blood volume of 88 to 110 millilitres per kilogramme body weight. For purpose of transfusion the volume is calculated as being between 40 and 50 millilitres per pound of body weight up to the age of 6 months, 600 millilitres at 1 year and approximately 2,000 millilitres by the age of 10 years.

Anæmia

Anæmia is a condition frequently seen in childhood. The usual causes are either a reduction in the hæmoglobin-carrying erythrocytes or red blood cells, or a reduction of hæmoglobin carried by each red cell. Sometimes a combination of these factors occurs.

Causes of Anæmia

The more common anæmias of childhood may conveniently be classified into the following groups:

Iron deficiency anæmia.

Hypoplastic anæmia.

Hæmolytic anæmia, due to excessive breakdown of red cells.
Secondary anæmia occurring in illnesses such as nephritis, acute rheumatism or rheumatoid arthritis.

Iron Deficiency Anæmia

Iron deficiency anæmia may be caused by inadequate iron intake due to dietary errors, prolonged illness such as gastro-enteritis and other infections, poor absorption or prematurity. This latter type is due to the fact that the fœtus obtains most of his iron in the last three months of pregnancy and stores it in his liver. Poor absorption causes the iron deficiency in cœliac disease. There may be either a reduction in the hæmoglobin-carrying erythrocytes or red blood cells, or a reduction of hæmoglobin carried by each red cell. Sometimes a combination of these factors occurs.

Age Incidence. Iron deficiency anæmia occurs most commonly between the ages of 3 months and 3 years. The condition frequently resolves itself as the child grows older, has a better balanced diet and eats more vegetables.

Signs and Symptoms. The child is noticed to become progressively more listless and pale over a period of time. He appears to get tired more easily than his playmates and is prone to colds and minor infections. His skin has a grey tinge and the lips and conjunctivæ are pale. On examination the child is often plump. Occasionally a mild cardiac murmur or an enlarged spleen is found and in the more severe cases puffiness of the extremities suggests slight œdema. There may also be tachycardia and a reduced pulse volume. Giddiness, blurred vision, headaches and irritability are all typical in the older child and, since these children are prone to infection, they have frequent periods of sickness due to colds, upper respiratory tract infections and sepsis. The blood picture will show a low red cell count and if the bone marrow increases the rate of production to compensate for this, immature cells (reticulocytes) appear in the blood.

Treatment. The underlying cause of the iron deficiency needs to be considered and treated. Anæmic children require extra rest with long hours of sleep at night. The diet should be varied and attractively served and adequate amounts of vitamin C, iron, copper, folic acid and vitamin B are essential. Artificially fed infants may be given proprietary foods containing extra iron in easily assimilated form, such as Farex. Older children will obtain all the essentials if the diet is sufficiently varied, but the following list of foods which are particularly rich in iron, may help the nurse to plan an attractive and suitable meal programme.

egg yolk	liver	cocoa	dried fruit
sardines	kidneys	Bovril	wholemeal bread
red meat	Marmite	chocolate	rye bread
green vegetables			
tomatoes			

Iron may be prescribed as iron and ammonium citrate, ferrous gluconate or ferrous sulphate. When administering iron in liquid form, the child should be given a drink of plain milk to follow in order to clear the teeth and mouth of iron. Alternatively the iron can be given through a straw, so as to avoid contact with the teeth as iron stains dental enamel brown. Occasionally a blood transfusion is required, or Imferon is given by intra-muscular injection.

Since overdosage of iron may have a toxic effect, the attractively coloured sugar-coated pills so often used in the home should be kept in a safe place out of reach of the inquisitive toddler.

Hypoplastic Anæmia

This is caused by failure of the bone marrow to manufacture erythrocytes correctly. Diagnosis in this case is established by bone marrow puncture and treatment consists in giving whole blood or packed cell transfusions in order to provide the mature red cells. These transfusions need to be given repeatedly and the consequent frequent admissions to hospital should be carefully considered. The child should be admitted to the same ward each time so that he returns to people and surroundings with which he is familiar and eventually comes to accept this process as part of his normal routine.

Hæmolytic Anæmia

Excessive breakdown of red cells is the cause of hæmolytic anæmia. This process takes place in the spleen and the reticulo-endothelial system. Treatment consists in replacing these cells by repeated blood transfusion. The following types of this anæmia are met with in childhood:

1. Anæmia following acute hæmolytic streptococcal infections.
2. Hæmolytic disease of the newborn. (For details see page 57.)

3. Acute hæmolytic anæmia, also known as Lederer's anæmia.
4. Acholuric jaundice.
5. Cooley's anæmia and sickle cell anæmia.

1. *Anæmia following Acute Hæmolytic Streptococcal Infections.* This form of anæmia is possibly the one most commonly seen in childhood. It often follows acute hæmolytic streptococcal tonsillitis and accounts for much of the debility which follows this illness. Foods which are rich in iron should therefore always be included in the convalescent diet and iron in the form of a medicine is frequently ordered. A certain amount can be achieved in the prevention of such infections by treating septic foci of infection such as diseased tonsils, teeth and sinuses.

2. *Hæmolytic Disease of the Newborn.* For details see page 57.

3. *Acute Hæmolytic Anæmia.* As the name suggests, this type of anæmia comes on rapidly and the hæmoglobin level falls to 20 or 30 per cent. and the red cell count to 1 to 2 million in the course of 2 to 3 weeks or less. The spleen is enlarged, petechial hæmorrhages may occur into the skin, mild pyrexia may be present, and the child is listless, fractious and acutely ill. Vomiting and diarrhœa may aggravate the condition. The illness is usually cured by blood transfusion, but may continue as a chronic, acquired hæmolytic anæmia which needs to be controlled by the use of cortisone.

4. *Acholuric Jaundice.* This condition is also called familial hæmolytic anæmia as it usually occurs in several members of a family. The cause of the hæmolysis is the unusual fragility of the red cells. The rapid breakdown of erythrocytes leads to jaundice because the bile pigments which result from the breakdown of hæmoglobin cannot be excreted sufficiently fast by the liver. They therefore remain in the blood stream and tissue fluids and give the patient's skin and conjunctivæ a yellowish appearance. The spleen is enlarged and firm. Latent periods and exacerbations occur. Crises are often caused by infections and at such times the jaundice deepens, the child may complain of severe abdominal pain, his general condition is poor and may even give rise to anxiety. Blood transfusion may be needed during crises. Once the diagnosis is established the spleen should be removed as this operation will prevent crises from recurring and produce clinical cure.

5. *Cooley's anæmia* (thalassæmia, Mediterranean anæmia) is a similar type of anæmia confined to Mediterranean races,

and *sickle cell anæmia* is seen only in negro races. Both are chronic conditions for which there is no known treatment and death usually occurs before the age of 10 years. Parents or brothers and sisters may be healthy although having a mild form of either disease—Thalassæmia minor or sicklæmia.

Acute Leukæmia

Acute leukæmia is a disease affecting the white blood cells. It is characterized by the presence in the circulating blood of immature leucocytes. In childhood the disease is acute and if untreated pursues a rapid downhill course. The more immature the cells which are circulating, the more advanced and acute is the condition. According to the blood count two types are described, although they seem to be merely phases of the same disease.

The Leukæmic Type. In this type, instead of the normal 5 to 10,000 leucocytes per cubic millilitre, there may be as many as 200,000. In *aleukæmic leukæmia* the white cell count is normal or even low. In both instances primitive cells are produced in excess in the bone marrow and there is proliferation of leucocytes. Deposits of cells are found in the liver, spleen and lymph tissues. The cause of the disease is not definitely known but it is thought that in some instances exposure of the fœtus to X-rays may be responsible for the disease in infancy. In others there is a history of a preceding infection such as tonsillitis or measles. The disease is more common after the age of 18 months.

Signs and Symptoms. These are the same for either type. Children suffering from leukæmia present a typical picture. They are listless and tire easily due to a severe anæmia, secondary to the disease. They are content to lie quietly watching others and are usually pathetically patient and grateful for a little extra love and attention. Their skin is extremely pale and usually has a yellow tinge and a wax-like, transparent quality. The temperature is of a characteristically swinging type and varies between 37·2° and 39·4° C. (99° and 103° F.). Anorexia, constipation and vomiting are common. There is a general tendency to bleeding. Large bruises and petechiæ appear on the skin and all over the body pain and tenderness may be caused by subperiosteal hæmorrhages. Hæmorrhage into the retina may interfere with vision and bleeding into the renal tubules causes hæmaturia. Bleeding from the gums, epistaxis, hæmatemesis and melæna are among the distressing symptoms. The mouth is sore and ulcerated, the lips cracked, the gums swollen and stomatitis may be severe in spite of careful oral toilet. The lymph nodes are enlarged and tender and the spleen is palpable. Towards the end of the illness the child is prone to secondary infections particularly of the throat. The diagnosis is confirmed by a blood count and by a bone marrow puncture.

The *prognosis* remains hopeless at present, though repeated blood transfusions and modern drug therapy may make the child more comfortable by lessening the symptoms. Remissions of several months may be expected.

Drug Therapy. Steroids, cytotoxic drugs, folic acid and 6-mercaptopurine are all used. Some of these drugs cause a severe depression in antibody and white cell formation and for that reason exceptionally rigid infectious precautions have to be observed to protect the patient. Temporary improvement may be striking and immediate. The child regains his appetite, feels better and more energetic and discharge home in a comparatively satisfactory state of health often becomes possible for several weeks at a time. Readmission for blood transfusion and reassessment of drug therapy is necessary and thoughtful management will arrange for the child to return each time to the ward and nursing staff he already knows. Despite the temporary improvement a fatal outcome must still be expected.

Special Investigations. Those which are commonly carried out include blood picture and bone marrow puncture. The procedure for bone marrow puncture is similar to that carried out on adults but the site of the puncture is usually the crest of the ilium rather than the shaft of the tibia or the body of the sternum. The child should be told what is going to happen and a sedative or light basal anæsthetic, such as rectal Pentothal is usually given. The procedure is frightening and the child's own nurse should accompany him to the theatre or treatment room where it is her duty to keep him warm and comforted while holding him firmly during the procedure.

Nursing Care. The nursing of children suffering from acute leukæmia calls for a high degree of skill, observation and gentleness. It is the nursing of a helpless child, who is restless and listless, to whom movements are often painful and who is disinclined to eat or play. The sudden and frequent epistaxes are frightening to the child and to any relatives who may be visiting. The nurse must be careful to remain calm and to remove any traces of blood and change the bedclothes as quickly and gently as possible. The child is best nursed in a semi-recumbent position or else sitting up well supported by pillows. His position should be changed from time to time, supporting him in the lateral position alternately. If he is to remain in bed for any length of time a water pillow or air ring will add to his comfort. *Oral toilet* needs to be carried out with special care and gentleness and, when bleeding has occurred, saline or a weak solution of sodium bicarbonate or hydrogen peroxide can be used. In many cases it is advisable to clean the teeth with cotton wool swabs securely held in a pair of forceps rather than to use a toothbrush, as the gums are inclined to bleed and become very sore. The lips should be kept from cracking and be protected from crusts of blood by the application of a little petroleum jelly several times a day.

A daily blanket bath should be given as it may induce rest and will refresh the patient who has a high temperature and is inclined to perspire. Care must be taken when lifting or turning the child to avoid bruising, easily caused even by slight pressure. The child should also be protected against bruising himself by restless movements of the arms, on the sides of his cot or bed-table.

A special diet is not required but the child's nurse should take the trouble to find out what he particularly likes in order to encourage him to eat. Loss of appetite may be countered by offering him small, frequent and attractively served meals, extra milk drinks and special treats. Adequate fluid should be given and extra vitamins may be prescribed in order to try and prevent infections and to raise the general standard of health.

Diminished urinary output and hæmaturia should be reported and a fluid balance chart is helpful. Fluids and fresh fruit in the diet will help to prevent constipation in a child who is confined to bed but, if it does occur, glycerin suppositories or a small olive oil enema may have to be given. In addition to the specific drugs iron may be ordered (page 188). Drugs given to relieve pain and to induce rest and sleep include codeine, phenobarbitone and Nepenthe. (Nepenthe 0·06 millilitres (1 minim) per year of age.)

As the illness advances admissions to hospital will become more frequent and the mother should be encouraged to visit as freely as possible. She should also be encouraged to help with feeding, mouth toilet and other nursing care as in this way she will feel less helpless and may be able to nurse the child at home for a time if this seems desirable. As the child's condition deteriorates, the mother will feel less anxious about his welfare in hospital if she herself has always been made to feel welcome and has been treated with courtesy and sympathetic consideration. Although the doctor will see the parents with regard to the prognosis and the ward sister will see them regularly, the student nurse may well be approached with questions about the child and his progress and condition. Such requests must be carefully answered and should usually be referred to the sister or staff nurse. The importance of the correct approach to patient and parents in a hopeless illness is discussed in Chapter 22.

Methæmoglobinæmia

Methæmoglobinæmia is caused by the absorption of aniline dye from unfixed marking ink or from ingestion from some marking pencils and paint removers.

The *signs and symptoms* are cyanosis with a greyish tinge and in severe cases respiratory difficulties, muscle twitching and low blood pressure.

Treatment is by intravenous injection of methylene blue (5 milligrammes), but prevention by washing all newly marked garments before use and by keeping paint removers well out of reach of children, is the only sure way of averting a tragedy.

Purpura

Purpura may be a sign of an underlying disease rather than a disease in itself. Characteristic, spontaneous hæmorrhages appear in the skin and mucous membrane of the body, causing bruising, petechiæ and frank bleeding of the gums, renal tubules, intestinal tract, conjunctivæ and the brain. *The causes of purpura* in childhood may be classified under three main headings.

1. Purpura due to primary or secondary platelet deficiency.
2. Purpura due to damage to the capillary system.
3. Purpura due to lack of essential constituents of blood plasma, such as prothrombin.

Purpura due to Platelet Deficiency

A. *Idiopathic thrombocytopenic purpura.* This is a primary purpura caused by gross reduction of the number of blood platelets. The condition may be acute or chronic and in the great majority of cases the prognosis is favourable. Blood transfusion and cortisone therapy are used in severe cases, and the more chronic cases respond well to splenectomy.

B. *Symptomatic thrombocytopenic purpura* is a toxic manifestation and occurs in leukæmia, severe infections, aplastic anæmia, rubella, diphtheria and some malignant diseases. The purpuric hæmorrhages clear when platelets reappear in the blood in adequate numbers.

C. *Familial thrombocytopenic purpura.* One of the causes of hæmorrhage in the newborn is familial thrombocytopenic purpura. Apart from giving blood transfusions from time to time there is no known treatment in infancy but when the child is a little older splenectomy is done and gives good results (see also Hæmolytic Disease of the Newborn (page 57)).

Purpura due to Damage of the Capillary System

This again may be primary or secondary. In primary cases it is thought that an allergic factor may be present which causes a temporary abnormal permeability of the capillary walls. Henoch-Schoenlein's purpura is the most common in this group. Among the secondary types the causes include scurvy and meningococcal meningitis and intolerance to drugs.

Purpura due to Lack of Essential Constituents in the Blood Plasma

This occurs in hæmorrhagic disease of the newborn and obstructive types of jaundice. (See also chapter on Diseases of the Newborn.)

Henoch-Schoenlein's Syndrome (Anaphylactoid Purpura)

Henoch-Schoenlein's purpura, which is one of the collagen diseases (see page 183), is seen fairly commonly in childhood, but rarely before the age of 3 years. The small purpuric hæmorrhages seen on the skin are at first of a purple colour but later they turn a dusky red and still later brown, until they gradually disappear. A faint urticarial rash is usually present. The areas most commonly involved are the legs, the back of the elbows and arms, the lumbar region and buttocks. Any pressure, such as sitting on a bed pan, may cause localized purpuric spots. If the hæmorrhages involve the intestinal tract, there may be severe abdominal pain of a colicky nature which may last for several hours. This may be followed by the passage of bright blood or a melæna stool. The child may be shocked and occasionally an intussusception may complicate the picture. For that reason there is a certain danger in giving drugs such as pethidine to relieve pain, as this may mask symptoms which should urgently be recognized. The Henoch-Schoenlein syndrome may also involve the large joints causing pain and swelling although there is no actual hæmorrhage into the joint itself. As different joints become involved, pain flits from one site to another but it never leaves permanent damage or stiffness.

Often no specific treatment is considered necessary and with bed rest the child gradually improves and the rash fades after about 2 or 3 weeks. Steroids may, however, be given if the erythrocyte sedimentation rate is high or if there is albuminuria. There is a tendency to recurrence.

Complications. These include nephritis and intussusception, which are dealt with in the usual way (see pages 274 and 222).

Nursing Care. This is symptomatic. Relief of pain for the affected joints may be given by applying pads of warmed cotton wool and in case of severe abdominal pain a well-protected hot water bottle might be used with special permission from the ward sister. Gentle massage may bring some comfort. A painful limb may be elevated on a small pillow and a bed cradle should be used to take the weight of the bedclothes. Pressure from the rim of a bed pan should be excluded by padding the bed pan, e.g. with an air ring or by using a rubber pan.

Hæmophilia

Hæmophilia, a blood disease which occurs only in males, though it is transmitted by the female, causes prolonged bleeding. The coagulation time is increased and even minor knocks, injuries or operations may take on unusually serious proportions. Bleeding may occur into joints and eventually lead to deformities. The need to lead a sheltered life and the inability to play games and take part in sports with other children and the constant fear of disabling hæmorrhage, as well as repeated admissions to hospital, may have a bad effect psychologically on the patient.

Christmas Disease

Christmas disease is a hæmorrhagic disease, very similar to hæmophilia. The condition is inherited in the same way as hæmophilia but is not confined to male sufferers. Heterozygous females may be affected in the same way as males. The condition was first described in 1952 and was named after the first patient in whom the condition was recognized. Treatment consists in giving transfusions of blood, plasma or serum.

13

DISEASES OF THE ALIMENTARY SYSTEM

Daily oral toilet is as important in young children as in the older ones and as in the case of adults. The popular belief that the first teeth are unimportant as they will soon be replaced by the permanent ones is erroneous, and the nurse should make it her duty to teach the child—and through him the mother also—good habits with regard to dental care.

Cleaning the teeth with an attractive toothbrush and nice-tasting toothpaste can be a pleasant part of the morning and evening toilet. Very young children are often reluctant to open their mouth, and make effective cleaning impossible. It is therefore often best to let the child chew a piece of raw apple at least once a day as soon as the first teeth have come through—a most effective way of keeping the teeth healthy and clean.

The Mouth

Intelligent observations on the condition of a patient's mouth will often assist in diagnosis and treatment. Of special importance are the following points:

1. *Dry lips and tongue.* These will be present in mouth-breathers and in those with high fevers and dehydration. At the same time the tongue will often be thickly coated.
2. *Herpes.* This is often seen in patients with colds, high fevers and pneumonia. These small vesicles, grouped on a patch of inflammation around the mouth, are sometimes also called fever blisters.
3. *Pallor of the lips.* This is caused by anæmia and may be a sign of loss of blood.
4. *Cyanosis.* This signifies lack of oxygen and is seen in congenital heart disease, respiratory tract infections or obstruction and in some instances in newly born babies.
5. *An abnormally large tongue.* This is characteristic of cretins.
6. *A constantly moving tongue.* This occurs in chorea.

Important odours which a nurse should recognize include:

A sweet smell, where acetone is present.

The smell of stale blood in cases of bleeding from the tonsil bed or from the stomach.

Offensive smells. These may be due to the presence of pus, as in retropharyngeal abscess and bronchiectasis.

A fæcal odour in intestinal obstruction.

A urinary smell in uræmia.

A foul smell from the mouth occurs in the late stages of leukæmia.

Specific smells when poisons have been swallowed.

Treatment of any of these symptoms depends on their cause, but in all cases of sickness careful mouth toilet is an essential of good nursing.

Infections and Inflammatory Conditions

Herpes Simplex

Herpes simplex is a virus infection which causes eruptions of vesicles. A common site is the lips in febrile illnesses causing swelling and blisters. The latter dry off and leave thick, uncomfortable crusts. The lesions are best treated by drying them up with dusting powder or applying Neocortef ointment. Dabbing the blisters with methylated spirit is painful and for that reason particularly unsuitable for children.

Catarrhal, Aphthous and Ulcerative Stomatitis

These are varying degrees of generalized inflammation of the mouth.

There is swelling and inflammation of the gums, coupled with ulcers on the mucous lining of the mouth. The tongue is coated and there is a foul smell. The patient seems ill, the temperature is often raised by two or three degrees, he refuses his food and shows intense misery. Frequently these children are debilitated and come from poor homes.

A swab is taken to determine the causative organism which may be streptococcus, staphylococcus or Vincent's organism. In many cases of aphthous stomatitis, the cause is the ultramicroscopic virus of *herpes simplex*.

Treatment. The mouth is treated with gentian violet in a 1 per cent. aqueous solution and frequent mouth washes are given if the child is old enough. For Vincent's angina a weak preparation containing arsenic may be prescribed. Penicillin injections may be beneficial.

Nursing Care. As these children dribble saliva because

swallowing is so painful, the chin should be protected by applying petroleum jelly. A dish or a piece of absorbent material can often be arranged to catch the saliva. Very young children may have to have their arms splinted to prevent them from putting their fingers in their mouths. It is usual to carry out barrier nursing.

Bland, cool fluids containing plenty of glucose should be given at first and later the diet should contain extra milk and nourishment. Vitamins are important, but concentrated orange juice should be avoided as it stings on the open lesions. Groats are often enjoyed and can be fortified by addition of an egg. Convalescence in the country may help to prevent a recurrence and build up the child's resistance. Teeth and tonsils should be inspected and, if necessary, treatment or tonsillectomy carried out, to eliminate septic foci.

Gingivitis

Swollen, bleeding gums, may be present in general oral infections. They occur in ulcerative stomatitis, scurvy and in leukæmia, but sometimes may merely be due to poor oral hygiene. Careful mouth toilet and a well-balanced diet are essential. Certain drugs taken over a long period may also cause gingivitis.

Stomatitis

Stomatitis is fairly common in childhood and may vary in severity from simple swelling of the gums due to teething, to extensive inflammation and ulceration. The child is usually reluctant to swallow during the acute stages owing to the pain caused by the inflammation and ulcers, and there is therefore danger of aspiration pneumonia from inhaled saliva. Drainage of saliva during sleep should be encouraged by raising the foot end of the bed at night. Occasionally this has to be done also during the day, the saliva being allowed to drain into a kidney dish or a piece of absorbent material.

Teething

Gentle mouth toilet should be carried out. Half a Disprin tablet (0·15 G.) may be ordered for relief of pain and there is no point in withholding this simple analgesic. A little comforting and nursing will help to soothe these children. Teething rings, which the infant can bite on, relieve the discomfort and there is nothing against them, provided they are kept clean and safely tied to the cot to prevent them from falling on to the floor.

Thrush

This is caused by the fungus *Candida* (*Monilia*) *albicans*. It is mostly seen in bottle-fed babies and is a highly contagious condition. White or grey patches appear on the inside of the cheeks and lips, on the roof of the mouth and on the tongue and cannot be removed without damaging the mucous membrane. The baby will be reluctant to take his feed.

Thrush can be prevented by scrupulous cleanliness, especially with regard to feeding utensils, and by keeping the mucous membrane moist in cases of high fever or dehydration. Babies on broad spectrum antibiotics are particularly prone to thrush because the drug kills the organisms which are normally present in the mouth and which can control the antibiotic resistant *Candida albicans*. Vitamin B should always be given with these antibiotics.

Treatment. Strict barrier nursing is essential. Feed bottles must not be returned to the common feed kitchen until sterilized. Milky feeds should be followed by a small drink of plain boiled water, in order to clean the mouth. The infection is treated by giving an oral antibiotic called nystatin. The usual dose is 1 millilitre (100,000 units) four times a day until all signs of thrush disappear. The solution can be added to the infant's feeds or dropped directly on to the tongue. It is important to know that nystatin should not be used for more than 7 days after it has been dispensed. If treatment exceeds this period a newly prepared solution should be ordered. Other means of treatment are: painting the mouth with a 1 per cent. aqueous solution of gentian violet or Bradosol, or a ½ per cent. solution of stilbamidine. The treatment is done three times a day.

Complications. Infection may spread throughout the gastro-intestinal tract and cause thrush septicæmia, a very serious condition. Vomiting may set in and a fungus pneumonia develop. Severe cases are treated by giving hydroxystilbamidine in a solution of glucose and saline by intravenous infusion.

Nurses can assist in the prevention of thrush by teaching mothers adequate, easy methods of hygiene in infant feeding. Breast-fed babies rarely have thrush.

THE CAUSES OF VOMITING IN CHILDHOOD

Causes	*Age*	*Content of the vomit*	*Remarks*
Underfeeding	0—3/12	Recently taken feed.	The hungry infant cries, swallows air and gulps the feed when offered.
Indiscretion in Diet	All ages	Undigested food.	Milky curd in infancy.
Congenital Abnormalities (e.g. Hiatus Hernia)	Infancy	Milk, mucus.	Effortless or projectile.
Pyloric Stenosis	2 weeks to 4 months	Curd, mucus, occasionally blood.	Projectile.
Cardiospasm	Late child-hood	Undigested food.	Alkaline reaction: soon after meals. Effort-less.
Gastritis	All ages	Food, mucus, blood.	Colicky pain often pre-sent.
At the Onset of Fevers	Young children	No characteristic.	Accompanied by rise in temperature.
Acute Appen-dicitis	All ages	Food at first. Bile later.	Associated with ab-dominal pain.
Toxic Illness	All ages	Food, gastric fluid.	Quickly causes dehy-dration.
Whooping Cough	All ages	Food and mucus.	During or just after meals. After attack of coughing.
Diabetes Mellitus	All ages	Food.	Heralds impending coma.
Renal Diseases, (e.g. Uræmia)	All ages	Fluid gastric contents.	Mostly in late stages of the illness.
Poisoning	All ages	Gastric contents.	Must be saved with special care.
Intolerance to Drugs	All ages	Gastric contents.	e.g. Salicylates. The drug may have to be discontinued.
Nervous Conditions	All ages	Watery.	Excitement, anxiety, habit.
Cyclical Vomiting	After age of 2 years	Food at first, later gastric fluid only.	Severe, general distur-bance. Ketosis, may last several days.
Mechanical	All ages	Gastric contents.	May result from finger sucking, enlarged tonsils, mucopus in nasopharynx, air swallowing.
Œsophageal Reflux	Infancy	Feed, mucus, sometimes blood.	e.g. Hiatus hernia. No nausea.

THE CAUSES OF VOMITING IN CHILDHOOD—*contd.*

Causes	*Age*	*Content of the vomit*	*Remarks*
Intracranial Pressure	All ages	Not related to taking food.	Gastric contents. Projectile. Without warning. If associated with meningitis, constipation is often an accompanying feature.

The Œsophagus and Stomach

Vomiting

Vomiting in the neonatal period should never be treated lightly. If it is persistent, recurrent, forceful or copious, admission to hospital should be arranged at once. Immediate operation for an obstruction may be necessary, and expert observations may prove life saving. In childhood the causes of vomiting are very varied and some children seem to vomit at the slightest provocation and show little or no concern about it. None the less the nurse should remember that vomiting in most cases entails considerable effort and the child may feel dizzy, faint, cold and miserable. The nurse should always remain with the child. She should protect the bedclothes, place the patient in a comfortable position and, if possible, put screens around the bed. The patient may find it comforting if the nurse holds her hand on his forehead and supports any recent abdominal wound. When the attack is over, the patient should be given a mouthwash, or have his mouth cleaned, and be left comfortable. Persistent vomiting may cause considerable loss of fluid and replacement by a parenteral route is sometimes necessary.

The vomit should always be inspected before it is discarded and an entry should be made on the patient's chart. The amount should be measured, the reaction tested with litmus paper, and the time and relation to meal times recorded. The nurse should notice whether the vomit is effortless, or forcible and projectile in nature. The presence of curds, blood, excess mucus, bile or foreign bodies should be reported at once. The odour may also be of importance in arriving at a diagnosis.

Cyclical Vomiting

Cyclical vomiting is a distressing condition occasionally seen in a children's ward. The child affected is as a rule tall for his age and thin, his posture is poor; he may be highly strung, inclined to sleep-walking, car-sickness and vomiting due to excitement, and frequently he is above normal intelligence.

Children usually outgrow cyclical vomiting at puberty but some develop attacks of migraine at that time.

Signs and Symptoms. Attacks start very suddenly. The child complains of severe headache and abdominal discomfort. He is irritable at first but soon becomes drowsy. Anything taken by the mouth, including plain water, is vomited immediately and signs of dehydration develop rapidly. The scanty amounts of urine are loaded with ketone bodies and the breath smells of acetone. The temperature may rise by one or two degrees. Head retraction and convulsions occur in the more extreme cases.

This alarming state of affairs may continue for three to four days and may recur with regularity as often as once a fortnight or merely once or twice a year. In spite of the apparent severity, there is no serious danger and the distressed parents can be reassured.

Nursing Care. The child should be treated with firm sympathy. He is best nursed in a darkened room and sedatives should be given as soon as an attack is suspected. Glucose may be given either in fluids or in the form of barley sugar. If fluids taken by mouth are retained, they are best given as frequent sips of fruit juice and glucose in a saline solution. A rectal infusion of ten per cent. glucose in sodium bicarbonate may be ordered, after the lower bowel has been emptied by an enema. Acidosis is severe, that is to say, the carbon dioxide (CO_2) combining power is greatly lowered and blood may have to be taken to estimate the carbon dioxide combining power (normal 45 to 60 vol. per cent.) and the sodium chloride levels. Intravenous fluids are given accordingly to correct the blood chemistry and replace fluid loss. On recovery the child is given a light diet with restricted fat. Glucose, toast, honey and sweetened tea are particularly suitable.

General Points. These children should be allowed extra rest in their daily routine. They should go to bed early and avoid undue fatigue. On the other hand, as little attention as possible should be drawn to the condition and the child should be kept fully occupied and his intelligence used to the utmost in order to keep him from self-centred interest.

The diagnosis of cyclical vomiting is usually made with great caution and such conditions as appendicitis, intestinal obstruction, pyelitis, meningitis and diabetic crisis have to be most carefully excluded. Vomiting due to excitement, as for instance before birthday parties, return to school or before an examination, are not true cyclical vomiting even though they may recur with a certain regularity.

Gastritis

The causes of gastritis range from unsuitable diet, swallowing infected material, e.g. pus from sinusitis, or dental caries causing incomplete mastication, to intolerance of drugs, swallowing an irritant such as a poison, gastro-enteritis or chronic dilatation, as in pyloric stenosis.

If old enough, the child may complain of discomfort or even pain, nausea and vomiting. The tongue is furred and the appetite is poor. The vomit may contain mucus, pus or altered blood. Vomiting frequently relieves the distension and discomfort.

Treatment. As gastritis is as a rule a symptom of some other disturbance, the underlying cause must be found and appropriately treated. In order to give the stomach a rest ordinary diet is omitted for a few days. Bland fluids and bengerized milk are well tolerated. Lightly boiled eggs, soups, mashed potatoes, jellies and ice cream, toast and honey are all light, and suitable as soon as the child is ready to have solid food. The return to a full diet should be gradual. Severe or long-standing cases may benefit from gastric lavage. The mouth toilet should receive particular attention.

Congenital Hypertrophic Pyloric Stenosis

Pyloric stenosis develops soon after birth and symptoms are first noticed at the age of 2 to 6 weeks. Mild cases or those which show late symptoms may improve spontaneously at the age of about 4 months, but early and severe cases require medical or surgical treatment. The condition is most common in first-born children and boys are more frequently affected than girls.

The condition is due to the thickening of the pyloric sphincter, causing a narrowing of the lumen. Signs of obstruction, gastritis and malnutrition develop.

Diagnosis is often delayed as varying feeds are tried in an attempt to stop the baby from vomiting. At each change a temporary improvement takes place but vomiting and loss of weight soon recur and eventually the presence of pyloric stenosis is suspected.

Signs and Symptoms. The infant's appearance is typical. He is wizened and pale and has large, anxious and hungry-looking eyes. The skin is dry and the fontanelle sunken. The lips and mouth are red and dry but remain clean despite the vomiting. Even though there is marked wasting he remains bright and very active.

In the early stages vomiting may occur once or twice a day only, but soon it follows every feed. Curd from previous feeds may be present in the vomit. As gastritis develops, mucus and specks of blood are noticed. Vomiting may at first resemble regurgitations but it soon becomes projectile, that is to say it occurs suddenly and with so much force that it is rarely seen on the baby's pillow or bib but usually hits the floor. Starvation and dehydration make the urine dark and concentrated and the stools are small and constipated. They may be infrequent and are often green "hunger stools".

The loss of chlorides in the vomit has a serious effect on the blood chemistry. Plasma bicarbonates are high and there

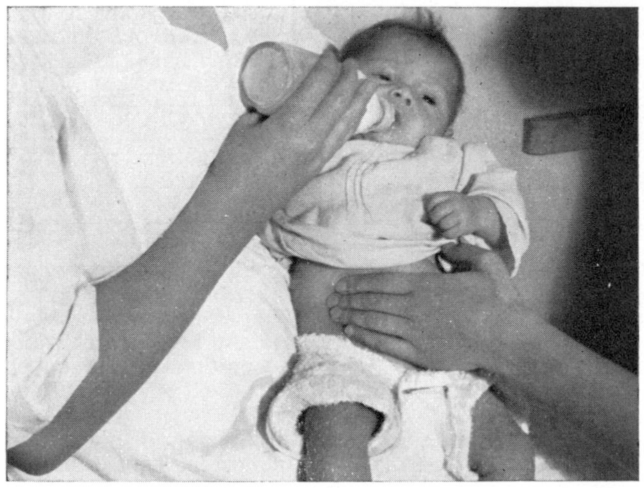

Fig. 41. PYLORIC STENOSIS.

The doctor is feeling the tumour and watching for visible peristalis. Note the relaxed position and the way in which the abdomen has been exposed by the nurse, although the rest of the baby is being kept warm.

is an increase in the non-protein nitrogen in the blood and urine. This toxic state is known as alkalosis and must be rectified without delay.

Examination of the Patient. For examination by the doctor, the baby should lie on the nurse's knees in a relaxed position while taking a feed (Fig. 41). After the baby has taken an ounce or two, peristaltic waves, resembling the movements of a golf ball, may be seen passing across the abdomen, just underneath the ribs and from the left to the right side. This is known as visible peristalsis. At the same time, the examining fingers can feel the hardening of the pylorus (the feel resembles that of the tip of the nose) immediately beneath the liver margin to the right side of the rectus muscle. A barium meal may help to confirm the diagnosis.

The treatment of choice may be medical in mild cases and sometimes in late cases if the child comes from good home conditions. Frequently, however, surgical treatment is preferred, though the baby usually remains in a medical ward under the care of the pædiatrician.

Medical Treatment

The principal points adopted in medical treatment of these children are:

1. A radical reduction of feed volume is made in order to reduce the vomiting from the start, and this is coupled with gastric lavage. For this normal saline is used.

2. A muscle relaxant drug of the atropine group is given 15 to 20 minutes before feeds. These include:

Eumydrin (atropine methyl nitrate 0·6 per cent. alcoholic solution) given from a pipette or dropper direct on to the tongue at the back of the mouth. Three to six drops are the usual dose.

Note that Eumydrin is an unstable solution and should never be kept longer than a maximum of 4 weeks.

Pylostropine (0·08 milligrammes) and Skopyl are comparable preparations. Pylostropine is dispensed in the form of lamellæ, which are placed underneath the baby's tongue. The lamellæ easily stick together and care should be taken to give only one at a time and to ensure that the baby does not spit it out.

As vomiting ceases, the feeds are gradually increased to the amounts appropriate to the infant's age and requirements. Another scheme in common use is here given in some detail. It is sometimes referred to as a Medical Pyloric Ladder Diet.

Medical Pyloric Ladder Diet. The relaxant drug is Skopyl. This is given 4-hourly for 6 doses or 3-hourly for 6 doses omitting the midnight and 9 p.m. doses. Dosage, 0·06–0·18 mg.

Feeds are as follows: Begin with 2 drachms of 5 per cent. glucose water 2-hourly. Increase by 2 drachms at alternate feeds until 1 oz. is given at each feed. Then alternate 5 per cent. glucose water with ½-strength Frailac (or feed ordered) continuing to increase by 2 drachms on alternate feeds until 2-oz. feeds are reached. Then all feeds are ½-strength 2-oz. 4-hourly for 6 feeds or 1½-oz. 3-hourly for 8 feeds and these feeds may be increased to 3-oz. 4-hourly for 6 feeds. The strength of the feeds is gradually increased by 1 drachm Frailac per day until full strength is reached (1 in 10).

Surgical Treatment

Rammstedt's Operation (division of the pyloric sphincter). Thorough preparation of the patient for this operation is essential. Blood is taken for analysis and any abnormality in the blood chemistry is corrected by subcutaneous or intravenous infusion of the appropriate fluid. The baby is often admitted one or two days prior to the operation. During the pre-operative period, gastric lavage may be done once or twice daily and again before the operation. The wash-out not only serves to clear the stomach of stale milk, curd and mucus, but also helps in assessing the type of curd and the severity of the gastritis as well as forming part of the treatment. It is of vital importance to obtain completely clear fluid at the end of the pre-operative wash-out as any stale material left behind in the stomach would pass into the intestine once the obstruction is relieved and might cause enteritis.

The usual feeds can be given up to 3 hours before operation, but it is desirable that the baby should rest for a time before going to the theatre and preparations should be complete one hour before operation.

The umbilicus is inspected and thoroughly cleaned. The baby's extremities may be loosely bandaged in cotton wool and a "cotton wool vest" placed over the shoulders. Most wards keep a special set of woollies (vest opening in the front, matinée coat, leggings, bonnet, bootees and mittens) for these babies, but as overheating the baby may be as dangerous as exposure to cold, discretion must be used when dressing them for the theatre.

A destructible napkin is used and the corners are tucked in so as to eliminate the need for a safety pin. The baby is then bandaged on to a well-padded pyloric splint. A knitted operation stocking may be pulled over the baby's legs and the splint, for additional warmth and neatness.

Usually the operation is performed under a local anæsthetic and pre-operative drugs are not required. Chloral hydrate or an injection of papaveretum may, however, be ordered to keep the baby drowsy. Some surgeons like a Ryle's tube passed and left *in situ* during the operation to facilitate aspiration and the escape of gastric gases, should this be necessary.

A sterilized container with two gallipots with glycerin sterile swabs, some port wine or brandy and a dummy or stuffed teat is taken to the theatre with the patient.

During the operation the nurse sits at the head of the table in the place of the anæsthetist and comforts the baby with the dummy dipped into the glycerin and brandy. This helps to relax the abdominal muscles. At the same time the nurse watches the patient's general condition. The clothes are folded back to allow access to the abdomen and the skin is cleaned with an antiseptic lotion and sterile towels draped over the patient and around the site of the operation. 8 to 10 millilitres of a solution containing 3 minims of adrenaline 1 in 1,000 to 1 per cent. procaine are injected to act as local anæsthetic and to help control any tendency to bleeding. A small incision, either in the midline or just below the right costal margin is made and the stomach delivered through the wound. The thickened pyloric sphincter can usually be plainly felt and seen. A nick is made in the surface of the muscle and with a blunt instrument (some surgeons use the blunt end of the handle of the scalpel) the muscle is divided right down to the mucosa but not through it. The mucous coat of the intestine can be seen bulging through the split. Muscle will later close around the bulge but the obstruction will be permanently relieved. The stomach is then returned into the abdominal cavity and the muscle and peritoneum stitched up in layers in the usual manner. The entire operation may last only eight to ten minutes.

After the operation the baby is placed in a warmed cot and taken off the splint. He is nursed flat. Overheating should be avoided at all stages and the temperature is taken in the groin at hourly intervals. The cotton wool is removed from one limb at a time to regulate the temperature. It is important to handle the baby as gently and with as little disturbance as possible.

Post-operative Feeding. Details of feeding vary from one

hospital to another but the fundamental principles remain the same. In uncomplicated cases feeding is started within 2 hours of return from the theatre and one drachm of half-strength saline and 5 per cent. glucose may be given. The feeds are given every hour and each feed is increased by a drachm until the feed volume reaches between 4 and 8 drachms according to the speed with which it is intended to return to normal feeding. This depends on the amount of gastritis present preoperatively and on the history of the illness. About 6 hours after operation, milk is introduced. The feed the baby is used to is diluted to $\frac{1}{4}$ strength for three feeds, to $\frac{1}{2}$ strength for the next feed and so on until full strength feeds have been reintroduced. It is usual to omit at least one feed during the night or to space the feeds to 2-hourly intervals to give the baby some rest. Amounts and strength of feed are increased in this manner until the baby is back to his accustomed feed by the third post-operative day.

Breast-fed babies and those with a short history can usually progress more rapidly than artificially-fed ones and in some cases it is possible to put the baby to the breast 4 hours after return from the theatre allowing him to suck for 2 minutes and increasing the time and the intervals between feeds on the same lines as described above. Breast-fed babies are test weighed to give some idea as to how much they are receiving.

Complications. Hyperpyrexia, vomiting, cross infection and inflammation of the wound edges are among the complications which may arise. Hyperpyrexia can often be relieved by adjusting the clothing and the room temperature, or by giving a small subcutaneous infusion to relieve post-operative dehydration. Vomiting may be due to residual gastritis and may have to be treated by one or two daily wash-outs during the first post-operative days. Diarrhœa, pneumonia and wound infection occur occasionally in these debilitated babies and the danger from them is one of the reasons for the earliest possible discharge. Inflammation of the wound edges is sometimes due to the local anæsthetic and this is rarely very serious.

The *prognosis* is excellent when the patient is in experienced hands. Babies often start to gain weight on the second post-operative day and rapidly reach the norm for their age. Discharge is often possible on the third day, or even sooner, and the baby is brought back for removal of sutures and a check-up. This lessens the risk of the infant picking up infection from other children. There are few pædiatric conditions that offer greater satisfaction and opportunities for skill in nursing than congenital pyloric stenosis. As the babies are often breast-fed, every attempt should be made to admit the mother with her baby. This gives greater opportunity for the hospital staff to comfort and reassure the young mother, who is bound to find the thought of an operation on her baby distressing. There is no reason why the mother should not assist with the care of the baby and her own confidence and peace of mind will help to maintain a good supply of breast milk for her child.

While the nurse should be careful to prevent the parents from taking too grave a view of the condition, she should always remember to ascertain in advance whether the baby has been christened and, if desired, should arrange for a minister of religion to christen the infant in the presence of the parents.

Gastric Lavage. The equipment required for gastric lavage in young children differs from that used for adults only in some minor detail. As the œsophageal tube can as a rule be connected directly to the funnel neither extra length of tubing, nor a glass connection are needed. This eliminates extra weight to manipulate. To stop the flow the tube is often doubled back on itself instead of using a gate clip and the rate of flow is regulated by raising or lowering the tube and funnel. Instead of the open-type funnel a cylindrical, upright glass funnel is used and any gastric contents or lavage-fluid should be allowed to run back into the funnel and not emptied direct into a receiver or bucket. In that way a comparison can be made between the amounts run in and returned. This is important on account of the small amounts involved and the danger of causing distension and colic if too much fluid is allowed to run into the stomach or to accumulate there. A measuring jug should also be used. Suction is never employed (as e.g. by aspirating with a syringe or a Senoran's pump) but instead the fluid is syphoned back by quickly lowering the funnel and tube just before the last fluid disappears at the juncture of glass funnel and rubber tubing.

Gastric lavage in children is as a rule less upsetting than in adults but babies and young children should be securely wrapped in a blanket to avoid any struggle (Figs. 22 and 42) as little cooperation can be expected. The tube should be measured from the bridge of the nose to the lower end of the sternum to give an idea how far the tube needs to be passed in order to enter the stomach. The point is reached when the mark made on the tube after measuring, reaches the level of the dental arch.

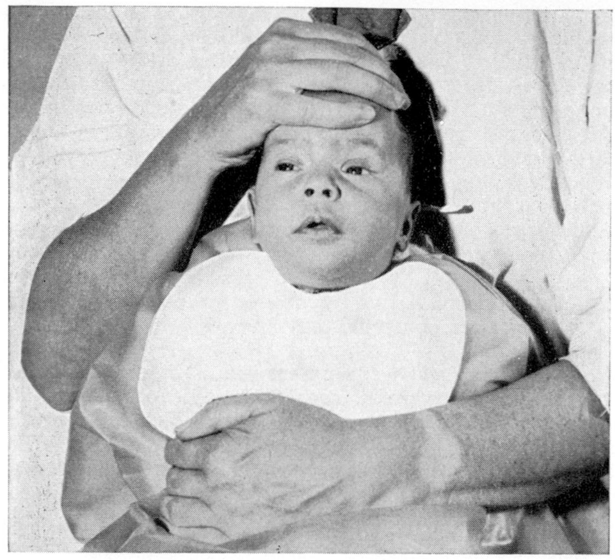

Fig. 42. A Convenient Way of Holding a Baby for Examination of Mouth or Throat.

Also helpful when passing tube, e.g. for gastric lavage.

Children cannot be expected to assist with the passing of the tube by swallowing or deep breathing and it is best to feed the tube gently, but firmly along the floor of the mouth after lubricating it with a little sterile water or glycerin. The assisting nurse may steady the child's head (Fig. 42) or support the chin as this helps to reduce the tickling sensation and excessive retching. After seeing gastric residue rise in the funnel, or after testing some resting juice which has been obtained by syphon action for reaction on litmus paper, fluid (e.g. normal saline at a temperature of 37·2° to 37·8° C. (99° to 100° F.) is run into the stomach. The amount will vary according to the age and size of the patient but in the majority of cases it is satisfactory to allow one funnel full to run in at a time and then to syphon the fluid back. Gastric lavage in children should always be supervised by a trained nurse who will be able to give advice from her own experience as to the correct quantity of fluid which should be used. By raising or lowering the funnel, fluid can be syphoned back. At the end of the procedure the nurse should make sure that no fluid is left in the stomach.

When giving a feed by tube the technique and equipment are essentially the same but at the end of the feed the funnel should be allowed to empty down to the juncture of the funnel and rubber tube, before adding a small amount of plain water. This reduces the mixing of plain fluid and feed to a minimum and also ensures that the baby really gets all the feed. If the tube is withdrawn before it has emptied completely as much as half an ounce of feed may be lost, a considerable proportion of the total if the small amounts sometimes involved in infant feeding are considered. Furthermore, as long as there is any fluid in the tube, there is always a danger that some may be aspirated into the trachea as the tube passes the larynx when it is withdrawn. As an additional safety measure and in order to prevent this from happening it is considered wise to pinch the tube whilst withdrawing it. The tube should always be withdrawn fairly quickly but in one steady pull.

The Intestines

Constipation

Infrequent bowel actions are unlikely to be harmful provided the stools are soft and passed without causing pain or distress. Few pædiatricians are in favour of giving enemata or aperients and the "weekly dose" is a deplorable custom which should be strongly discouraged. No medication is satisfactory unless used intelligently and as the need arises, and it is obvious that giving an aperient on a set day once a week cannot be classed as either an intelligent or a necessary measure. It is far more likely to cause resentment and a family scene if, for instance, Friday evening is set aside for the giving of an aperient, than to contribute to good health and good bowel training of the child.

True constipation, that is to say dry, hard fæces passed with difficulty, may be due to a long list of causes including those mentioned below.

In Young Babies. Underfeeding due to inadequate fluid or calorie intake or to failure of lactation. Insufficient sugar added to artificial feeds.

Congenital Abnormalities. These may hold up the food or fæces or inhibit peristalsis; among such conditions are congenital pyloric stenosis, intestinal atresia; stricture of the anus; Hirschsprung's disease; cretinism, mental deficiency and atonia due to muscular dystrophy or debility.

Types of Stools in Infancy and Childhood: their characteristics and significance

Description	*Usual occurrence*	*Colour*	*Odour*	*Consistency*	*Frequency*	*Composition*	*Reaction*
Meconium	First 2–3 days after birth	Tarry, changing to greenish-black	None	Semi-solid	3–6 daily	Normal	Neutral
Changing Stools	Approx. 3rd –6th day of life	Dark green changing to yellow	None	Soft	5–8 daily	Normal	Acid
Breast-milk stools	In breast-fed babies	Mustard colour	Characteristic	Soft homogenous	5–6 daily	Normal	Acid
Cow's-milk stools	In artificially fed babies	A pale yellow-grey	Musty	Semi-formed bulky	4–5 daily	Normal	Alkaline
Mixed Feeding	In toddlers	Brown	Slight	Formed	1–2 daily	Normal	Varies
Buttermilk Feeding	In infancy	Olive-green	Characteristic	Soft	5–6 daily	Normal	Acid
High protein content	In infancy	Grey	Sour and offensive	Dry and crumbling	1–2 daily	Excess protein	Alkaline
High fat content	e.g. Cœliac disease	Grey, clay coloured	Offensive	Bulky greasy	Several daily	Excess fat deficient in bile	Acid
High carbohydrate content	In infancy	Green	Slightly offensive	Relaxed frothy	Frequent	Fermented fæces	Very acid
Soapy stools	Digestive disturbances	White	Offensive	Pasty	Several daily	Excess fat or deficient in bile	Neutral

Melæna	Swallowed blood, intestinal bleeding	Tarry-black	Characteristic sweet	Soft	Varies	Blood	Alkaline
Intestinal hurry	Gastro-intestinal infections	Bright green	Characteristic offensive	Fluid relaxed	Many times daily	Unconverted bile	Neutral
Hunger stools	Infancy	Dark green	None or sour	Small dry	Frequent	Large proportion of mucus-bile	Acid
Over-feeding	Infancy	Bright green	Offensive	Frothy fermenting	Frequent	Excess fat and carbohydrate	Very acid
Intestinal Infections	Gastro-enteritis	Pale green	Characteristic offensive	Soft or liquid	Very frequent	Partially digested food, mucus	Varies
Fresh blood	1 Anal fissure 2 Ulcerative colitis 3 Dysentery 4 Rectal polyp	Bright red	1 none 2, 3 offensive 4 none	1 hard 2, 3 liquid 4 normal	1 infrequent 2, 3 frequent 4 normal	1 normal 2, 3 mucus, bile, blood 4 normal and streaks of blood	Alkaline
Red currant jelly stool	Intussusception	Bright red	None	Jelly-like	1 or 2 isolated stools	Mucus, blood	Neutral
Pea-soup stool	Typhoid	Green	Offensive	Liquid	Very frequent	Mucus, pus, blood	—
Pus, mucus	Pelvic abcess	Normal or green streaked with pus	Offensive	Relaxed	Once after rupture of abcess into bowel	Pus, mucus	—

Painful Defæcation. This may be due to local causes, e.g. anal fissure, which makes the child hold back the stool to avoid pain.

Parenteral Causes. These include tuberculous meningitis and nephritis with œdema.

Psychological Factors. These, or faulty habit training, may lead to infrequent bowel actions and so cause hard stools and painful defæcation. Such psychological factors include maternal anxiety.

Treatment. Laxatives may occasionally have to be used for short periods until a regular routine has been re-established. In early infancy a teaspoon of milk of magnesia, given three times a day may be ordered. For older children syrup of figs, 2 to 15 millilitres daily, or Senokot, ½ to 1½ tablets daily, are suitable. Liquid paraffin should not be given as it interferes with vitamin absorption and because there is some danger of lipoid pneumonia from inhalation. Severe cases of long standing, may need initial treatment by colon lavage or enemata. Special points arise in the case of:

Anal Fissure. The severe pain experienced on defæcation should be minimized by keeping the fæces soft by giving the correct diet and mild laxatives. Witch hazel ointment may be applied to the anal region and a small piece may be introduced into the anus several times a day. This assists the healing of the torn mucosa and relieves pain. Alternatively an anæsthetic ointment such as amethocaine may be used.

Constipation with Overflow. This is a term used for leakage of decomposed fæces around a mass of impacted fæcal matter. These cases can be very persistent. Tedious toilet training, enemata, purgatives and, on occasion, manual removal of the fæcal mass under an anæsthetic may prove necessary. For treatment to be successful it is important to find out the underlying cause. In the meantime the patient's mother, exasperated by the constant soiling of clothes will need support and sympathy in order to gain her patient cooperation in treating the condition.

Complications of True Constipation. True constipation can be responsible for a number of symptoms such as furred tongue, anorexia and vomiting, poor general circulation and sluggishness, restless sleep and bedwetting.

As constipation is a symptom rather than a disease in itself, the underlying cause should be found and treatment given accordingly. Dietary adjustments may be all that is necessary. For infants this may mean additional sugar in the bottle feeds or drinks of boiled water in between ordinary feeds as well as extra orange juice. In older children a diet rich in roughage and adequate exercise and regular habit training should be encouraged. Allbran, wholemeal bread, fresh fruit, green vegetables and prune juice are palatable, suitable high roughage additions to the daily dietary. Occasionally it is found that constipation has developed because the lavatory in the child's home is situated in a cold, dark, or isolated part of a tenement building or at the bottom of the garden, so that the child is frightened of going there on his own. Alternatively, the toilet seat may be too high and, as the child's feet cannot reach the ground, he is frightened of falling in. Lack of time before leaving for school may be another, easily remedied cause of chronic constipation. Lack of exercise leading to poor circulation and muscle tone should be corrected. Driving and television viewing have contributed to physical inactivity in recent years and all types of sport should be encouraged as a healthy counterbalance.

Observation of Fæces

Although the observation of fæces is an important duty of every nurse it is of immeasurable value in pædiatric nursing. Children are often unable to describe symptoms accurately and the abnormal stool, preserved for inspection by an experienced ward sister or medical officer may frequently lead to the establishment of a previously doubtful diagnosis. The nurse should note such points as the colour, consistency, the odour, shape and frequency of the stools. Any abnormal constituents such as blood, mucus or foreign bodies should be noted and any complaints of pain on passing the stool treated as being significant.

Collection of Specimens. The collection of fæcal matter for investigation does not differ from that in adult nursing but, in the case of 24-hour specimens for very young children, a specially constructed chair may have to be used (see Hiatus Hernia Chair, Fig. 13), or the napkin lined with thin plastic or cellophane. The type of colostomy bag known as a "Chiron" disposable bag can sometimes be fixed to the buttocks and the child allowed to run around without restriction while the fæces are being collected.

The handling of bedpans and pots should at all times be reduced to a minimum. Soiled napkins should be saved with the corners tucked underneath the part on which the stool lies when first taken off the baby, placed in a receiver and covered with a glass plate. It is now ready for easy inspection. Any doubtful stool should always be saved and kept available during the pædiatrician's round (see page 38).

Infantile Gastro-enteritis

At one time gastro-enteritis was one of the killing diseases of infancy. To-day, in this country, the illness remains serious but the majority of patients can be expected to make a good recovery even though the illness may be a prolonged one with an anxious period for all concerned. Gastro-enteritis now occurs throughout the year, in contrast to the one-time high incidence during the summer months which gave the illness the name of summer diarrhœa. Premature babies are particularly prone to gastro-enteritis, but it is rarely seen in breast fed babies or in any babies before the age of a month or after the age of 2 years.

The infection is as a rule due to various strains of *Escherichia (Bacterium) coli*, salmonella or dysentery bacillus, and possibly to some as yet unidentified virus. Other types are secondary to infection outside the gastro-intestinal tract such as middle ear infections, meningitis or the common cold. Symptoms similar to those caused by infective gastro-enteritis may be due to dietetic errors.

Signs and Symptoms. The symptoms of gastro-enteritis in infancy may vary from slight frequency of the bowel actions, relaxed stools and an occasional vomit, to a severe illness with gross dehydration and generalized disturbances. For the purpose of this chapter a severe, fully established case is described.

The infant with severe gastro-enteritis presents a pitiable picture. He is limp and lethargic, although often restlessly moving his head and beating his arms around. His cheeks may be flushed and his eyes sunken and surrounded by dark rings. The fontanelle is depressed. The abdomen is often distended and the infant draws his legs up as if in pain. The skin is dry and inelastic and feels hot to the touch. The temperature may be raised to 39·4° C. (103° F.) and the pulse is rapid and of poor volume. In severe cases convulsions are common.

The mother will explain that the infant has had increasingly frequent, loose and explosive stools with a characteristic, offensive smell and that his buttocks are becoming sore. She may have noticed traces of blood or mucus in the stools, or she may have seen bits of curd and free fluid. The colour may be green or bright orange. An observant mother may even have noticed that her baby is passing very little and rather dark urine, a sure sign of severe dehydration. She will say that the baby is wakeful, restless and constantly whimpering. Although he appears to be thirsty and to want his feeds, he is often unable to retain them and the vomiting may be forceful and copious and occur during or immediately after taking a feed. Vomiting, however, is not a constant feature and in many cases it is absent or develops as a late symptom. As he gets worse, the baby may refuse his feeds. It is obvious that loss of weight will be rapid and severe, and that all the signs of dehydration and loss of electrolytes will soon be present.

Investigations. A thorough examination of the child is essential in order to exclude any parenteral cause of the illness. Blood is taken for biochemical analysis and any electrolyte imbalance corrected without delay. In vomiting, chlorides are lost to the body and diarrhœa causes loss of sodium and potassium. These deficiencies must be made good by giving intravenous fluids urgently, as young infants deteriorate very rapidly. It is often necessary to start treatment without waiting for the result of the laboratory tests. The acid-base upset may be severe and is usually corrected by giving modified Ringer-Lactate (Hartmann's) solution or Molar Lactate solution. Serum protein deficiencies and anæmia may have to be corrected by blood transfusion. Anæmia may be severe, though hæmoglobin readings may at first be high, due to hæmoconcentration; the blood urea will also be raised.

A rectal swab is taken and it should be sent to the laboratory while fresh. Some hospitals like the swab to be moistened by dipping it in sterile broth solution, as used for blood cultures, before insertion into the rectum.

Special Observations. It is important that any complication should be noticed early because no time should be lost before appropriate treatment is started. Any change in the infant must be reported without delay and its significance understood. Starvation will be obvious through loss of weight, weakness, the appearance of ketone bodies in the urine and a hard, palpable liver. Deep, rapid respirations are characteristic of acidosis, and an increase in the vomiting, spasms and convulsions are often signs of severe alkalosis. A diminished urinary output is a sign of impaired renal function or dehydration. Abdominal distension may be marked and is caused by gas formation in the intestines; pallor may be a sign of anæmia.

Treatment aims at eliminating the underlying cause and replacing lost fluids and electrolytes; also at introducing suitable feeds very gradually after resting the gastro-intestinal tract. Pyelitis, otitis media and any other parenteral infections are dealt with in the appropriate manner and the giving of an antibiotic is usually part of the treatment.

Drugs. Neomycin, a broad spectrum antibiotic, or framycetin are at present the drugs of choice. They can be given in high dosage as they are not absorbed but remain in the bowel. Their use not only serves to shorten the course of the illness and reduce mortality, but by sterilizing the stools also helps to reduce the risk of spreading the infection. Brandy and nikethamide may be ordered in severe cases with threatening collapse. Opium derivatives are not as a rule well tolerated by very young infants.

Once the electrolyte and serum protein losses have been corrected by intravenous therapy, oral feeding can be started and it is now rarely necessary to continue with intravenous or subcutaneous fluids for longer than 36 hours. If subcutaneous fluids are ordered, they are usually given with hyaluronidase to assist absorption but even so this method is rarely satisfactory if dehydration is severe, as the peripheral circulatory failure precludes absorption from the tissues.

The *prognosis* of severe infantile gastro-enteritis has recently changed completely, due to the better understanding and management of blood chemistry. Most infants can now be expected to make a good recovery.

Nursing Care. Strict precautions against spread of infection must be observed and where other infants are nursed in the same unit, ideally no nurse attending a case of infective gastro-enteritis should handle these or be allowed into the feed kitchen. Although lack of ideal conditions does not preclude excellent nursing care, the following facilities and equipment should be available whenever possible.

A cubicle equipped with a swing door, running water and good ventilation, two buckets or pedal-bins (one for napkins and one for clothes), a rubber apron, two barrier gowns, their outsides plainly marked and hung on coat hangers when not in use, an adequate supply of masks, facilities for preliminary sterilization of feed bottles (e.g. a bowl of Milton solution 1 in 80), separate toilet equipment, stethoscope, auriscope, pencils for charting observations and a pulsometer. Some hospitals use only materials which can be easily boiled for bed linen, blankets and clothing. Cotton is ideal and with good heating and ventilation which excludes draughts, entirely adequate from the point of view of warmth. Separate cleaning utensils and materials must also be provided.

In addition, nurses should be meticulous in the care of their hands and finger nails and a hand lotion should be provided to avoid rough or cracked skin due to frequent hand washing.

Bearing in mind the symptoms of the disease and the complications already mentioned, the nurse will closely observe the following points: The infant's attitude in his cot and the degree of restlessness or lethargy. The condition of the skin, whether hot or cold, dry or clammy, pale, flushed, inelastic or even jaundiced. She will note whether the fontanelles are depressed or bulging and whether the mouth is dry, the lips cracked, the tongue unusually red or coated, and whether there are signs of thrush. She will watch to see whether the eyes are anxious, staring, sunken and only semi-closed during sleep and whether the abdomen is distended or sunken. She will make further observations on the state of the buttocks which may be raw and excoriated and of the extremities which may be blue and cold. She will note the amount of urine passed and the degree of its concentration and the number, frequency, size, colour and odour of the stools and she will watch for the presence of blood, mucus or free fluid.

The infant's eagerness or reluctance to feed is an important guide and, when temperature, pulse and respirations are taken, full observations should be made. The infant should be weighed daily even while parenteral fluids are being given and to make this possible the intravenous tubing should be long enough to allow for lifting the infant on to the scales. At first the gain in weight will be large, as hydration improves, and this gain should not be regarded as an absolute gain. When the intravenous infusion is discontinued there may be a temporary slight loss of weight or at least no gain until the body has regained its normal balance of hydration and until adequate intake by mouth and general improvement cause a real gain which will eventually be maintained.

Rectal temperatures should never be taken, as the irritation of introducing the thermometer into the rectum may cause unnecessary bowel actions. It is always necessary to correlate these observations and to judge the condition of the patient as a whole, when deciding on treatment and diet, instead of noting only the number and frequency of the stools.

Complications of Gastro-enteritis. It is sometimes difficult to distinguish between the primary-parenteral illness which causes gastro-enteritis and the complications which result from the illness and the low resistance of the infant. Inhalation of vomitus causing pneumonia, inflammation of the middle ear and mastoiditis from vomitus tracking up the short, straight Eustachian tube are examples. Other complications include sore buttocks, thrush, convulsions, meningitis and circulatory failure.

The Diet. In all but the mildest cases, milk feeds are discontinued for 24 to 36 hours and are replaced by boiled water and glucose 4·3 per cent. dextrose in $\frac{1}{5}$ strength normal saline solution. If the baby is being treated at home, a suitable mixture may be made by using one tablespoon of sugar to $\frac{1}{4}$ tea spoon of salt in one pint of boiled water. This gives a solution of approximately 5 per cent. sugar in a $\frac{1}{4}$ strength normal saline. The amount of fluid required is based on the principle of giving $2\frac{1}{2}$ to 3 ounces of fluid per day for every pound of body weight and allowing up to 10 ounces extra daily to make up for loss of fluid. Skimmed or half cream milk in dilution is gradually introduced until the infant's usual feed has been re-established. Expressed breast milk may be invaluable in some cases. Sugar is at first omitted and the fat content of the feed should be low as fat is not easily tolerated. Lactic acid milk, whey and Benger's Food are often very suitable. Arabon added to the feeds makes the stools more solid. Tea and apple diet may yield very good results (see below). Saccharin can be used as a sweetening agent and should not be withheld while the feeds are diluted, as most babies object to unsweetened feeds and refuse them even though they may appear to be eager when they first start sucking.

Except in the case of planned schedule feeding, time should always be allowed to observe the effect of various stages of the diet and, as a rule, changes should be made once in 24 hours at the most.

Tea and Apple Diet. Raw, ripe dessert apples are pulped and sieved, allowing approximately $2\frac{1}{2}$ ounces per pound of body weight per day. The pulp is added to an infusion of tea (half a teaspoonful of tea to half a pint of boiling water, allowed to stand for two minutes). Saccharin may be added as a sweetening agent.

Disinfection of Feeding Bottles. After use, feeding bottles are rinsed under the cold tap and placed in a solution of Milton 1 in 80 in the infant's cubicle until the next feed. Care should be taken to fill the bottles to capacity with the Milton solution before immersing them. The presterilized bottles are then dealt with in the usual way. Teats are rinsed under cold, running water and kept in a special teat jar filled with a disinfectant lotion such as Milton 1 in 80, in the cubicle.

Disposal of Napkins. Napkins used by gastro-enteritis patients should be soaked; Formalin 1 in 250 or Milton 1 in 80 solution are suitable disinfectants. After one hour, the napkins are rinsed and wrung out by a nurse wearing protective rubber gloves and apron and are then disposed of in the usual way. Some hospitals allow these napkins to go to the laundry untreated, on the theory that this particular infection is not dangerous to the adult laundry workers. In this case special arrangements for transport are made. In other hospitals, destructible napkins are used; these can be placed in paper bags immediately they are taken off the baby and bag and napkin burned in an incinerator in the ward sluice.

Intestinal Obstruction

Intestinal obstruction in childhood may be due to congenital abnormalities, strangulated hernia, intussusception, volvulus, a swallowed foreign body or pressure from a tumour. The classical symptoms are the same as in adults, namely vomiting pain, absolute constipation and abdominal distension. Urgent operation to relieve the obstruction is necessary otherwise there is danger that the constriction of the blood supply may lead to gangrene of the strangulated portion of gut, and the continued vomiting result in dehydration and loss of electrolytes. A Ryle's tube is passed and the stomach contents aspirated before giving an anæsthetic and an intravenous infusion will be necessary.

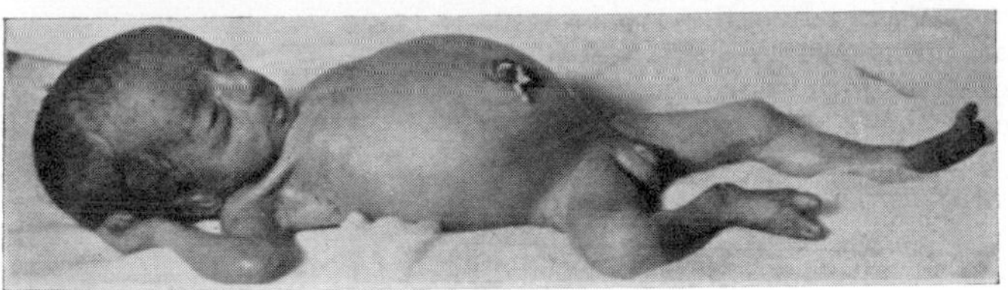

Fig. 43. AN INFANT WITH ABDOMINAL DISTENSION DUE TO ACUTE INTESTINAL OBSTRUCTION.

Volvulus

A different kind of obstruction occurs in volvulus when a loop of bowel gets twisted round causing complete obstruction, but symptoms and treatment are similar to the ones described above. After opening the abdomen the site of the volvulus is sought and the gut untwisted and anchored to the peritoneum. Resection and anastamosis are rarely necessary.

Intussusception

Intussusception is one of the most urgent emergencies of early childhood, though on occasions repeated attacks occur, which rectify themselves. Acute intussusception is seen usually at the time the infant starts on a weaning diet and it is probable that irritation of the bowel causes a small area of inflammation and œdema in the ileocæcal region which is the starting point of the telescoping of the bowel. A portion of the bowel becomes invaginated and is dragged onwards towards the rectum by peristaltic movement.

Signs and Symptoms. The infant is as a rule a well-nourished, healthy baby of nine months to two years. The mother will explain that he suddenly seemed to have severe abdominal colic which made him draw up his legs and that these pains had been recurring at intervals, during which the baby seemed normal and contented. At first the pain may recur every hour or half-hour but it soon becomes more frequent and its severity causes shock, with pallor, sweating and a cold, clammy skin. The baby soon becomes exhausted. At first a normal stool may be passed but this is followed by complete constipation due to the obstruction, except for the passage of blood stained mucus—the typical "red currant jelly stool". Vomiting may occur but is not a constant symptom.

On *examination* a sausage-shaped tumour may be felt over the colon, while the right inguinal fossa feels empty as the cæcum is drawn into the colon—the "Sign de Dance". On rectal examination the apex of the intussusception may be felt.

Operation. The child is prepared as for any other operation but sometimes a gastric tube is passed and the stomach contents aspirated to avoid inhalation of vomited food. An intravenous infusion may be started to treat the shock and to restore the electrolyte balance. The abdominal skin, the umbilicus and the groins are washed with soap and water or the child is bathed, if his condition permits.

No time is lost in starting the operation as the invaginated section of the bowel causes obstruction of the blood supply and if left too long would result in gangrene and toxic symptoms. A laparotomy is done, the intussusception found and the invaginated bowel gently drawn out, with a "milking movement". After reduction the bowel is sometimes stitched to the peritoneum to prevent recurrence. Special care is taken to ensure that the bowel is viable and that the blood supply is capable of complete recovery. Occasionally resection of gut is necessary.

Post-operative Care. This is usually straightforward. Fluids are given in small amounts—some hospitals start on a "pyloric schedule"—but in most cases the child can return to a light, normal diet within three or four days. Any vomiting, the passage of flatus and the first stool are reported as they are an important guide to treatment. The wound is often left exposed or covered with a small dressing and the stitches are usually removed on the 8th and 10th day respectively.

If the diagnosis is doubtful, a barium enema may be ordered to confirm the diagnosis and on occasions this has the effect of reducing the intussusception so that operation becomes unnecessary.

Acute Appendicitis

There are few conditions in childhood that present a more confusing picture than acute appendicitis. Among the conditions which may lead to this diagnosis erroneously are tonsillitis, mesenteric adenitis, urinary tract infections, pneumonia, diaphragmatic pleurisy, meningitis, anaphylactoid purpura, dysentery, gastro-enteritis, and premenstrual pain. Assessment of all symptoms and sometimes a period of careful observation will, however, establish the correct diagnosis. Because of the extensive examination that is necessary to establish the correct diagnosis the nurse may have to be prepared for an ear, nose and throat and a neurological examination, a rectal swab, a clean specimen of urine, blood picture and possibly a lumbar puncture and chest X-ray.

Signs and Symptoms. Acute appendicitis is rare before the age of 2 years and most common at 5 to 12 years. The onset may be insidious with anorexia, listlessness, nausea or one or two attacks of vomiting and constipation. Alternatively the child may become acutely ill with little warning. The temperature may rise to 37·2° to 38·4° C. (99° to 101° F.), the pulse become rapid and the expression anxious. The tongue is furred and there is halitosis. The child is irritable and resents being touched or examined. If the appendix lies deep in the pelvis—pelvic appendix—the symptoms may include frequency of micturition and diarrhœa due to irritation, and if the appendix is retrocæcal the abdominal signs will be masked and diagnosis made very difficult.

Pain may be vague at first and may be intermittent to begin with but it gradually moves to the para-umbilical region and within twelve hours settles in the right iliac fossa.

On *examination* there is guarding and tenderness, and rectal examination causes the patient to flinch or cry out in pain as the finger points towards the right side. Abdominal rigidity may be caused by cold or general protest and for that reason it is particularly important in children that the doctor's hands should be warm and that a moment or two should be spent in gaining the child's confidence. Occasionally a sedative has to be given before a satisfactory examination can be carried out. If a white cell count is done, it is found to be raised to as much as 30,000 white cells per cu. mm. (mainly polymorphonuclear cells).

Once diagnosis has been made, operation should not be delayed. Peritonitis occurs readily as the poorly developed peritoneum is less resistant to infection in a child than in later life, and infection does not localize well in childhood. The appendix wall is thin and the appendix perforates more often than in adults with more serious results. Operation and aftercare are the same for children as for adults and in an uneventful case the child can be expected to be up for bedmaking on the first day and playing happily in the wards on the second day after operation.

Complications

1. *Perforated Appendix.* Acute appendicitis which cannot be diagnosed or treated in time may lead to perforation and set up peritonitis or form a pelvic abscess. When perforation has occurred, there may for a time, appear to be some improvement in the child's condition. The pain subsides, he seems more relaxed and may fall asleep. After a few hours, however, it is evident that he is now seriously ill and in spite of operation, complications have now become unavoidable.

2. *Peritonitis.* Peritonitis may be caused by surgical emergencies such as a ruptured appendix, perforation of the bowel due to ulcerative colitis, by ascending infection from the vagina and by infection in the blood stream. In newly born babies the infection may enter via the umbilicus. The causative organisms include the staphylococcus, *Escherichia* (*Bacterium*) *coli*, the tubercle bacillus, gonococcus and pneumococcus.

In the case of a perforated appendix the causative organism is usually the *Escherichia coli* and the fluid in the peritoneal cavity soon becomes infected. The onset is mostly very acute. The temperature rises to 39·4° to 40·6° C. (103° to 105° F.), the tongue is furred, the child vomits and complains of abdominal pain or draws up his legs. In very young patients this pain may not be localized as it is in older children. Respirations are rapid and shallow, the diaphragm being immobilized as the movements of the abdomen cause pain, but the arms are thrown out above the head in order to increase the respiratory capacity. The colour of the skin is grey, with a malar flush and the eyes bright but sunken and surrounded by dark rings. The legs are drawn up in "frog position" in an attempt to relieve abdominal pain. Free fluid will be present in the abdominal cavity and the abdomen is rigid. The entire picture is that of severe toxæmia.

Nursing Care

Children suffering from such a serious illness need expert and continuous nursing care. The mouth will have to be treated frequently, the position changed and pillows turned in order to encourage rest and sleep. Pressure areas need most careful attention. For bedmaking the child should be lifted rather than rolled from side to side so as to keep the intraperitoneal fluid localized. The upright position is adopted for the same reason and at the same time this will encourage deep respirations (Fig. 44). Hot fomentations may relieve abdominal pain and rigidity. Open windows and the use of electric fans help to reduce hyperpyrexia. Fluid balance charts are kept as well as 4-hourly temperature and accurate observation charts. The room or ward should be well ventilated and provided the child is warmly covered and that draughts are excluded only good can come from opening a window.

With the help of a stethoscope, the bowel sounds should be checked as the absence of peristalsis, flatus and bowel actions are signs of intestinal obstruction. A small blood transfusion is sometimes given to correct anæmia. It may also help to build up the patient's general strength and resistance.

At times the free fluid in the abdomen may fail to absorb and become infected. A generalized septicæmia may develop or in more favourable cases, the pus will localize and form a pelvic abscess. Adhesions may form between the convolutions of the bowel and later give rise to colic and obstruction.

3. *Pelvic Abscess.* This rarely requires surgical interference. The pus localizes and in the majority of cases the abscess

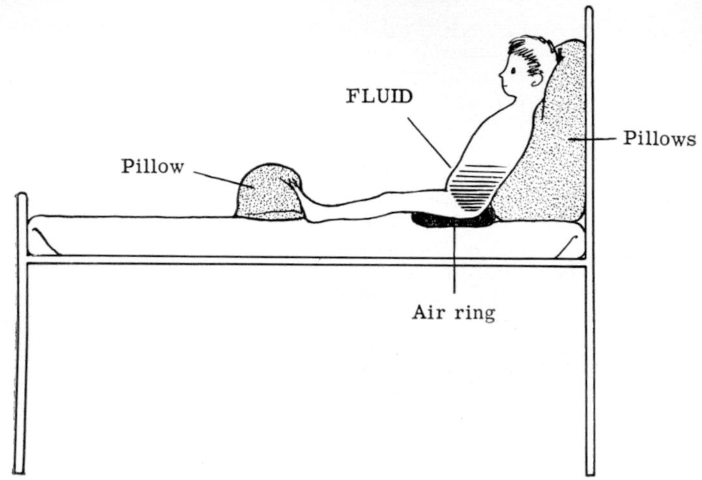

Fig. 44. PERITONITIS, WITH FREE FLUID IN THE PERITONEAL CAVITY.
Sitting the patient in the upright position helps with drainage and localizes the fluid in the pelvic cavity. Children move around far more freely than adults so that danger from the use of pillows causing thrombosis of a deep vein is negligible.

eventually ruptures into the rectum. Pus and mucus are passed when the child has his bowels opened. This complication delays recovery by a week or two but is rarely very serious although the child may have considerable pain.

A far more serious complication, *paralytic ileus*, arises when the bowel has had to be handled a great deal at operation or when peritonitis is generalized.

Paralytic Ileus

Peristalsis ceases and there is complete constipation; no flatus is passed and the abdomen is distended and resonant when tapped. Vomiting may be severe and continues even when the normal stomach contents have been vomited and the vomit consists only of gastric and intestinal secretions mixed with bile.

Treatment. This consists of resting the bowel completely until peristalsis is re-established. Continuous gastric suction (Fig. 45) or frequent aspirations by syringe through a Ryle's tube are carried out until there is no more aspirate and bowel sounds can be heard through a stethoscope.

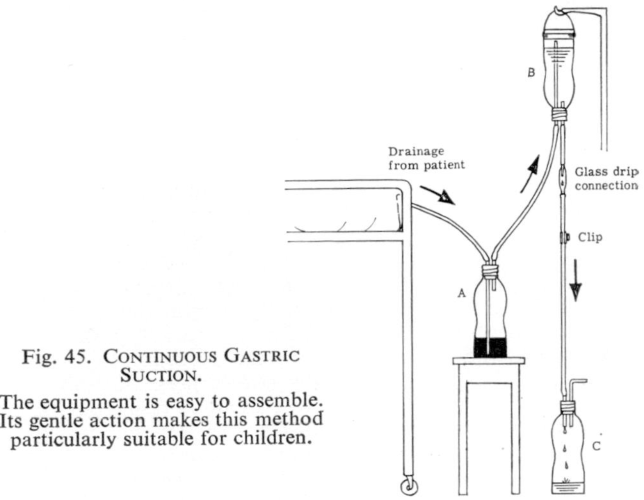

Fig. 45. Continuous Gastric Suction.

The equipment is easy to assemble. Its gentle action makes this method particularly suitable for children.

Fluids are given only by the intravenous route until peristalsis is once more present. The child will need a good deal of nursing attention. He is usually restless and needs comforting. Hands and face should be sponged from time to time, the mouth treated regularly, the position of the limb into which the infusion is running adjusted and supported by small pillows and the hands restrained to prevent him from pulling out the aspiration tube. Thirst may be troublesome and occasionally it is permissible to give sips of water even though they may have to be aspirated again. Sedatives will probably be needed to ensure adequate rest. Once peristalsis has started again, recovery is rapid and the child is as a rule eager to have his meals and gains strength rapidly. Despite the serious manifestations of paralytic ileus, prognosis is good.

Drugs. Since the advent of modern drugs, particularly the broad spectrum antibiotics, most patients suffering from appendicitis with complications are now successfully treated. The causative organism can often be determined by blood culture or from a discharging wound and laboratory tests show which antibiotic is most effective against it. Sulphonamides, streptomycin, a broad spectrum antibiotic or a combination of any of these drugs may be used.

Rectal Prolapse

Rectal prolapse is a common occurrence in children of about nine months to three years. There are several underlying causes and each will have to be treated before improvement can be expected from either medical or surgical therapy. The following are the *usual causes*: poor muscle tone as in diseases of the nervous system; malnutrition and wasting disease in which the supporting fatty tissue is absent; stress from coughing, as in whooping cough; long-standing diarrhœa causing irritation of the lower bowel; general mismanagement, behaviour problems, poor toilet training, long periods spent sitting on the pot and finally mental deficiency.

Treatment. When a rectal prolapse occurs it should be dealt with calmly and the prolapse gently reduced. In most cases it can easily be pushed back by steady pressure with a piece of damp cotton wool while the patient is lying on his back. Alternatively, very young children can be held up by their legs when gravity may cause the prolapse to reduce itself. It may help if, after reducing the prolapse, the nurse holds the child's buttocks together for a few minutes, while she distracts his attention, by telling a story or playing with him.

Patients who have had prolapses over a long period of time may have to learn to defæcate in a recumbent position. Good, consistent toilet training is a very important part of the treatment, but young children should not be allowed to sit on their pots for long, nor should undue importance be attached to daily bowel action. A day or two missed will rarely be of consequence and is preferable to fussing over this point.

Operation. Intractable or long standing cases may have to be treated surgically. This is either done by threading a piece of chromic catgut around the anal sphincter immediately underneath the skin, and so tightening the anal orifice, or by injecting a fibrosing agent, such as phenol 5 per cent. in almond oil, into the wall of the rectum. The fibrosed tissue causes some constriction and gives support to the rectal wall. In either case there is no pre-operative treatment although some surgeons may order a rectal wash-out before the patient is sent to the theatre. Postoperatively the buttocks may be strapped together for four or five days and extra fluids, a roughage free diet and liquid paraffin given, to ensure soft stools and easy bowel action without straining.

Special Points. All young children are inclined to focus much attention on their excreta and the anal region. This is an entirely natural thing. It is, however, important to manage rectal prolapse and the attendant treatment with as little fluster as possible and to ensure that the discomfort accompanying the operation should not be regarded as a punishment by the young patient.

At times, a strong psychological factor is involved and the child of overanxious or overprotective parents may learn to produce a prolapse at will, in order to call forth demonstrations of concern. In such cases the parents require reassurance and help. They should be told that the condition is a relatively harmless one and that their expressions of interest in the child should be directed into other channels. Proof of the psychological nature of the disturbance is that these children rarely have a prolapse in hospital.

Jaundice

Jaundice is a symptom and not a disease in itself and there are several causes, some of which are dealt with in the appropriate chapter in greater detail. The main causes of jaundice in childhood can be grouped under the following headings.

1. *The hæmolytic types.* These are due to excess destruction of red cells, i.e. at a greater rate than the liver can deal with. As these bile pigments are not excreted by the kidneys but are eliminated by the liver, stools and urine retain their normal colour. Examples are:

(*a*) Hæmolytic disease of the newborn (see page 57).
(*b*) Acholuric jaundice.
(*c*) Transfusion jaundice.

2. *Obstructive jaundice.* This is caused by an obstruction in the bile ducts so that bile pigment cannot reach the duodenum. Stools are pale or even colourless but the urine is heavily coloured, and the skin is tinged yellow to olive colour. Examples are:

(*a*) Congenital obliteration of the bile duct (see page 69).
(*b*) Obstruction from pressure of a tumour or a choledochus cyst.
(*c*) Very rarely by gall-stones or roundworms.

3. *Jaundice due to sepsis.* The principal examples are infection spreading from the umbilicus of the newborn or general infection spreading via the blood stream and causing liver damage. In these instances the jaundice is rarely very deep.

4. *Infective or acute virus hepatitis.* As the name suggests an as yet unidentified virus is thought to be responsible for this illness which frequently appears in epidemic form. Serum hepatitis comes under this heading and this is caused by contamination with virus-infected blood or needles used for injections and blood tests. The urine is dark while the fæces are pale or colourless. There is a similar neonatal "giant cell" hepatitis. Other conditions accompanied by jaundice are congenital syphilis, galactocæmia, cystic fibrosis of the pancreas, physiological jaundice and Weil's disease.

Infective Hepatitis (Epidemic Hepatitis, Virus Hepatitis, Catarrhal Jaundice)

Children are frequently admitted to hospital suffering from infective hepatitis and whole epidemics may sweep through schools and nurses' homes, as the long incubation period (2 to 6 weeks) makes the control of the infection difficult. The virus is present in the fæces and carriers may harbour the infection for many months.

Signs and Symptoms. The onset of an attack may follow one of several patterns. It may be acute, the temperature quickly rising to 38·4° to 39·4° C. (101° or 103° F.) and the patient feeling very ill. Alternatively there is a low pyrexia coupled with mild gastro-intestinal disturbances, malaise and gradually developing jaundice. In yet another variety there are few symptoms apart from general malaise, the first indication of the illness being the appearance of dark urine.

In the most typical cases of infective hepatitis the mother will have noticed almost complete loss of appetite, mild gastro-intestinal upset with occasional vomiting, a furred tongue, abdominal distension and possibly some diarrhœa (though constipation is an equally common feature). The child may complain of vague abdominal pain and tenderness particularly on movement and when lying on the right side. He is irritable and feverish and wants to be left alone. After 3 to 4 days the urine turns brown and shortly after that the temperature starts to subside. The fæces are now pale and constipated; the skin takes on a yellow tinge and the conjunctivæ become jaundiced.

The child may complain of feeling cold, his pulse is sluggish and there is marked irritability and lethargy. This is due to the circulation of bile salts through the nervous system. As the jaundice becomes established, these symptoms usually improve. Irritation of the skin is not a common feature in children. Bile pigments are present in the urine in the earliest stages of the illness and often diagnosis can be confirmed by a urine test.

Nursing Care. Pædiatricians differ in their wishes concerning the isolation of these patients. As a sound principle however, barrier nursing should be observed for five days after the onset of jaundice and the excreta disinfected for approximately three weeks.

The patient is kept on bed rest and the clothing should be warm, though wool next to the skin should not be worn as it may cause unnecessary irritation. Any itching may be treated with calamine lotion or ordinary dusting powder. Observation charts will mention particularly the colour of the stools and urine, the degree of jaundice present and the quality of the pulse. A specimen of urine is saved daily so that comparison of colour can be made throughout the course of the illness.

Diet. In the early stages of the illness there is almost complete anorexia. Fruit juices and abundant glucose (as much as half a pound a day) are given. Few pædiatricians prescribe a rigid, fat-free diet and as a rule the best guide in the matter is the patient himself, who will accept fat as soon as he feels ready for it. Where a more definite diet is prescribed, tea, toast and honey or golden syrup, jellies, fat-free broth and skimmed milk dishes are offered. Adequate fluid intake should be ensured. Occasionally high protein intake in the form of Casilan or Complan may be ordered and often these have to be camouflaged skilfully to make them acceptable to the patient. Loss of weight may be severe during the acute stage of the illness but is often made up rapidly during the convalescent stage

The first signs of improvement may start a few days after the onset of the jaundice. The stools and urine gradually regain their normal colour. The patient feels better and the appetite returns and may soon become voracious. The child should, however, be kept in bed until all jaundice has cleared and is not discharged until all liver tenderness has subsided. Fatigue may persist for some time and extra rest and a period of convalescence before return to school is highly desirable. Some pædiatricians make a rule that convalescence should be double the time spent in bed. The total recovery may take from one to three months. The outlook is as a rule good, but patients may have to have treatment and be careful with fat intake for several weeks. On occasions permanent liver damage is caused and very occasionally necrosis of the liver, followed by death, may ensue. For this reason, the illness should never be treated lightly and adequate rest and treatment must be given, and the patient followed up until the serum bilirubin level has returned to normal.

Drugs. On the whole little drug therapy is employed. Occasionally, if constipation is obstinate, saline aperients are ordered. In chronic cases or when there is recurrence of symptoms, cortisone therapy may prove of value. Avomine 12·5 mg. (for 6–10 years old) given three times a day or chlorpromazine (Largactil) 1 mg. per Kg. body weight given three times a day may lessen the feeling of nausea and reduce vomiting.

Complications. Severe attacks of hepatitis or recurrent attacks may lead to permanent damage of the liver structure. The prognosis of chronic hepatitis and cirrhosis of the liver is always grave although compensation in the liver function may simulate permanent recovery. The symptoms of cirrhosis include jaundice, pale stools, the presence of bile pigment in the urine, portal hypertension, the formation of varicose veins in the œsophagus, hæmatemesis, ascites and mental changes. The breath takes on a sweet, fæcal odour. Coma is common and eventually leads to death of the patient.

Intestinal Parasites

Threadworms (*Oxyuris vermicularis*)

Threadworm infestation is exceedingly common in children and entire families may be affected. It is thought that about 70 to 80 per cent. of all children of school age may have threadworms.

The threadworm normally inhabits the large intestine but the female migrates to the anal region where she deposits her eggs. Irritation, particularly during the night, causes the child to scratch and reinfect himself through his finger nails. Sharing beds and towels is an obvious way in which infection is spread to others.

Signs and Symptoms. The most general symptom is itching and this in turn may cause restless sleep and irritability. Scratching and irritation may cause inflammation of the perineum, vulvovaginitis, bed-wetting and occasionally diarrhœa or rectal prolapse.

The tiny worms may first be noticed in the course of a toilet round, although the worms remain on the surface of the stool only momentarily and then disappear into its substance. Alternatively the mother may describe symptoms which suggest the diagnosis.

Diagnostic Test. In order to prove the presence of threadworms a simple test can be done. A piece of Sellotape (adhesive cellulose tape) 1 inch wide and 3 inches long, is placed, sticky side down on the perineum immediately on waking. It is then transferred to a microscopic slide, again sticky side down and labelled and sent to the laboratory. The threadworm ova are obvious under the microscope. As the procedure is such a simple one it can easily be carried out by an outpatient's mother.

Treatment. Careful hygiene is the first essential. Finger nails should be kept short and hand washing before meals be enforced. Pyjamas should be worn in preference to night gowns and both pyjamas and day knickers should be washed and boiled daily. At night cotton mittens can be worn to prevent infecting the finger nails. An enema given immediately before bedtime sometimes clears the lower bowel, and so reduces irritation. The local application of an analgesic ointment is useful.

Drug Therapy. Piperazine hydrate (0·25 grammes to 2 grammes twice daily for seven days) may be given. More recently a new preparation has become available. This is Pripsen, a granular compound containing piperazine phosphate and standardized senna, as Senokot. It is effective when given in one single dose. However, in order to exclude possible reinfestation during the first two days after treatment, when occasional ova may still be present, a second dose is often given after a week or ten days.

Tapeworms (Tænia saginata)

The sight of long lengths of tapeworm may cause justifiable disgust and alarm to parents and they should be reassured about the comparatively harmless nature of the infestation.

Treatment can be carried out successfully as an out-patient by giving an oral dose of dichlorophen with a drink before breakfast on two successive mornings. The dose is from 2 to 4 grammes and the drug is well tolerated. Segments are secreted over a period of time so that a cure cannot be achieved for 8 to 10 weeks. Mepacrine 0·05 to 0·3 grammes according to body weight and followed by a saline purge three hours later is another effective form of treatment. Occasionally, however, there are side effects such as gastro-intestinal irritation, nausea and malaise.

Roundworms

The roundworm has a complicated life cycle and the fully

grown worm can survive a number of years inside his human host. Roundworms resemble earthworms in shape and size and stools should be watched for their appearance, as this is the usual means of proving the diagnosis. Other signs and symptoms are uncommon, though furred tongue and halitosis may be present and in rare cases the worms cause intestinal obstruction or may even be vomited, or reach the lungs and cause collapse of a lobe and jaundice due to blocking of the bile duct. Worms which have died within the host, may cause convulsions due to liberated toxins. Treatment with piperazine is usually successful. The dose is the same as for threadworms.

Hirschsprung's Disease

Hirschsprung's disease is due to absence of the parasympathetic ganglia in that part of the bowel which lies between the rectosigmoid junction, or sometimes even higher up than that, and the anus. As peristaltic action is initiated and maintained by these nerve cells, normal bowel movements do not take place and the intestine above the affected part becomes grossly dilated, while the rectum is as a rule empty, smaller than usual and frequently in spasm.

The disease is present at birth but diagnosis is sometimes delayed, as symptoms may at first be attributed to other causes.

Signs and Symptoms. From birth, bowel actions are infrequent and there may be delay in the passage of meconium. The introduction of a finger or small catheter or even a small enema may be needed to remove the meconium from the lower bowel. The abdomen is distended and the baby may be reluctant with his feeds and inclined to vomit. Once the rectum is emptied these symptoms disappear and general progress may be good for a time but symptoms reappear as soon as constipation starts again. The diagnosis is confirmed by radiography or biopsy.

As the disease becomes established, thin ribbon-like stools are passed at infrequent intervals. The abdomen becomes distended with gas and visible peristalsis is caused by the attempt of the colon to move the bowel contents through the aperistaltic lower intestine. Occasionally a plug of fæcal matter becomes lodged at the lower end of the rectum and may necessitate manual removal, sometimes under an anæsthetic. At intervals the stagnating bowel content putrifies and for a day or two highly offensive, loose stools are passed.

Babies suffering from Hirschsprung's disease are unlikely

to thrive; they usually look toxic and wasted and are prone to intercurrent infections.

Surgical treatment consists in removing the abnormal segment of the intestine and anastamosis of the healthy portion of the colon to the anal canal. Rectosigmoidectomy is at present the treatment of choice. As the operation is a major one, an attempt is usually made to tide the infant over the early months of life by giving him a temporary colostomy.

Prior to operation a course of phthalyl-sulphathiazole is given to sterilize the bowel. Any anæmia is treated and blood taken for grouping. The immediate pre-operative preparation is the same as for any other major operation. An intravenous infusion is set up.

Operation consists in trans-secting the transverse colon and bringing both ends to the surface, thus making a double transverse colostomy. The colon and lower bowel are then allowed to rest for several months and during that time the bowel returns to its normal size and regains its tone. The child's general condition usually improves and he gains weight. After some 4 to 6 months the child is readmitted. Another course of phthalyl-sulphathiazole is given and the distal end of the bowel between colostomy and rectum is irrigated with a solution of phthalyl-sulphathiazole, or a cream containing sulphaguanidine is injected into the bowel. At operation the abnormal segment of intestine is removed and the normal colon and the anal canal anastomosed: rectosigmoidectomy.

Colostomy

The colostomy is usually retained for a further 2 or 3 weeks to allow for healing. It is then closed at a third, minor operation. Following closure, careful regular bowel training is necessary at first and enemata and laxatives may have to be given for a time. The ultimate prognosis is however excellent and complete cure may be expected. Rectosigmoidectomy is a major operation and the preparation and after-care include all points associated with major surgery, shock and inter-abdominal surgery. In addition both parents and patient will have to adjust to the existence of a colostomy and the mother should be carefully instructed in the care of the colostomy before the child is allowed home.

General management of a colostomy in children differs little from that in an adult. In the immediate post-operative period there is danger of bleeding from the bowel and this is best stopped by the application of a firm bandage and a gauze pad soaked in a solution of adrenaline 1 in 1,000.

Occasionally the protruding bowel becomes strangulated and the opening in the abdominal wall has to be enlarged. A loop of bowel may prolapse through the incision and if this happens a pack of warm, sterile saline is applied until the patient can be taken back to the theatre. The delicate skin of children needs particularly careful attention. The surrounding area and buttocks should be washed frequently and no soiled pads left on longer than necessary. A barrier cream should be applied. The protruding bowel is protected from damage by a layer of tulle gras. If wash-outs are ordered they are done with a very soft catheter for fear of perforating the bowel.

With care the bowel can be so regulated as to produce a semi-formed stool which is easily passed but not too messy, and bowel actions can be reduced to twice daily. Extra nourishment and vitamins should be given, keeping in mind the fact that absorption can take place only in part of the length of the digestive tract.

The *psychological aspect* of a colostomy is of little importance in children but it is important to remember the effect such an operation may have on the mother. As a rule she can be reassured that the colostomy is merely a temporary measure. Permanent colostomy, performed for a congenital abnormality of the lower bowel will of course cause greater distress to the parents and they will need a long period of adjustment and sympathetic support. Children with a permanent colostomy can be fitted with a colostomy belt and a normal life should be possible.

Medical Treatment. In cases with mild symptoms or symptoms which develop in the older child, medical treatment is sometimes preferred. Frequent enemata and high rectal lavages are necessary, in many cases as often as three times a week. As the dilated bowel is capable of holding large quantities of fluid and absorption is rapid, isotonic saline should be used to prevent intoxication. Regular administration of purgatives may be ordered and strict toilet routine must be encouraged.

When flatulence and distension cause colic, discomfort and refusal of food, relief can sometimes be given by passing a flatus tube and applying warmth to the abdomen.

Because of the constant treatments and the chronic nature of the disease these children frequently become self-centred and take an unusual interest in their symptoms. They need special guidance, plenty to interest them and should be helped to lead as normal a life as possible.

As the onset of Hirschsprung's disease is often insidious, it is through nursing observations and good reporting that the diagnosis is frequently made. Accurate recording of the number of bowel actions and the nature of any stools passed will bring abnormalities to the notice of senior medical and nursing staff at an early date. The putrified smell often associated with bouts of diarrhœa, and the abdominal distension which causes the umbilicus to evert and the abdominal veins to be unusually prominent are often first observed through daily handling and nursing care of the patient.

The infant may be reluctant with feeds as the distension causes pressure on the stomach and an associated feeling of fullness. For this reason small feeds of high calorie value should be given in preference to the usual mixtures. Prosol, Casilan and Complan are all suitable preparations. Later a well-balanced diet can play an important part in maintaining the patient's health and minimizing discomfort.

Bouts of diarrhœa or sudden evacuation following rectal examination and removal of a fæcal plug may cause great change in intra-abdominal pressure accompanied by shock. A tight abdominal bandage applied without delay may assist with the usual treatment given for shock.

Since the use of surgery, the prognosis has improved considerably and in many cases complete cure may be expected.

Idiopathic Megacolon

The difference between idiopathic megacolon and Hirschsprung's disease has only recently been recognized. In the former the anal canal is short and rectum and colon are grossly dilated. Treatment is conservative. Olive oil enemata and large doses of purgatives are given. Manual removal of impacted fæces may become necessary and strict toilet routine should be enforced.

Umbilical Hernia

Umbilical hernia is a very common condition of childhood. It is entirely harmless although it is unsightly but may cause parents much worry and may be thought by them to be the cause of such disturbances as wind and colic. The defect consists of a small, oval-shaped weakness in the linea alba through which a loop of gut protrudes, and in the majority of cases it disappears spontaneously during the first year of life. Small umbilical herniæ rarely call for treatment but larger ones resolve more rapidly if efficient treatment is given. Trusses, pennies, adhesive strapping and elastic bandages are useless, but the following method carries a high rate of rapid cure.

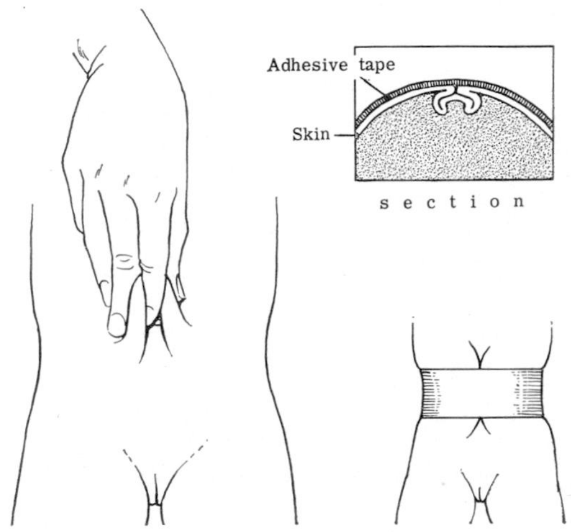

Fig. 46. Reduction of Umbilical Hernia by means of Non-stretch Adhesive Strapping.

Treatment. Two strips of 3-inch-wide adhesive tape are cut long enough to reach to the umbilicus and overlap by approximately 2 inches. A slit is cut across the end of one, while the end of the other is cut to the shape of a tongue. The strips are carried from within 2 inches of either side of the spine forward, to within 3 inches of the umbilicus. The skin over the hernia is then pinched into a fold by a second nurse and the strapping pulled taut by passing the tongue of one through the slit of the other. A piece of strapping may be stuck over the two ends for additional support. A second, somewhat similar method is shown in Fig. 46. In either method the underlying skin may be painted with compound tincture of benzoin to reduce skin irritation and to make the strapping more adherent. The baby can be bathed and the strapping is not taken off for a matter of weeks.

In the rare cases in which this treatment is not effective,

operation may be advised. This is a simple repair of the hernia and can be done as a minor operation in outpatients or as a day case.

Inguinal Hernia

Inguinal herniæ are due to a developmental weakness in the abdominal wall and are usually first seen when the child cries, strains at stool, or coughs (particularly during the paroxysms of whooping cough). A small lump appears just lateral to and above the crest of the pubic bone. Occasionally this lump spreads down into the scrotum. It usually disappears when the child is at rest, or if he is held with shoulder and head lower than the rest of the body. Occasionally the hernia is very small and easily controlled by a truss, but in the majority of cases operation is the treatment of choice. The operation is a minor one, consisting of locating and excising the hernial sac, and can be carried out in an outpatients' theatre, or the child admitted as a day case. Post-operatively the child is allowed the freedom of the cot as soon as he feels like it, and he can be allowed up on the day after the operation.

Inguinal herniæ occur more frequently in boys than in girls due to the fact that before birth, or in some cases during infancy and early childhood, the testes migrate through the inguinal canals into the scrotum. There is therefore a certain weakness in the abdominal wall in boys due to the fact that the inguinal canal is patent and the track through which the testes descend has not become obliterated. If either of the testes remains undescended it has to be brought down into the scrotum by a surgical operation (orchidopexy) or by hormone therapy. Often at operation for undescended testicles, a hernial sac is also found and a herniotomy performed.

If an inguinal hernia is sufficiently large or the neck of the hernial sac too narrow, the hernia can become *irreducible* and there is a danger of intestinal obstruction. As the child draws up his legs in pain and cries, the abdominal pressure increases and so aggravates the state of affairs. A sedative should be given and the buttocks and foot end of the cot raised. Occasionally the child is put into a warm bath or is nursed in a gallows-type of extension. Alternatively an ice bag is suspended over the area to reduce the engorgement caused by the constriction of the gut in the inguinal canal. As the child relaxes, gravity causes the intestinal loop to slip back into the abdominal cavity and the hernia reduces itself. Once this kind of situation has arisen, operation and repair should be carried out at an early date. If the hernia cannot be reduced by any of these methods, an operation should be carried out before a *strangulated hernia* occurs. If this happens the blood supply to the loop of gut is cut off, and this leads to gangrene of the loop.

14

DISORDERS OF METABOLISM AND ABSORPTION

Rickets

High standards of living and nutrition and a well developed welfare service have caused rickets—once known as the English Disease—to become a rare condition in the British Isles. The few cases seen occur as a rule in over-crowded, industrial cities where little sunlight penetrates the atmosphere and where children are often kept indoors while their mothers go out to work.

Active Rickets. This is often due to dietary deficiencies and occurs between the ages of 3 months and 3 years. It is caused by lack of vitamin D, which is essential for the utilization and storage of calcium and phosphorus in the body. The deficiency may also be produced by prematurity, rapid growth, lack of exposure to sunshine, faulty diet and inability to absorb the fat soluble vitamin D in diseases such as cœliac disease.

Signs and Symptoms. In severe cases the entire bony system of the body can be involved. The sutures and fontanelles of the skull are late in closing and together with bossing of the forehead give the skull the so-called hot cross bun effect. Thinning of the cranial bones causes a resilience known as *craniotabes.* Dentition is delayed and the teeth are defective. The affected infant sits up and walks late, the bones are soft and arms and legs are bent and the epiphyses enlarged. Respiration causes sucking in of the softened ribs where there is no resistance offered by the underlying liver and spleen. This results in a horizontal groove, known as *Harrison's sulcus*, running round the anterior aspect of the chest. At the same time beading at the juncture of the ribs and sternal cartilages forms the *rickety rosary.* The pelvic bones may become flattened and the angle of the neck of the femur on its shaft alters and eventually leads to limping and in girls to obstetric complications in later life.

Children with rickets look ill in spite of being fat and they are usually flabby (Fig. 47). The abdomen is protuberant and there is a tendency to respiratory tract infections, sweating, and diarrhœa and vomiting. The child is miserable and sleeps little. Tetany, carpopedal spasm and laryngismus stridulus are rare complications which can often be demonstrated by simple, specific tests, but are of too little importance in this country to merit full description.

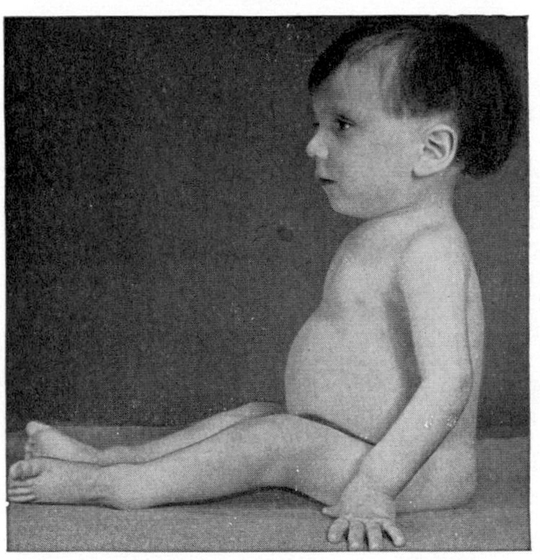

Fig. 47. CHILD WITH WELL-DEVELOPED RICKETS.

Treatment. This consists of giving adequate amounts of vitamin D and minerals in the diet which should be rich in milk, dairy butter, fortified margarine, fresh eggs, green vegetables, meat and oily fish.

The diet should be supplemented by vitamin D concentrates. Daily doses of 5,000–50,000 I.U. (international units) of vitamin D or of calciferol by intramuscular injection or by mouth may be ordered in the active, acute stage. Ultra-violet ray therapy may assist treatment where access to natural sunlight is difficult.

General Care. This aims at improving the child's health. Plenty of fresh air and sensible clothing, and a well balanced diet are often all that is needed. The wearing of thick napkins should be avoided as they may cause bowing of the femora by holding the legs apart. Deformities are prevented by restricting walking and crawling in the acute stages and by nursing the infant on a firm flat mattress. If admission to hospital is necessary the risk of cross infection is minimized by admitting these children to cubicles.

It is important that the correct dose of vitamin D should reach the child. Oily preparations are given on a spoon or from a dropper but never added to a feed as the oil may cling to the bottle so that the patient receives less than the intended dosage.

If splints are worn, they are taken off daily and the skin washed and powdered to avoid pressure sores.

Late Rickets

Defective absorption of vitamin D and its attendant symptoms may occur later in life. They may be caused by metabolic diseases which interfere with absorption or cause excess excretion of calcium and phosphorus. Among these conditions is *cœliac disease*, in which instance the disturbance in the digestion of fats impedes the absorption of the fat soluble vitamin. In *renal rickets* the impaired kidneys cannot excrete phosphorus so that it is retained in the blood. In consequence calcium is withdrawn from the bones to balance it—again causing manifestations of rickets.

Points of Interest

Up to recent years it was thought to be impossible to give harmful amounts of vitamins. This theory, however, was recently disproved when a condition known as hypervitaminosis D was described. The symptoms are seen in very young infants who have been given fortified dried milk foods and fortified baby cereals as well as the usual amounts of vitamin D preparations, such as cod-liver oil.

The manifestations are anorexia, failure to thrive, constipation, abdominal colic and eventually renal failure leading to death. The blood calcium level is greatly raised.

Although infant foods are now carefully controlled, the possibility of this condition developing should never be overlooked.

Scurvy

Like rickets, scurvy is now rarely seen in the United Kingdom, as the Government provides concentrated orange juice at a low price; better wages mean generally better nutrition including greater consumption of milk and fresh fruit, and more housewives know how to cook vegetables correctly.

Scurvy occurs somewhat later than rickets because infants seem to have a small store of vitamin C, and breast milk also contains an adequate amount.

Signs and Symptoms. These are due to abnormal permeability of the capillary walls, causing subperiosteal bleeding. bruising, hæmaturia, anæmia and in extreme cases cerebral hæmorrhage. The gums may be swollen and bleed when touched and occasionally teeth may become loose and drop out. At times there is bleeding into the kidneys, bowels and the orbits of the eye.

The exquisite tenderness of the limbs makes the child lie perfectly still so that it is easy to mistake the condition for a form of paralysis. The hips are abducted and the lower legs partly flexed. Any movement, jarring of the cot or picking up causes the child to scream with pain. There may be moderate fever, pallor and listlessness.

X-ray pictures show up the subperiosteal hæmorrhages and occult blood may be found in the stools and red cells in the urine. A vitamin C absorption test confirms that an abnormal amount of the vitamin is absorbed. The test is based on the knowledge that vitamin C taken in excess of normal storage is excreted in the urine. 3,000 milligrams of vitamin C are given orally. Urine is collected in a bottle made of dark glass and the amount excreted is analysed and compared with the test dose.

Prognosis. Scurvy responds rapidly to treatment and cure is complete. Treatment consists of giving vitamin C both in its natural form and as ascorbic acid. It may be given by mouth or by intramuscular injection and there is no known toxic effect.

Nursing Care. This aims at reducing any handling to a minimum on account of the pain. The infant is washed and fed in his cot, clothing should be of a pattern that makes changing without much movement possible and small, soft pillows are used to support the swollen limbs. As the gums are tender and inclined to bleed, the diet should be soft and should of course have a high vitamin C content.

All artificially fed babies should have vitamin C in the form of orange juice* or other preparations such as rose hip syrup or ascorbic acid tablets. Milk should be brought to the boil

*30 to 90 millilitres of fresh orange juice or 15 millilitres of the "government" orange juice.

in a double saucepan but not allowed to continue to boil. Green vegetables, tomato juice, fresh fruit and fresh orange juice should be introduced into the diet as soon as the child is old enough to be weaned. A dish high in vitamin C content and at the same time soothing to the gums and easily prepared is creamed potato. The floury part of the potato and particularly the part underneath the skin is mixed with milk and butter after baking the potato in its jacket. The meal is usually greatly enjoyed and several potatoes can be given daily in this way.

Phenylketonuria
(Phenylpyruvic Oligophrenia)

One of the most exciting discoveries of recent years is the existence and treatment of phenylpyruvic oligophrenia as a cause of mental deficiency as it points, perhaps for the first time, to the possibility of early recognition and successful treatment of mental diseases on a chemical or metabolic basis. In England about 1 in 40,000 of the population suffers from this inborn error of metabolism in which phenylalanine cannot be metabolized. Instead it accumulates in the blood plasma and eventually causes poisoning of the brain cells. Phenylalanine is normally present in all protein foods and is an essential amino-acid, and needed for normal growth and development. It can therefore be only partly dispensed with.

As up to 30 times the normal amount of amino-acids may be excreted in the urine of patients suffering from this disease, a simple urine test is carried out to determine the diagnosis. The test is so simple that it has been suggested that prophylactic tests might be carried out on every one month old infant in order to detect the presence of phenylketonuria and commence treatment before any brain damage has taken place and symptoms appear. The test should certainly be done in every case where there is already known to be an older brother or sister with the disease. Many local health authorities already do that.

The Test. A few drops of ferric chloride 5–10 per cent. solution are added to 5 millilitres of acid urine, and if the result is positive an opalescent, deep green colour develops within two minutes, and fades again on standing. A very simple alternative test can be done with the help of Phenistix. Although the test is usually accurate when squeezing the stick between a wet napkin, fresh liquid urine should be used whenever possible. The test should be carried out at the ages of 2, 4 and 6 weeks as it sometimes takes as much as 6 weeks for the test to become positive.

Signs and Symptoms. Children suffering from phenylpyruvic oligophrenia present a typical picture. They are fair and blue-eyed. Their heads are small and they have large alveolar arches and widely spaced teeth. Their growth is stunted, they sit up late and spinal curvatures are common. Profuse perspiration causes skin eruptions and sepsis. A musty peculiar odour can be noticed. Minor convulsions occur frequently and all these children are grossly mentally defective and often difficult to manage.

Treatment. This should be started without delay and consists of giving a diet which is almost free from phenylalanine. The diet is both complicated and expensive and as it is unpalatable may be difficult to persevere with. An initial loss of weight must be expected. Improvement may be marked within 6 to 8 months and with early treatment these children may become educable instead of adding to the 2–3 per cent. of patients now in mental institutions due to phenylpyruvic oligophrenia.

The Diet. In order to exclude phenylalanine from the diet, all the usual proteins have to be eliminated. For infants two special preparations are available: Minafen (Trufood Ltd.) and Cymogran (Allen & Hanbury). Both can be made into a milk-like feed and can be given by bottle.

Later the following foods are allowed:

Bread made from gluten free wheat starch.

Breakfast cereals with a low protein content (Weetabix, cornflakes).

Fruit, vegetables, kosher margarine, honey, jams, boiled sweets.

Small amounts of milk, best given as double cream may gradually be introduced. There are special vitamins on the market suitable for these patients (Paynes & Byrne Ltd) which should be included in the diet. Fish, meat, eggs, butter and cheese must not be given. As the diet which can be offered contains little solid food, the child should be given raw apple and whole raw carrots to chew in order to develop the teeth and dental arches normally.

Both the special foods and the vitamins are expensive but they can be obtained on a National Health Service prescription. Any lapses in the diet are easily detected in the urine and this should be tested at regular and frequent intervals.

Galactosæmia

Galactosæmia is a familial disease caused by an inability to metabolize galactose and so leading to intoxication of the body and brain cells. The result is mental deficiency, cataract and cirrhosis of the liver. The baby fails to thrive, is drowsy, refuses his feed and vomits. Jaundice may be present from the first day of life. Œdema may give a false impression of a satisfactory gain in weight. The stools are loose and the liver becomes enlarged. The death rate is a high one.

Treatment must be started at once if it is to be effective. It entails substituting all feeds containing galactose by special preparations such as Nutramigen or Galactomin. Where these are not available, soya bean "milk" to which Casilan, cane sugar, coconut oil, minerals and vitamins can be added, may be given.

Diagnosis. Whenever there is a familial history of the disease a simple test can be carried out on the cord blood, or alternatively a urine test will show the presence of glycosuria. Any finding of sugar in the urine must always be reported at once so that more specialized laboratory tests can be carried out.

Glycogen Disease
(Von Gierke's Disease)

Glycogen disease affects both sexes equally. It is a familial condition, due to an abnormality in the metabolism of glycogen. The first symptoms usually appear in the first 2 years of life.

Signs and Symptoms. Glycogen is deposited in the heart, liver and kidneys causing signs of heart failure, cardiac murmur, a large firm liver and ketonuria. There is no sugar present in the urine and the fasting blood sugar is low and does not rise when a test dose of adrenaline is given. Hypoglycæmia convulsions may occur.

Treatment. There is no known cure and treatment remains symptomatic.

Prognosis. Although most of these children lead invalid lives, death may not occur for many years.

Disorders of Lipoid and Glycogen Storage

This group of diseases includes such rare conditions as xanthomatosis, Schüller-Christian syndrome, Gaucher's disease, Niemann-Pick disease and lipoidosis. In the last, abnormal amounts of various lipoids are stored in the reticulo-endothelial system. The chief damage is in the brain cells, but in spite of this, diagnosis can be confirmed by a simple rectal biopsy involving approximately 1 centimetre of full thickness bowel wall.

Agammaglobulinæmia

Agammaglobulinæmia is a rare condition mostly seen in boys and the principal manifestation is a marked tendency to infections, as the lack of gamma globulin prevents antibody formation.

Treatment. Gamma globulin is given by weekly injections and in some cases prophylactic antibiotic treatment is ordered.

Steatorrhœa

Steatorrhœa is a symptom rather than a disease in itself and by it is meant the passage of fluid or excessively soft stools containing an unusual amount of fat.

Steatorrhœa may be caused by some disturbance in the function of the small intestine and the amount of fat present in the stools may vary from amounts so small that they are only found in the process of careful analysis to visible, oily globules on the surface of the stools.

Causes include the following:

Absence of bile salts as in obstructive jaundice and infective hepatitis.

Absence of pancreatic enzymes as in fibrocystic disease of the pancreas.

Disorders of absorption as in cœliac syndrome.

Tuberculous peritonitis and mesenteric adenitis.

Ulceration of the bowel.

Lamblia intestinalis infection.

Some young infants suffer from mild fat intolerance causing fatty diarrhœa but this is readily treated by dietary measures and not necessarily due to disease.

Signs and Symptoms. The stools have a characteristic, highly offensive smell. Their appearance is putty-coloured, unformed and bulky and their frothy quality suggests the presence of fermentation. Occasionally fatty globules can be seen on the surface. The frequent loose evacuations may alternate with periods of constipation. Abdominal distension, redness around the anus, excoriated buttocks and rectal prolapse often accompany the steatorrhœa.

The abnormal fat losses and frequent stools may cause secondary symptoms such as a voracious appetite and tetany due to loss of calcium, which in turn results in a low blood calcium level, dehydration, stunted growth and lassitude.

Investigations. These depend on the suspected, underlying cause and may include:

Mantoux test and X-ray of abdomen (tuberculosis).

Barium enema and X-ray (congenital abnormalities affecting the gut).

Glucose tolerance curve (this is a flat one in cœliac disease).

Analysis of duodenal secretions and stools for tryptic activity (fibrocystic disease of the pancreas—see page 254).

Sweat tests (fibrocystic disease of the pancreas—see page 255).

Examination of stools for ova, cysts, starch granules and excess of fat.

A fat balance will probably be done as one of the investigations.

Method. The fat balance is as a rule done over a period of 8 to 12 days. During that time a diet containing a known quantity of fat is given. At the end of the first 3 days a so-called marker is given (e.g. a capsule of indigo carmine) which colours the stools red. All stools are saved from the time the first coloured stool appears and the fat content estimated and analysed in the laboratory.

Not even the smallest amount of fæces must be wasted and it is useful to line the bedpan with cellophane paper or plastic material during the test period. The stool can then easily be lifted out and sent to the laboratory without wastage. The same can be done with a baby's napkins without causing much discomfort. Good ways of collecting fæces in infants are given on page 215.

Care must be taken to ensure that the child has nothing by mouth beyond the prescribed diet (e.g. no chocolate brought in by visitors) and the parents' cooperation is essential where daily or unrestricted visiting is the practice. Any food not eaten, must be returned to the diet kitchen (including left-overs on the plate) and the fat content estimated and taken into account in the calculations. In a healthy individual 90 per cent. of fat should be absorbed.

The Cœliac Syndrome

The cœliac syndrome usually becomes established in the first year of life, frequently at the time of weaning. It is caused by malabsorption of food from the intestines and there is an abnormal sensitivity to gluten, found in wheat and rye. At the same time the absorption of fat is impaired and large amounts of split fats may be excreted in the stools.

Signs and Symptoms. Children with cœliac syndrome are stunted in growth and underweight and X-ray examination reveals osteoporosis (rarefaction) and immature development of bone due to poor vitamin absorption and calcium deficiency. Excess gas formation caused by fermentation of malabsorbed food causes abdominal pain and vomiting. The patient has a large, protuberant abdomen. The buttocks are wasted and the

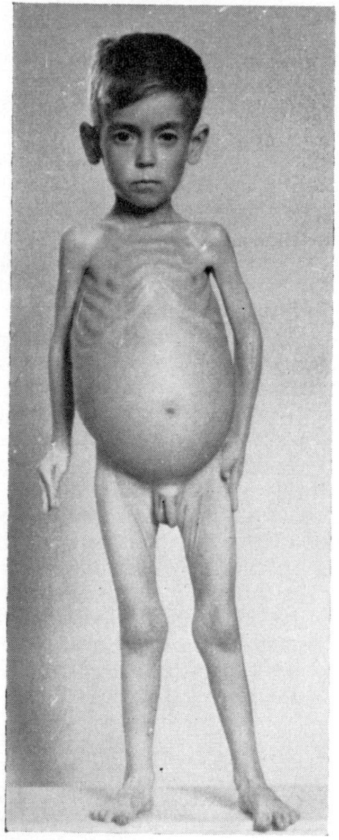

Fig. 48. Coeliac Disease.

Enlarged abdomen, wasting of muscles and loss of subcutaneous fat. Right hand in typical position of tetany. Severe cases of this kind are rarely seen now.

skin hangs in loose folds. The stools are bulky, putty coloured, unformed and greasy and have a characteristic, putrified smell. The child may have his bowels opened several times a day.

The child himself looks frail, stunted, pale and wizened, and usually utterly miserable, though the face may at first look round and well. The hair is sparse and dry, the limbs thin as drum sticks and cold to the touch. Poor muscle tone reflects itself in bad posture and rectal prolapse is common. Anæmia is a usual feature and sometimes a small blood transfusion or a course of Imferon will improve the child's condition considerably.

The appetite is very poor and capricious. These children often have the strangest whims and their feeding may tax the ingenuity and patience of the nurse to the utmost. The patient may insist on a special way of being served, on being fed by a particular person and on always having the same plate and feeding utensils. He may "order" a particular dish and refuse it when it arrives. The slightest change in the accepted routine may cause a complete refusal of meals. These little patients are negative in every way and often take an almost morbid interest in their illness. They are emotionally unstable, unhappy, and both apathetic and irritable at the same time.

Treatment. Relapses are now uncommon if parents can be persuaded to follow a diet free of gluten.* The child rapidly becomes happier, more comfortable and therefore less temperamental and the figure takes on normal lines and proportions. At first fat intake is restricted and extra protein is added to the diet. However, if all foods containing any product made from wheat and rye are omitted, a normal amount of fat can soon be taken. Gluten free bread, cakes and rusks can be obtained and gluten free flour can be made into cakes, bread, biscuits and puddings. A satisfactory diet can, however, be given without much extra work if foods made of maize (corn), oats, rice, sago and tapioca (not semolina) are substituted for those made of wheat and rye.

Investigations. Analysis of stools, fat balance (see page 249), a complete blood count, a glucose tolerance test (which will show a flat curve), a xylose excretion test and jejunal biopsy may all be performed. The jejunal biopsy is done with the aid of a Crosby Capsule (Fig. 49) and may reveal characteristic changes in the mucous membrane.

*Birkett and Bostock of Stockport, Cheshire, supply flour, bread, biscuits and rusks by post. Gluten free flour can also be obtained from Energen Food Co., London, N.W.10.

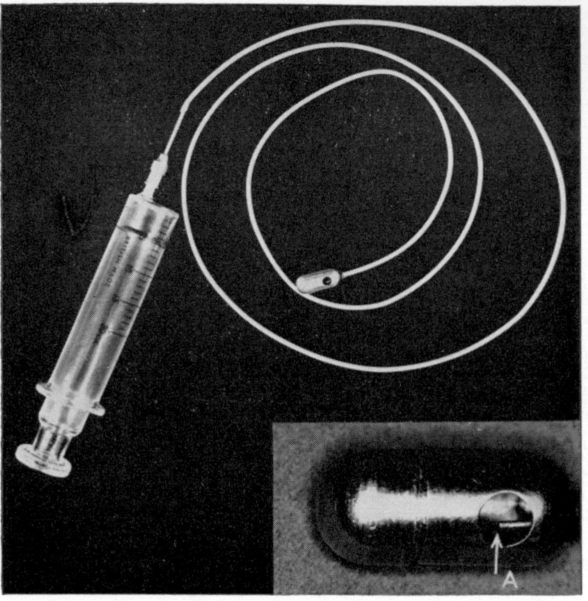

Fig. 49. A Crosby Capsule, used to Obtain Small Specimens of Intestinal Mucosa.

Prognosis. With modern treatment, the prognosis should be favourable and improvement may be rapid. The stools soon become less bulky and offensive, the appetite improves and the child gains in weight and is happier. Wheat products can often be reintroduced after 2 years' successful treatment, but this must be done tentatively and may have to be discontinued if symptoms reappear.

Complications. These include intercurrent infections, œdema due to low serum protein; rickets and tetany due to impaired absorption of the fat soluble vitamins.

As excess amounts of potassium and fluids are lost in the large stools "cœliac crises" due to electrolyte depletion occasionally call for urgent action. The child suddenly becomes severely dehydrated, lethargic and collapsed. The temperature may rise by several degrees. Intravenous therapy may be necessary to correct both the blood chemistry and the dehydration.

Nursing Care. Admission cannot always be avoided but the stay in hospital should be cut to a minimum while investigations are carried out and treatment is established.

Occasionally these children are acutely ill and during that time need careful nursing care. Because of emaciation, skin and mouth require special attention. Mouth toilet is carried out frequently and pressure areas are treated four-hourly. Even slight wrinkles in the sheet, crumbs or a damp bed may cause bed sores which do not heal easily. After a bath the skin should be dabbed dry and a good dusting powder applied to the skin folds. The child should never be left sitting on a pot longer than is necessary, for fear of causing pressure sores and encouraging rectal prolapse.

Much can be done to reduce the bulk of the stools by adding a 5 per cent. solution of Arobon in water to the food and chlorophyll tablets, taken orally, diminish their unpleasant odour.

As soon as possible, these children should be allowed to get up and lead a normal life. Schooling or play therapy are important in stimulating interest and speedy recovery. Frequent visiting will not only help the young patient but will also teach the mother much about the handling of her child and about the special diet. The mother must be told that even minor deviations from the prescribed diet may cause a serious relapse.

Fibrocystic Disease of the Pancreas (Mucoviscidosis)

Fibrocystic disease of the pancreas may be present at birth or develop during the first weeks of life. Several children of one family may be affected and the outlook is poor.

In this condition the ducts leading from the pancreas to the duodenum are blocked by thick, tenacious mucus, and as the disease progresses these are replaced by fibrous tissue and cysts. As a result of the blockage, the pancreatic enzymes cannot reach the digestive tract and the normal digestion of protein, fat and carbohydrates cannot take place.

A similar process may affect the lungs, where patches of collapse, emphysema, bronchiectasis and cysts occur. Repeated infections seriously interfere with the child's progress and these are the cause of the high death rate.

Occasionally the disease is well established at birth and causes a condition known as *meconium ileus.* Bowel actions may be completely absent or, if meconium is passed, it is almost solid. Complete obstruction may follow and urgent surgical intervention is then the only way of saving the baby's life.

Signs and Symptoms. Unlike the child suffering from cœliac disease, children with fibrocystic disease of the pancreas are friendly, easy-going little people. The appetite remains good in the absence of general infection but in spite of this there is failure to gain weight, growth is stunted, the abdomen is distended and the child may have a barrel-like appearance. The stools are pale and bulky, bowel actions are frequent and the smell is characteristically offensive.

Investigations. As pancreatic juice is known to digest gelatin, by the action of the trypsin present, diagnosis can be confirmed by obtaining a specimen of duodenal juice for testing in the laboratory.

Alternatively, stools are analysed for the presence of trypsin, or sweat may be collected for the estimation of electrolytes, as the sodium and chloride contents of sweat are increased in fibrocystic disease of the pancreas (see page 255).

Treatment. This aims at correcting the pancreatic deficiency and the lack of pancreatic enzymes is to some extent corrected by the giving of enteric-coated pancreatic granules before the main meals. The granules can be given in cold milk or with cereal. They have a strong taste but the children soon get used to this. There are several preparations of pancreatin dispensed in varying strengths. Particular care should be taken to verify that the preparation for which the dose is prescribed is being used. One of them is Pancrex V Forte 1 to 3 grammes for infants, 10 to 15 grammes for older children, given before meals. Occasionally some irritation of lips, chin and buttocks occurs. The dose should then be reduced for a short period.

At the same time an attempt is made to reduce the risk of chest infections by encouraging a healthy, open-air life away from unnecessary crowds, a nutritious diet and, in some cases, by giving regular dosages of antibiotic drugs over a period of years.

As the defective absorption from the bowel may cause vitamin deficiencies, this is corrected by giving adequate amounts of vitamin concentrates. Iron may be prescribed to prevent or correct anæmia.

Nursing Care. When intercurrent infection or the carrying out of tests necessitates admission to hospital, a bed in a "clean ward" or cubicle should be chosen. Fresh air is beneficial. Oxygen therapy is frequently needed to relieve respiratory distress. The humidity of the tent may be increased by the use of a nebulizer through which compressed air is driven. Plain water is used or, alternatively, preparations such as Alevaire or Acetylcysteine ordered. These help to liquefy the mucus and ease expectoration.

Remembering the chronic nature of the illness, general attention will be given to the mouth and pressure areas. The meals should be attractive and with some ingenuity, the nurse can think up many methods by which to camouflage the addition of concentrated proteins.

Fatty and starchy foods are given in reduced amounts but extra glucose is added to the diet. Honey is very suitable and often much enjoyed.

Sweat Test

To prove the diagnosis of fibrocystic disease of the pancreas sweat from the patient is collected for analysis. This is done by placing the child's fingers on a specially prepared surface containing silver nitrate and potassium chromate in a petri dish. If there is an excess of chlorides in the sweat, as in fibrocystic disease of the pancreas, the impression shows up clearly as a grey finger print.

Duodenal Intubation

This test is no longer done as a routine, now that far simpler sweat tests are available. The procedure, if ordered, is as follows: a Ryle's tube is passed into the stomach and from there manœuvred into the duodenum. Specimens are taken at frequent intervals and tested with litmus paper. A change from acid to alkaline reaction indicates that the tube has passed through the pyloric sphincter. Duodenal juice can now be withdrawn, and a minimum of 3 millilitres is immediately sent to the laboratory. The aspirate must be kept cold on ice whilst in transit.

15

DISEASES OF THE ENDOCRINE SYSTEM

Diseases of the endocrine system are comparatively rare in childhood but where they occur they may have a serious effect on mental and physical growth and maturation.

Those diseases which are so rare that they are unlikely to concern the nurse in general training are omitted in this text.

The Thyroid Gland

Thyrotoxicosis

Over-secretion, causing thyrotoxicosis is very uncommon in childhood. If it occurs, thiouracil, Neo-Mercazole, Lugol's iodine or potassium perchlorate and surgery are employed in its treatment, in much the same way as for adults. Treatment by irradiation or radioactive iodine is considered unsuitable in children.

Cretinism

Under-secretion of the thyroid gland causes cretinism in children. The condition, though congenital, is sometimes missed at birth as the infant carries a small amount of thyroid secretion from the maternal circulation. As the amount decreases, general metabolism is slowed down and symptoms appear.

Signs and Symptoms. All cretins have certain, typical characteristics. Their skin is cold, coarse and dry with a sallow appearance. The hair is brittle, sparse and lacks lustre and the hair line grows low down on to the constantly puckered brow. A broad, flat nose with a depressed bridge lies between the small widely spaced eyes. The lips are thick and as the tongue is apparently too large for the mouth, it protrudes. The abdomen is large, and constipation and umbilical hernia are common features. Pads of fat over the clavicles make the neck appear short. As bony development is retarded, the fontanelles are late in closing, the head seems disproportionately large and the first teeth are late in coming through. The entire appearance is heavy, coarse and dull. As general metabolism is suppressed, the temperature is subnormal and the pulse rate slow. Anæmia is common. Speech develops late and some cretins achieve only an elementary vocabulary. The voice is croaky and unmelodious. All milestones are late and, if left untreated, the child will be mentally severely subnormal, unable to look after himself.

Although not all these characteristics are noticeable at birth, a nurse will soon learn to recognize cretins at an early age. She may first notice the umbilical hernia and the constipation and, if she is alert and well-informed, may link these symptoms with the low temperature and sluggish pulse. Most cretins are poor feeders, at least partly due to the abnormally large tongue which makes sucking difficult and also causes attacks of suffocation. An observant nurse or midwife can contribute greatly to a good prognosis as early treatment is the key to success.

Investigations. The ones likely to be carried out are: blood cholesterol and serum lipoid levels, both of which tend to be raised, creatinine and protein-bound iodine levels, which are abnormally low, X-ray of bones to estimate the bone age, electrocardiogram and blood picture. The basal metabolic rate is difficult to estimate in children but, if done, shows readings much below the normal.

Treatment. This should be started without delay and will have to be continued throughout life in order to replace the thyroxine which the abnormal gland cannot produce. Treatment may be so successful that the child develops normally and cretins have been known to reach scholarship level. However, a great deal depends on the age at which treatment is begun. The treatment consists in giving thyroid extract in dosages just below the point at which signs of intolerance appear. The initial dose for infants is probably 15 to 30 milligrammes daily and this is increased until tachycardia, diarrhœa and wakefulness suggest that the dosage has passed the tolerance level. Tolerance may be higher during the cold season than in the summer months. The maintenance dose is fixed slightly below the maximum reached during the stabilizing period.

Nursing Care and Observations. During the initial stage nursing care is symptomatic. The infant should be kept warm and the nurse feeding the baby will have to be both experienced and very patient. Suppositories or milk of magnesia will have to be given for the constipation and the skin should be kept supple with baby creams or lotions. Care must be taken when the baby is placed in his cot and it is safest to lie him on his side to guard against the danger of respiratory obstruction caused by the large tongue.

Once thyroid therapy has been started the nursing observations will be the principal guide in determining the maintenance dosage. Signs of response, such as an increased pulse rate and a rise in the body temperature, are all due to an increase in the metabolic rate. There is an improvement in the infant's colour and activity and a drop in weight due to the disappearance of the excess fat. The bowels will start to act regularly. The infant will begin to look around and play and will become more interested in his feeds.

The nurse should keep full and accurate observation charts. The feeds may have to be large for a time to satisfy the newly found appetite and to supply adequate nourishment for the sudden progress. As growth is rapid, extra vitamins should be given. It is well worth while to arrange for a little extra attention by mother or nurse to encourage every attempt at play and to help the infant develop his activities and mental achievements.

The Pituitary Gland

The chief importance of the pituitary gland is probably its influence on the other ductless glands. Abnormalities of the anterior lobe cause gigantism if there is over-secretion, dwarfism if there is under-secretion. Abnormalities of the posterior lobe cause *diabetes insipidus.*

The abnormalities may be congenital or may be caused by pressure from intracranial tumours or by inflammatory conditions such as encephalitis. None of these conditions are sufficiently common to warrant description in a small handbook and the reader is referred to larger text books for greater detail.

The *hormone activity* of the gland, however, is of great interest. The pituitary gland produces adrenocorticotrophic hormone (ACTH) which makes the adrenal cortex produce hormones with three effects:

(1) on carbohydrate metabolism;
(2) on mineral metabolism affecting blood electrolytes;
(3) on growth and maturity including masculinization if there is excess in the female.

In addition excessive amounts can damp down inflammatory reactions by interfering with antigen-antibody reactions and can cause the production of ACTH to be lowered.

Cortisone or similar preparations such as prednisone,

prednisolone or Triamcinolone can be given by mouth and hydrocortisone by injection for the following purposes:

(*a*) to make up for deficiency of the adrenal activity as in shock or in Addison's disease;
(*b*) to suppress the production of ACTH in cases of precocious sexual development of a masculine type;
(*c*) to prevent antibody production or reaction, as in rheumatic fever, rheumatoid arthritis, some types of nephritis, asthma and hæmolytic anæmia.

ACTH may be given by injection for the last purpose (*c*) but would be useless in (*a*) and harmful in (*b*). If any of these drugs are given it may be necessary to counter their effect on mineral metabolism by giving potassium or calcium.

The Adrenal Glands

Diseases of the adrenal and suprarenal glands are extremely rare in childhood and are usually due to tumours, injury at birth resulting in hæmorrhage, or infections such as tuberculosis. Both the diagnosis and treatment are difficult, though the discovery of cortisone has contributed much to the understanding of the diseases caused by over- or under-secretion of the glands.

Tumours of the medulla are often malignant and cause metastases in the liver, lungs and bone tissue. Surgery and deep X-ray therapy are usually attempted but rarely successful. In some cases long periods of remission may be brought about by a course of intramuscular injections of vitamin B_{12} (1,000 micrograms on alternate days). Surgery in the benign type of tumours however carries a hopeful prognosis. The adrenal medulla produces adrenaline and noradrenaline which, like cortisone, have a place in the treatment of asthma and shock.

Over-activity of the adrenal cortex leads to sexual precocity in both sexes and to virilism in the female. The over-activity may be present before birth and in this case causes pseudohermaphroditism (see page 260). In the young child over-activity causes sexual precocity and virilism and if the anterior pituitary gland is secondarily affected, Cushing's syndrome will result. The signs and symptoms of Cushing's syndrome are similar to those in the adult and a text book on general medicine should be consulted, should the nurse come across one of these cases in childhood.

Pseudohermaphroditism

Sometimes children show features of both male and female sex development and in the newborn it may be extremely difficult to make a definite decision about the sex. It is, however, possible to determine the sex by examination of the chromosomes in certain cells. Buccal smears are taken for the purpose. Polymorphonuclear leucocytes also show sex characteristics.

The condition will naturally be distressing to the parents on account of its implications and the complex problems involved. Great understanding and tact are needed in explaining the condition to them and in helping them to adjust to the peculiarity of their child. Nurses should see to it that these children are not subjected to unnecessary examinations by curious students or young medical staff who wish to see such unusual cases, as even very young children may be sensitive to repeated examination or handling of the genital area.

Cortisone therapy and plastic surgery may help these unfortunate patients.

The Parathyroid Gland

Low activity of the parathyroid gland causes tetany, convulsions, osteoporosis and fractures, due to a drop in the blood calcium level. The condition is sometimes caused by a tumour of the gland and surgery may relieve the symptoms.

Diabetes Mellitus

Even new-born infants may occasionally suffer from diabetes, and apnœic or cyanotic attacks in premature or ill-nourished infants should always be investigated. The disease, however, is very rare under the age of 2 years. In about a quarter of all cases there is a family history of diabetes. The basic cause of the disease is similar to that in adults. Insulin has to be given in most cases as severe dietary restrictions may impede the normal growth of the child, even in mild cases. The disease is frequently severe and dangerous fluctuations in blood sugar levels due to variable activities and childhood illness are common.

In children, the onset of diabetes may be very sudden and, although never actually responsible for the disease, infections such as tonsillitis or measles, and emotional stress seem to act as the trigger starting off the symptoms.

Signs and Symptoms. Most obvious, and therefore often

first noticed, is the sudden excessive thirst coupled with frequency of micturition or the onset of enuresis in a previously clean child. The output of urine is large but in spite of this it is of high specific gravity. The child grows listless and fractious. As dehydration occurs, his skin becomes dry and he is constipated. The breath may smell of acetone. The tongue is dry but, as a rule, it remains clean and abnormally red. Loss of weight may be rapid and considerable and a proportion of children develop an unusual appetite.

The penis or vulva are often red and irritating due to the high sugar content of the urine, and the child may complain of abdominal pain. As ketosis increases, vomiting sets in and may hasten the occurrence of diabetic coma. The urine contains sugar and acetone.

Investigations. These include testing of urine, blood sugar estimation and glucose tolerance tests, similar to those done for adults. If possible, tests involving pricks and fasting should be spaced and not all done the first day after admission, as it is important to preserve the young patient's confidence since he will probably be starting on a lifetime of daily insulin injections. In testing for acetone, many physicians prefer the ferric chloride test to Rothera's test as the latter is extremely sensitive. If the ferric chloride test is positive for acetone there is a definite danger of diabetic coma. A quick alternative test can be done with Acetest tablets. It is important to remember that the tests may appear positive if aspirin has been taken.

Treatment. Some specialists like to treat these children as out-patients as they feel that the child should be assessed and stabilized under his usual living conditions. The majority feel, however, that the child should be admitted to hospital so that the investigations and the initial stabilizing can take place under controlled and known conditions. The fact that in hospital the child's activities are of necessity restricted should always be borne in mind. The mother should be asked about the child's normal routine and exercise should be given so that the child's usual energy output is maintained. He may for instance be allowed to accompany the ward orderly on errands. Diabetic children should never be kept in bed unnecessarily. From the start, a healthy attitude and interest should be fostered and any special diet should be accepted as a natural part of the young diabetic's routine. It is interesting to note how upsets such as home sickness can cause variations in the blood sugar levels and also that acetone is most frequently found in the urine of children who have failed to settle down happily at boarding school or in hospital.

Insulin Therapy. The dose of insulin will have to be re-adjusted until the condition is stabilized. This may not happen until some weeks after discharge home. Adjustment will usually become necessary when the child has an infection or any severe emotional upset, as he grows and increases in weight and especially at the time of puberty. The aim is to find the dose which will enable the child to live a normal life on a diet adequate for growth, energy and enjoyment of life. Requirements will depend on the patient's temperament and activities. There should always be a little sugar in the urine.

Operations such as tonsillectomy or even major surgery can be safely carried out providing they are done under controlled conditions. Glucose, equal to the normal diet in carbohydrate value, is given at any time when a meal has to be omitted.

Cortisone, owing to its action on carbohydrate metabolism is not a suitable drug for use in diabetic patients.

It is here assumed that the reader has already a sound understanding of the types of insulin available and of the

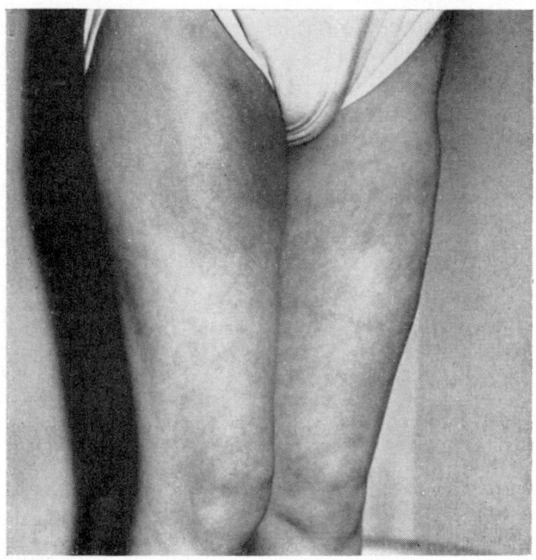

Fig. 50. Fat Atrophy of Legs following Injections of Insulin over a Period of Time.

Atrophy is very marked on the left upper thigh.

various syringes and their marking, as well as of the principles involved in insulin therapy. In these aspects there is no difference when dealing with young diabetics as compared with adults, but the approach to the problem of diabetes in childhood is important and specialized.

Both the parents and the child should be taught how to give injections and test the urine and, as far as they are capable, they should be taught to understand the principles involved. They should also be taught confidence and the child himself should take a healthy interest in his illness. By the age of 10 years it should be possible to teach a sensible patient to give his own insulin and to draw up the dose himself, even if it is still checked by his parents.

The site of the injections should be as varied as is possible in order to prevent thickening of the tissues and local fat atrophy which, though harmless, causes unsightly depressions and irregularities in the contours of the limb. The injection should be given fairly deeply with the needle almost at right angles to the skin. Alternatively, a Palmer mechanical injector, shaped rather like a pistol, can be used.

General Points. Both the young patient and his parents should be helped to come to grips with the disability and the latter not allowed to make the child into an invalid by misplaced solicitude. Both the parents and the child, once he is old enough, should be taught the fundamentals of the illness and should be allowed to practise urine testing and the giving of injections well before discharge, so as to gain confidence and dexterity in so doing.

It is a good plan to allow the child to experience one or more insulin reactions while still under supervision in hospital so that after his discharge he will be able to guard himself in good time against any serious hypoglycæmic reaction.

Most diabetic children can attend normal schools provided the teachers know of their condition. Hypoglycæmic reaction is often heralded by naughty or unusual behaviour, and glucose or a lump of sugar may correct the hypoglycæmia without much disturbance. Teachers should have sugar or glucose available, but as soon as he is old enough the young diabetic should be made responsible for recognizing and dealing with a hypoglycæmic reaction by taking sugar from his own supply. It is possible to allow diabetic children to have the usual school meals, as the high carbohydrate content of school puddings supplies the extra amount needed during the exertion of the afternoon games period.

For holidays, under controlled conditions and supervision,

the Diabetic Association runs holiday camps which have the added value, that the children meet other diabetics, often learn much from each other and come to realize that they are not alone with their abnormality.

Parents should be advised to let the child carry a card or disc with his name and address, particulars of his disease and the emergency treatment required. Undesirable food or sweets should be kept out of temptation's way but on the whole a normal outlook and existence should be encouraged.

Hyperglycæmic or Diabetic Coma

The signs of oncoming coma are essentially the same in children as in adults, but a child's behaviour may differ according to his age. Thus a very young child may demand to be put to bed or may curl up in a corner and fall asleep. Shock and dehydration often come on very rapidly and both may be severe.

Hypoglycæmic or Insulin Coma

Insulin coma comes on even more suddenly than diabetic coma. It often happens that the child is hard to wake in the morning and, when roused, looks pale and apprehensive and shows a peculiar emotional behaviour.

Points of Importance. If there is any doubt about the nature of the reaction, the child should be given some glucose as little harm can be done by hyperglycæmia, while insulin coma may require urgent relief. It is useful to remember that 2 slightly heaped teaspoonfuls of sugar in water equal approximately 10 grammes of carbohydrate.

The Diet. With the present-day insulins, which are very stable and long acting (e.g. the Lente group), the child, once stabilized, can be kept free from reactions by allowing his appetite to regulate his blood sugar levels. It will be found that if he has been unusually energetic he will also be very hungry, and if he has sat quietly for a time his appetite will decrease. Periodic tests to estimate the serum cholesterol levels are done. If the level rises, foods containing cholesterol are omitted from the diet (e.g. eggs) as a persistently raised serum cholesterol level predisposes to vascular changes in later life.

16

THE GENITO-URINARY SYSTEM

The kidney excretes waste products of metabolism, and acts as a filter and reabsorbs certain substances necessary to the body. A nurse who understands the importance of any abnormalities in the urine and who uses her powers of observation to the full should not find the toilet round a boring routine but will appreciate her responsibility in this respect. Her careful reporting may help the physician who relies on the accuracy of her reports and tests.

Observations should be recorded clearly and accurately on the patient's chart and abbreviations should be avoided as they may easily lead to misinterpretations or misunderstandings. The presence of albumen for example should be charted as being a trace, a moderate, or a large amount and not merely charted as one, or several + signs.

Methods of Collecting Clean and Ordinary Specimens of Urine

It may be difficult to collect urine from babies and toddlers. The container should be of appropriate size for the amount of urine collected (e.g. 10-millilitre bottles are quite adequate for babies). Special plastic urine collecting bags may be used both for boys and girls (Fig. 51). Where these are not available the following techniques can be used:

Baby Boys. Urine may be collected by strapping a test tube or Paul's tubing to the penis. If the specimen is for bacteriological investigation, an aseptic technique should be used. A tray with receivers and sterile cotton wool swabs, saline or a mild antiseptic solution, such as 1 per cent. cetrimide, a sterile test tube or Paul's tubing, and four lengths of ¼-inch strapping is required. The penis is well cleaned, where possible the foreskin retracted and the glans gently swabbed before fixing the tube in position. Paul's tubing, previously sterilized, is easy to use and very effective.

Baby Girls. Baby girls present a much more difficult problem. It may be advisable to wash and swab the buttocks and genitalia carefully before commencing a feed and then to sit the baby on a sterile receiver while she is feeding. Babies often pass urine during a feed.

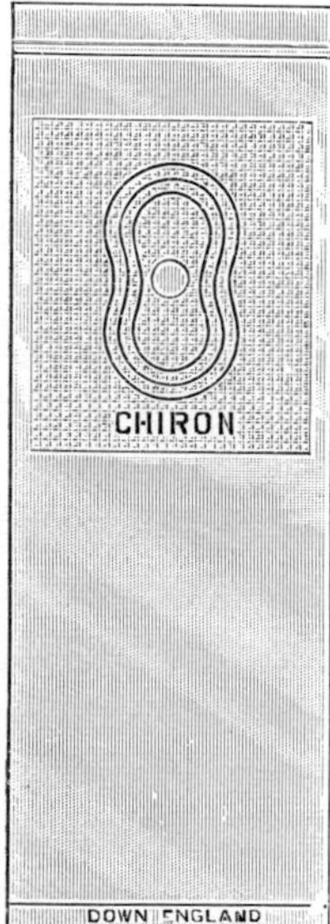

Fig. 51. Urine Collecting Bag as used for Little Girls.

Alternatively, a sterile receiver may be placed inside a well fitting air-ring and the baby nursed sitting upright over the opening. If these methods fail, the baby may be placed in a "Hiatus Hernia Chair" with a hole in the seat. (Fig. 13.)

Specimens obtained in this way, are usually accepted for bacteriological examination but sometimes a catheter specimen is required for absolute reliability. In some units where metabolic beds are available, these may be used when 24-hour specimens are required.

Catheterization

Catheterization may have to be carried out for diagnostic purposes, to relieve retention of urine, in preparation for operation and in certain post-operative cases. In the two last instances the catheter may be left *in situ* for several days.

Basically the requirements are the same for children as for adults. It is, however, essential to have at least one assistant who will ensure that the child maintains the correct position without struggling and who can reassure and talk to the child.

Little girls should have their buttocks raised on a sand bag. When the buttocks are thus elevated the catheter should be directed downwards rather than at right angles to the perineum, as it would be with an adult. As the urethra is short urine should be obtained after passing only 1 to 2 inches of the catheter. It is important to wash the groins, thighs and genitalia with soap and water before starting the actual catheterization. When the procedure is completed the surrounding skin should be carefully dried and powdered. A pot or bedpan should be offered as catheterization leaves the patient with a feeling of irritation and an apparent desire to pass urine.

Mid-stream Specimens. With older children, capable of co-operation and control in passing urine, this method can replace catheterization in many cases. After cleaning the genital area in the method described above, the child is asked to pass some urine in order to flush the urethra. After approximately an ounce has been passed the stream is interrupted and the remaining urine collected in a sterile container with clear indication that the specimen was a mid-stream one.

Twenty-four Hour Specimens. To estimate accurately the volume of urine passed in 24 hours, the following procedure is adopted.

The patient is asked to empty the bladder at 8 a.m. and this urine is discarded. All urine passed in the following 24 hours is then collected. The patient is asked to pass urine at 7.55 a.m. the following day and this specimen is added to the total collected.

Early Morning Specimen. Specimens of urine taken on waking are usually highly concentrated.

Addis Count. In preparation for this test, the fluid intake in the preceding 12 hours is restricted to one pint. The patient passes urine at 7 p.m. and at the same time has his last drink for the following 12 hours. All urine passed up to 7 a.m. the next morning is collected in a container provided. In the laboratory the number of red cells is estimated as is the amount of protein and casts. This count can give a valuable guide to the progress made in cases of nephritis. A count of below 500,000 red or white cells excreted in the 12-hour period is satisfactory.

Some Abnormal Substances which may be present in the Urine in Certain Diseases

Blood Hæmaturia	*Sugar* Glycosuria	*Albumin* Albuminuria	*Bile*	*Pus*	*Diacetic acid or Acetone* Ketonuria	*Hæmoglobin* Hæmoglobinuria
Nephritis	Diabetes mellitus	Nephritis	Infective hepatitis	Cystitis	Diabetes mellitus	Severe burns
Pyelonephritis	Low renal threshold	Pyelitis	Congenital obliteration of the bile duct	Pyelonephritis	Starvation	Severe infections
Tuberculosis	Excess carbohydrate intake	Cystitis			Severe vomiting	Incompatible blood transfusion
Calculi		Fevers			Infections	
Wilms's tumour		Congestive heart failure			Emotional causes	
Polycystic kidneys						
Trauma		In the presence of pus			After operations	N.B. There are no red cells present
Foreign body in the bladder		In the presence of blood				
Purpura		Orthostatic albuminuria				
Leukæmia		Emotional causes				
Hæmophilia						
Sulph. therapy						

N.B. Red urine may be caused by urate crystals in infancy, by certain sweets and by beetroot. Other abnormalities may occur but they are rare and are not included in this table.

Retention of Urine

This, irrespective of the cause, may produce restlessness in unconscious patients and may disturb sleep. Simple nursing measures may relieve retention. The nurse can partly fill the pot or bedpan with warm water, she can irrigate the pubic area with warm water, sit the patient in a warm bath, allow small boys to stand up while using a bottle, and run a nearby tap. Such nursing attention is infinitely worth while and may make painful, complicated measures such as catheterization unnecessary.

Investigations of the Urinary Tract

Intravenous Pyelography

Intravenous pyelograms are done to outline the urinary tract and demonstrate the efficiency of renal function. A light, low-residue diet is given for 2 days and fluids are withheld for the 12 hours preceding the test. An enema may be ordered to clear the bowel and in some hospitals a vegetable aperient is given. Charcoal biscuits or tablets may be given during the morning to help absorb gas in the intestine. Children tend to swallow much air and to have more intestinal gases than adults and it is often difficult to obtain a satisfactory pyelogram. The following scheme may be used with some success. The child is given a bottle of ginger beer and instructed to drink it through a straw. The fizzy drink tends to distend the stomach which in turn displaces the small intestine in a downward direction. A clear picture of the renal pelves and upper ureters can now be obtained. This procedure can be adopted with quite young babies without any harm, but it is obviously not useful if the lower portions of the ureters are to be shown up. If the child is well enough he should be allowed to be up and to run about as, together with abdominal massage, this may help to rid the bowel of stagnating gases which might obscure the X-ray picture. The patient should be asked to pass urine just before going to the X-ray department.

A straight X-ray picture is taken first, in order to ascertain that no gases will obscure the picture. If this is satisfactory a radio-opaque dye is then injected into a vein. As there may be general intolerance to iodine, the base of most of these dyes, the patient's sensitivity should be tested the previous evening by applying some tincture of iodine to the forearm and observing any skin reaction. In most cases the median basilic vein is chosen for the injection but with babies it may be necessary to use another vein or to give the dye intramuscularly. In that case hyaluronidase is used in conjunction with the dye, in order to speed up and facilitate absorption. The dye is rapidly excreted by the urinary tract.

Pictures are taken after 3, 8, 15 and 30 minutes, and the progress of the dye is watched. Any abnormalities in the filling of the renal tract or in excretion are demonstrated on the X-ray.

Cystoscopy

This procedure is exactly the same as with adults except that children are given a light anæsthetic. Cystoscopy is usually done to examine the bladder, urethra, and ureteric openings into the bladder, for congenital abnormalities.

Retrograde Pyelography

For this procedure a light anæsthetic has to be given but otherwise preparation is the same as for intravenous pyelogram, and the procedure similar to that used in adults.

Cystography

Cystography may be done in order to determine the capacity and outline of the bladder or to demonstrate the presence of urethral valves.

Urea Clearance Test

A comparison is made between the amount of urea present in the circulation and urine respectively. The test demonstrates the extent of healthily functioning substance in the kidney, following disease.

Investigation for Tuberculosis

For tuberculosis investigation, an early morning specimen of urine is sent to the laboratory on three successive days and injected into a guinea pig. Four to 6 weeks later the guinea pig is killed to see if it has developed tuberculosis.

Diseases of the Genito-urinary Tract

Vulvovaginitis

Vulvovaginitis is a fairly common condition, especially in little girls from 3 to 10 years old.

Causes. These include lack of cleanliness, strongly acid urine, diabetes mellitus, eczema, foreign bodies pushed into the vagina, threadworm infestation and gonorrhœa.

Signs and Symptoms. The child will frequently complain of soreness between the legs or alternatively the mother will notice reluctance to let her touch and wash this area. She may also notice that the knickers are stained with discharge. On examination the labia are found to be red and œdematous, they may be stuck together and there is a ropy mucoid discharge.

Treatment. This will depend largely on the underlying cause. The area should, however, be washed frequently, dried by gentle dabbing with a soft towel and well powdered. Antiseptic baths are soothing and speed up treatment.

General Care. The patient is frequently debilitated and efforts should be made to build up general health and to arrange for a period of convalescence. The mother may be given advice about general hygiene.

Barrier Nursing. It is usual to nurse these children with barrier precautions for the first few days until the discharge has cleared. A swab is sent to the laboratory to determine the nature of the infection. Gonorrhœa should always be considered, and treated if present.

Special Points. Despite their age, these little girls are often very sensitive about their condition. Examination should be reduced to a minimum and the nurse should be very gentle and tactful. Screens should always be used when treatment has to be carried out, in order to ensure privacy. Vaginal douching is considered unsuitable during childhood, mainly on account of the psychological trauma which may be caused.

Early symptoms of urinary infection in very young infants are easily overlooked. However, symptoms such as anorexia, fever, vomiting, apathy and failure to thrive should alert the doctor and nurse, and a clean specimen of urine should be sent to the laboratory. Catheter specimens are usually unnecessary and are to be deprecated (see page 267).

Pyelitis (Acute Pyelonephritis)

Pyelitis is essentially an infection of the pelvis of the kidney but in most cases other parts of the kidney become involved as well. The disease is a very common one in childhood, affecting girls rather more often than boys and it occurs frequently in very young infants.

Mode of Infection. The infection may reach the kidneys via the blood stream, from the bowel via the lymphatic system or as an ascending infection from the bladder and urethra. In many cases the infection is caused by a malformation in the urinary tract, such as a kink in one of the ureters which causes the urine to be dammed back, to stagnate and to become infected.

In about 70 per cent. of cases the causative organism is the *Escherichia* (*Bacterium*) *coli*, but streptococcal and staphylococcal infections also occur.

Signs and Symptoms. As a rule the onset of the disease is a very sudden one. One of the earliest symptoms is *vomiting*, soon followed by a rise in temperature to 39·4° to 40·6° C. (103° to 105° F.); rigors and meningism are common. The child is pale and ashen in colour, with flushed cheeks and dark rings round the eyes. She is irritable and there are signs that she is suffering from spasmodic, colicky pain, which is a constant feature. With young babies diarrhœa occurs and this together with the vomiting soon causes dehydration. The urine is scanty, strongly acid and may have a curious fishy smell. The tongue is dry and thirst is marked. If old enough to do so the patient complains of a burning sensation on micturition.

Complications. In extreme cases head retraction is present, a squint may develop and convulsions occur. It is in fact not always easy to distinguish the symptoms from those of meningitis on account of the meningismus, or of appendicitis on account of the abdominal pain and vomiting.

Investigations. Examination of a clean specimen of fresh urine under the microscope will reveal the presence of pus cells, albumen and organisms. The prognosis is as a rule a good one, recovery taking place in 3 days to a week. Recurrent cases are often due to malformations in the urinary tract and therefore X-ray investigations are carried out. The prognosis depends on the underlying cause.

Nursing Care. The nursing care in the case of an attack of pyelitis is mostly symptomatic. In order to reduce the temperature, the bedclothes are cradled and a fan may be used to cool and circulate the air. Tepid sponging is soothing but must not be done without medical permission. If the patient is incontinent the buttocks should be washed frequently as the acid urine is liable to excoriate the skin. Zinc and castor oil cream should be applied. The mouth easily gets dry and dirty, and careful mouth toilet is essential.

Temperature, pulse and respirations are taken and recorded 4-hourly and a strict intake and output record is important. The reaction of the urine is tested every time the patient passes urine, the aim being to keep the urine alkaline. If vomiting persists and dehydration becomes marked, fluids may have to be given subcutaneously or by rectal infusion.

Constipation may be marked and may have to be treated. Local applications of heat over the loins may help to relieve the pain.

Drugs. According to the sensitivity of the causative organism, sulphonamides, nitrofurantoin or streptomycin are prescribed. A prolonged maintenance course to prevent recurrent infection may be prescribed. Alkalies are rarely given.

Diet. The patient should be given liberal amounts of fluids especially while on sulphonamide therapy. For babies milk is withheld as long as vomiting persists. Once the acute stage of the illness is passed, the children quickly regain their appetite and no special diets need be given.

Cystitis

Cystitis is rarely seen as a primary disease but is frequently associated with inflammation in other parts of the urinary tract. The cause may be infected, stagnating urine as in paralyses, infection following catheterization or malformations of the bladder and rectum.

Signs and Symptoms. The child complains of frequency and of burning pain on micturition. The temperature may be raised. On examination the urine is found to contain pus, mucus and occasionally blood.

Treatment. The nursing care is similar to that for pyelitis. Alkali mixtures, sulphonamides and antibiotics may be given. Bladder wash-outs may be ordered and a liberal fluid intake is essential.

Orthostatic Albuminuria

Orthostatic or postural albuminuria is a harmless condition which often is discovered only accidentally, for example in the course of a School Medical Inspection.

Signs and Symptoms. The albumin is present only after the child has been in the upright position for some time, hence early morning specimens are free from albumin. Children with orthostatic albuminuria commonly show signs of generalized poor tone. They have poor posture, lordosis is common and they are thin and frequently suffer from chilblains.

Prognosis. Parents may be reassured about this condition and the child should be treated as normal.

Nephritis

Owing to the complicated nature of the disease and the slowly progressive stages seen, a variety of classifications of nephritis are used.

	Type 1	*Type 2*
Mode of onset	Very sudden	Insidious
Cause	Streptococcal infection 10–14 days previously in 75% of cases	History of preceding infection rare
Age group affected	Rare in infancy but common in childhood	Occurs equally in infancy and childhood
Hæmaturia	Present	Rarely present
Urinary output	Reduced	Variable
Albuminuria	Moderate degree	Present and considerable
Œdema	Slight œdema is present but clears readily	Present and persistent
Complications	Hypertension, renal failure	Intercurrent infections
Prognosis	Recovery in 90% of cases	Eventual recovery in 25–50% of cases
Blood pressure	Raised at onset	Not raised
Diet	Low salt if œdema present. Restricted protein	Low salt, high protein
Blood urea	Often raised to 80–120 mg.%	Not raised

Type 1 Nephritis

Type 1 nephritis is also known in the early stages as acute nephritis, acute glomerular nephritis, acute hæmorrhagic nephritis and in the later stages as subacute nephritis or chronic interstitial nephritis.

Pathology. Both kidneys are affected. They are red, swollen and congested and minute hæmorrhages can be seen. These small hæmorrhages cause blocking of the glomeruli and thus reduce the filtering capacity of the kidneys. Blood and albumin escape into the urine, while other constituents of normal urine are dammed back into the blood stream. Œdema may develop.

Cause. In about 75 per cent. of patients an attack of type 1 nephritis is preceded by a streptococcal infection such as tonsillitis, otitis media or cervical adenitis. Acute nephritis may also develop as a complication after severe burns. Occasionally the infection may have been so slight as to have escaped the mother's notice.

Signs and Symptoms. The first sign of the trouble may be the passing of blood-stained urine. In other cases the child has been off colour; he may have vomited and in the early morning there is puffiness of the eyelids and pendent parts. Very occasionally a convulsion may precede the other symptoms. The output of urine is normal or scanty and the urine contains a trace of albumin. It may be heavily blood-stained or merely darker than usual. The term used to describe the colour is "smoky". Laboratory tests will prove the presence of cells and casts (i.e. tubulous exudate shed by the inflamed renal tubules).

The temperature is raised by one or two degrees and the child may complain of headache and thirst. The tongue is furred and constipation is usual. Much later in the disease anæmia develops. The erythrocyte sedimentation rate is raised to twenty or more millimetres.

Course of the Illness. In uncomplicated cases improvement may begin after 3 or 4 days; œdema disappears and diuresis is noticed. The urine gradually returns to normal. The child feels much brighter and takes more interest in his surroundings.

Mild Complications. These are not uncommon. The erythrocyte sedimentation rate remains raised and a few casts and cells persist. A trace of albumin can still be found in the urine for some 6 to 8 weeks or longer.

Prognosis. Recovery is usual in approximately 90 per cent. of cases, the remaining 10 per cent. make an apparent recovery and may lead a normal life for many years, but hypertension and renal failure eventually supervene.

Investigations. These include daily ward urine tests with quantitative albumin estimation, laboratory tests for presence of cells and casts, full blood-picture, throat swabs and daily blood-pressure readings. X-ray of the sinuses and examination of tonsils and teeth are carried out in order to discover any foci of infection. The urine is examined microscopically at weekly or fortnightly intervals once frank blood has disappeared from the urine.

Treatment. Diet, rest and good nursing care are the main forms of treatment, though at times penicillin is prescribed for any latent streptococcal infection. Anæmia is treated by iron therapy. Sulphadimidine 1 gramme daily may be prescribed as prophylaxis to "reinfection" and sometimes, after a period of convalescence, tonsillectomy may be performed to reduce the risk of further streptococcal infections.

Nursing Care. Children suffering from nephritis are kept on bed rest. As they are very susceptible to chills they should be kept warm, but few pædiatricians now expect their patients to be nursed between blankets. If this is still done, a special narrow mackintosh and draw sheet should be used. The patient is nursed in the recumbent position on complete rest and the more severe case is not even allowed to feed himself. A second pillow is however permissible both for comfort and in order to make it easier for the child to watch the life of the ward if he is well enough to take an interest.

A daily blanket bath is given and pressure areas treated 4-hourly. Mouth hygiene is particularly important during the early days when the child may not be allowed solid food. If constipation is troublesome a mild aperient may be given.

Charts. Temperature, pulse and respirations are recorded 4-hourly. The fluid balance chart must be kept up to date and accuracy is of the greatest importance. Degrees of œdema present must be mentioned on the observation chart. During the first few days blood pressure readings are taken twice daily, charted and any rise reported without delay. A frequent check is kept on the child's weight this being a good guide to the amount of œdema present. It is useful to chart this in the form of a graph.

Diet. In order to rest the kidneys, the diet for the first 3 or 4 days consists of fruit drinks only, with added glucose. The amount allowed is as a rule 300 millilitres (10 ounces) above the previous day's output of urine.

Nurses should remember that fresh fruit drinks are preferable to "squash" and that a child will enjoy variety. Occasionally orange juice is not allowed on account of the relatively high potassium content. Hot drinks as well as cold ones should be offered to relieve the monotony of the fluid diet. Relatives are often glad to be told what they could bring at visiting times and many mothers may like to bring a bottle of freshly prepared orange juice when they visit. Boiled sweets are also permitted.

When diuresis occurs, a light diet is gradually introduced but protein is restricted until urine tests show improvement in the cell count. Milk, eggs and fish are the first, red meat the last protein foods allowed. Salt is allowed in moderation unless œdema is present.

Duration of the Illness. Bed rest may have to continue for weeks and the total stay in hospital may extend to several months. The nurse should make time to play and read with the child in order to lighten the monotony of prolonged bed rest and to ensure quietness for her patient. Later the child may be able to take part in the activities of the hospital school. In tedious diseases such as nephritis, it is of paramount importance to provide occupation and to keep the child's interests alive. In many cases it is possible for the mother to visit outside ordinary visiting times and so help to keep boredom at bay.

Type 2 Nephritis
(Subacute Parenchymatous Nephritis, Lipoid Nephrosis)

Type 2 nephritis is far less commonly seen in children than type 1 nephritis.

Pathology. The phrase "the large white kidney in the large white man" describes the case graphically. The kidney is large and swollen. There are marked pathological changes in the tubules and lipoid deposits may be found in the cortex.

Cause. Type 2 nephritis may follow an attack of acute nephritis but in many cases the predisposing factor remains unknown.

Signs and Symptoms. The onset of the disease is insidious. The mother will probably tell of the gradual onset of œdema spreading from the extremities to the face and eventually over the whole body. This is due to the loss of plasma proteins in the urine. The child is listless and fractious, he is disinterested in food and as œdema spreads to the peritoneal cavity (ascites) and the pleural cavity (hydrothorax) pressure may cause dyspnœa.

Œdema may be so gross that the child is unable to open his eyes and with boys the swelling of the penis and scrotum may become very distressing. The urine is loaded with albumin (as much as 10 to 25 grammes may be lost per day) but hæmaturia is absent. The urine is very concentrated and sometimes only very small amounts are passed. Anæmia becomes marked and together with the œdema, explains the peculiar pallor. The mouth is usually very dirty and despite careful mouth toilet halitosis is often present. The erythrocyte sedimentation rate is raised. The blood urea is as a rule normal (20 to 40 milligrams per 100 ml.) or it may be slightly raised.

Course of the Illness. Although the œdema may improve

for periods of varying length, the course of the illness may be chronic and downhill or show sudden vicissitudes. The blood pressure tends to rise, tachycardia develops and chronic cardiac failure becomes established. Albuminuria may decrease but the specific gravity of the urine becomes fixed at an abnormally high level.

With modern drug therapy (steroids) recovery may be as high as 85 per cent.

Investigations. These are similar to those described for type 1 nephritis, although renal biopsy may sometimes also be done.

Treatment. In addition to that already described for type 1 nephritis, treatment aims at getting rid of the œdema. *Paracentesis abdominis* may have to be performed if ascites is marked and pressure on the diaphragm causes respiratory embarrassment. This is done in the same way as for adults, but with children emptying of the bladder before starting the procedure and preventing shock from lowering of the intra-abdominal pressure as the fluid is drained off, is even more important. With young children the trocar and cannula are sometimes replaced by a Southey's tube connected to fine rubber tubing. Drainage of subcutaneous tissues by acupuncture or by Southey's tubes may be carried out for several hours or days and may have to be repeated periodically.

The treatment, though not a painful one, may at first be alarming for an older child, but he soon appreciates the relief obtained and is happy to co-operate. For very young children wrist restrainers may have to be used in order to prevent interference with the drainage tubes.

Drugs. To induce diuresis, mercurial diuretics and chlorothiazide may be ordered. In an attempt to bring about remission or even cure, steroids may be given in decreasing amounts over a period of 6 months, and if necessary continued in small doses indefinitely. It must, however, be remembered that the defences against inter-current infections are suppressed by the steroids. Every sign of sepsis, however small, should therefore be reported immediately, and prophylactic antibiotics given whilst the patient is on steroid therapy. When steroids are given, œdema may increase for a time before diuresis occurs.

In order to replace lost protein and to induce diuresis, plasma may be given intravenously. A blood transfusion is given occasionally to correct anæmia and to improve the child's general condition.

Nursing Care. This differs little from that given to children suffering from type 1 nephritis, but œdema may embarrass breathing and the nurse will have to use her ingenuity in making the patient comfortable with additional pillows. As a rule bed rest is enforced during the early stages only and a fairly normal life encouraged as soon as is possible. While on bed rest conscientious care of skin and pressure areas is important. Peripheral circulation is often poor and the œdematous limbs may be cold and discoloured. Warm blankets and woollen socks may help to keep the feet warm; particular care must, however, be taken not to use hot-water bottles as the œdematous limbs may be relatively insensitive and burns would occur very easily. As the child is unlikely to move much while œdema is present, small pillows and bed cradles should be used to prevent foot drop and to take off the weight of the bedclothes. An air ring or a Dunlopillo mattress may be valuable for additional comfort and for the prevention of pressure sores. Daily weighing is important as a guide to the amount of œdema present.

Since these children are very susceptible to intercurrent infections children with sore throats or upper respiratory tract infections should not be placed in neighbouring beds.

Diet. A low salt diet is indicated where œdema is marked and while the patient is having cortisone or ACTH he should have a low sodium (less than 2 grammes daily) intake as sodium is easily retained in the tissues. Potassium, which is lost in the urine, should, however, be given either in drug form or in the form of foods with a high potassium content such as Ovaltine. As a great deal of protein is lost in the urine a high protein diet may be ordered, provided the plasma urea level is normal. Repeated blood urea estimation is used as a guide to tolerance to this régime. If the blood urea rises the protein intake may have to be reduced. The fluid intake is restricted. Some pædiatricians allow 600 millilitres a day, others relate the fluid intake to the output by allowing the child to have 300 millilitres more fluid than the urine output of the previous 24 hours.

These children frequently suffer from anorexia, and the nurse's skill in presenting meals attractively may be taxed to the utmost. When a precise amount of protein is sent up from the diet kitchen, the amount of food refused should be recorded after every meal, so that the protein taken can be accurately estimated by the dietician.

Points of Interest. For unexplained reasons an attack of measles has at times been known to cause a long remission or even to bring about a cure of the disease.

Chronic Nephritis

Either type 1 or type 2 nephritis may pass into a state of chronic nephritis. Severe disturbances of body chemistry cause stunting of growth and such conditions as "renal rickets" or "renal dwarfism" develop.

The renal substance eventually becomes fibrosed and ceases to function. Headaches, visual disturbances, dry skin, vomiting, hypertension and albuminuria are all present. Systolic blood pressure may rise to 100 or 200 millimetres of mercury and blood urea levels to 200 or 300 per cent. Uræmia is common and the specific gravity of the urine is abnormally low.

As there is no known treatment, the child should be allowed to lead as normal and happy a life as possible but it should be remembered that a spoilt child is not always a happy one.

Renal Rickets

Renal rickets or dwarfism is a rare complication of chronic kidney disease. Renal inefficiency causes large amounts of calcium to be excreted in the urine and this in turn causes delayed and incomplete bone formation which resembles the lesions in rickets due to vitamin deficiency. Polyuria is marked and the urine is pale and of low specific gravity. It often contains albumin. The skin is dry and thirst may be troublesome.

Prognosis. There is no known treatment apart from keeping the child comfortable. Chronic ill health is followed by death within 5 to 10 years.

Uræmia

Uræmia is a poisoning of the body by waste nitrogen products. This poisoning may be caused by sulphonamide poisoning, obstructed urinary flow, incompatible blood transfusion, infantile gastro-enteritis, burns and renal disease. Spasm of the blood vessels may lead to cerebral œdema and this explains some of the symptoms which arise.

Signs and Symptoms. Lassitude, drowsiness, headaches, loss of appetite, vomiting, sore dry mouth, pyrexia, diarrhœa and convulsions are all common and may occur simultaneously or at different times. Blood pressure and intracranial pressure are high and there may be visual disturbances and retinal hæmorrhages. The pulse rate is rapid and the volume poor. Cheyne-Stokes type of breathing occurs in the terminal stage.

Prognosis. The condition is an extremely serious one and

presents an acute emergency which requires expert medical and nursing care even though the outlook is often hopeless.

Treatment. This aims at eliminating waste products by stimulating skin action, inducing diuresis and giving rectal lavage, for which hypertonic saline is often used. Lumbar puncture, venesection and peritoneal dialysis may be attempted. When the cause is a temporary one, as after an incompatible blood transfusion, the use of an artificial kidney may allow the kidneys time to recover.

When renal function is impaired, as little fluid as possible is given and all calories necessary may be administered by giving a mixture of peanut oil and glucose in a minimum of distilled water either by mouth or more usually by stomach tube: 1 pint is usually given per 24 hours.

If convulsions are present phenobarbitone is given orally or by intramuscular injection, and if this is not sufficient rectal Pentothal may be tried.

It is sometimes necessary to tide a patient over a temporary crisis which is interfering with renal function, so causing a dangerous accumulation of urea in the body. Peritoneal dialysis is one of the treatments which may be undertaken as a life-saving measure. In certain centres where artificial kidney machines are available, the patient is treated by means of this advanced therapy.

Surgical Conditions of the Genito-urinary Tract

In childhood the majority of operations performed on the genito-urinary system are done to correct congenital abnormalities. These are often the cause of recurrent urinary tract infections, colicky pain, and failure to thrive. In extreme, untreated cases, uræmia and death may result.

In all investigations and treatments of the urinary tract the danger of ascending infection must constantly be borne in mind. Catheterization, the use of indwelling catheters and bladder lavage are consequently only ordered if there is no other alternative. When drainage tubes are in use it is the task of the nurse to watch the tube carefully. Kinking or compression of the tube may lead to damming-back of urine and as a child is unlikely to voice his complaint it is the nurse's responsibility to appreciate that there is something wrong by noticing the patient's restlessness or by noticing an abnormal output of urine. Accurate measurement of the urinary drainage and output is most important if serious complications are to be prevented. Operations on bladder or kidney may result in bleeding and clot formation. Morphine may be given to lower blood pressure and relieve pain and lavage may have to be employed to dissolve clots and prevent the child from straining in an attempt to pass the clot per urethram. At operations which may be expected to cause post-operative bleeding, the surgeon usually stitches a drainage tube into the wound, the substance of the kidney or the bladder, to allow blood to escape. These tubes or drains call for careful nursing attention and vigilance.

Movement of the patient need not be restricted and change of position from side to side is helpful in promoting drainage and preventing chest complications.

Congenital Abnormalities and their Treatment

Agenesis of the Kidney

Failure of development of the kidney is as a rule unilateral. In that case the other kidney may hypertrophy and take over the total renal function and no treatment is necessary. Bilateral agenesis is incompatible with life.

Horseshoe and Double Kidney

A horseshoe kidney is formed by the union of the lower poles of the two kidneys. It occurs on one side only and may remain symptomless. The abnormality may be found accidentally in the course of a routine abdominal X-ray examination, or in other instances the child has recurrent urinary tract infections or attacks of pain and vomiting. A double kidney shows up plainly when pyelography is performed and it is often associated with double ureters. In long-standing cases hydronephrosis may develop. One of the ureters may have a kink or stenosis and if this is the cause of the recurrent infection or pain, it is removed.

Hydronephrosis and Mega-ureter or Hydro-ureter

Recurrent infections, obstructions and congenital abnormalities of urethra, bladder, ureters or renal pelvis may cause dilatation of one or both ureters or renal pelves. The obstruction may be due to abnormally situated blood vessels which press on the ureters, stenosis of the ureter, ureteric or urethral valves, obstruction in the bladder neck and neurological causes. The obstruction may be unilateral or bilateral. If the cause of the obstruction can be removed, the ureters may regain their tone and return to a normal size. If left untreated there is danger of uræmia developing. It is often possible to relieve the condition by cutting out the narrowed part and so achieving complete cure.

Urethral Valves

Urethral valves occur only in boys. They may obstruct the urinary outflow and eventually cause renal failure. The bladder becomes distended and in babies this may cause a grossly enlarged abdomen. There is a constant trickle of urine so that the napkins are wet all the time. This may lead to the condition being missed for some time. The baby may, however, be observed to strain on passing urine and later there is enuresis both day and night. A catheter can be passed quite easily as the valves merely act as an obstruction to the outflow.

The presence of valves can best be demonstrated by carrying out a voiding urethrogram. A catheter is passed into the bladder and a radio-opaque substance run in. After removing the catheter X-ray pictures are taken while the patient voids urine and dye and empties the bladder.

In some cases the urethra can be sufficiently dilated to relieve the obstruction, but often the valves have to be excised through a resectoscope or removed by diathermy.

Neuromuscular Inco-ordination of Bladder and Bladder Neck

Neuromuscular inco-ordination causes incontinence, back pressure of urine and eventually hydronephrosis. If the hydronephrosis is bilateral, it may be necessary to transplant the ureters into the sigmoid colon or rectum but unfortunately this operation is not always successful. The suture lines frequently break down and ascending infections are common.

Urethrocele

It sometimes happens that part of the mucous lining of the bladder prolapses into it and causes obstruction of ureteric or urethral openings. This leads to stagnation of urine, back pressure, hydro-ureters and hydronephrosis. Treatment consists of diathermy to the prolapsed mucosa through a cystoscope or cutting and re-emplanting the ureters.

Sclerosis of the Bladder Neck

In this condition the bladder neck is fibrosed and hardened and so interferes with the normal contractions of the sphincter and causes urinary incontinence. Excision of a wedge of muscle may bring about the desired improvement but often repeated dilatation of the urethra may still be necessary.

Ectopic Anus

Occasionally a child may be born with an anal opening in an abnormal position. Various types may occur, and one of the most severe and common of these is the type often referred to as rectovaginal fistula. In this anatomical abnormality the anus opens into the posterior wall of the vagina and just inside the vaginal orifice. Fæces may leak through the fistula but in rare cases there is a fairly satisfactory sphincter action. Treatment consists of plastic repairs which aim at producing as normal a function as possible. Although there is an ever present danger of infection, these patients can often lead a perfectly normal life in spite of their abnormality.

A comparable condition occurs in boys. The ectopic anus may open onto the skin surface at the juncture of penis and scrotum and in this case the condition is left untreated. Occasionally fæces are discharged per urethram. In these cases surgical repair is attempted but results are as a rule disappointing. Occasionally no apparent anal orifice can be found. This condition of imperforate anus is fully described on page 69.

Circumcision

Surgical removal of the foreskin is done either if it is abnormally tight (phimosis), for recurrent balanitis or for religious reasons. In the neonatal period the prepuce normally adheres to the glans penis and only begins to separate after some months. Attempts to retract the foreskin routinely at bath time should therefore not be made during the first year of life.

Circumcision should always be carefully considered. Some authorities believe that any operation in this area should be avoided if at all possible on account of the psychological implications. Postoperatively, severe hæmorrhage occurs easily and irritation of the glans, ulceration of the urethral opening from friction, ammoniacal dermatitis and meatal ulcers causing scarring and stricture are complications which result fairly frequently.

In young children the operation is often carried out in the out-patient or minor operations' theatre and the child admitted to hospital as a day patient only. He is discharged towards evening and the mother is instructed to call her own doctor or bring the child back to hospital in the event of bleeding or if the child fails to pass urine.

Postoperatively the wound edges are often covered with ribbon gauze soaked in compound tincture of benzoin and left in place for approximately one week. After that time it is soaked off in a bath and routine washing and dusting with some antiseptic powder are all that are required. Very occasionally the ribbon gauze has been put on too tightly and congestion and œdema of the glans result. This requires urgent relief by sitting the patient in a warm bath of potassium permanganate (2 crystals to each pint of water) and peeling the dressing off gently. Failure to do this may result in gangrene. Some surgeons leave the penis uncovered but spray the wound with Nobecutane, allowing the child to have a bath as usual from the second day. Others apply hexachlorophane ointment or powder instead.

During the immediate post-operative period these children are often very restless and miserable and chloral hydrate (sometimes combined with bromide) should be given. The mother or a nurse should be available to pick the baby up and comfort him as much as possible. In uncomplicated cases there is no difficulty of micturition but the first time the child passes urine should always be noted.

Paraphimosis

Occasionally children are brought to hospital with a grossly swollen or discoloured penis caused by a tight foreskin which has been retracted but could not be returned to its normal position. Relief is a matter of urgency as the blood supply is partly cut off. Cold packs or a bath may make it possible to reduce the condition and circumcision may be undertaken at a later date. Alternatively immediate operation may be necessary if other methods fail. The skin is divided and the constriction relieved. A watch should be kept for retention of urine.

Hypospadias

Malformation of the penis and urethra may cause the urethral opening to be somewhere on the undersurface of the penis and in extreme cases it may be at the juncture of penis and scrotum. Plastic surgery aims at straightening the penis and making a new urethra from flaps of skin. The operation is usually done in two or three stages. Œdema following operation may be severe and for that reason an incision is sometimes made on the dorsum of the penis to prevent constrictive swelling and the formation of a hæmatoma, by allowing for adequate drainage.

The stitches are as a rule left exposed and are kept dry by dusting with an antiseptic powder. Some surgeons secure the sutures with glass beads. During the second stage, when the urethra is newly constructed, the site of operation is kept dry by the use of an indwelling catheter which is passed into the bladder through the perineum immediately behind the scrotum. The catheter and tubing, leading to the underwater drain containing a mild antiseptic solution, should be watched for any kinking and drainage has to be carefully measured morning and evening. The drainage bottle is changed and replaced by a sterile one at least once in 24 hours to minimize the danger of ascending infection. Bladder lavage with a mild antiseptic solution such as potassium permanganate, sufficient to colour the sterile water pink, may be ordered. When the draining catheter is disconnected for treatment or for changing the bottle, it is spigoted off with a spigot which is boiled every time before use.

After 8 to 10 days the patient is allowed to pass urine through the urethra while the catheter is still in position, but spigoted, and as soon as he can do so satisfactorily the indwelling catheter is removed. The perineal wound heals without suturing.

Following any operation on the penis or urethra, the urinal should be boiled prior to offering it to the patient, until the wound can be expected to have healed.

All operations on the penis are extremely painful and distressing and every effort should be made to alleviate apprehension and discomfort. Sedatives should be given generously, penis and scrotum carefully supported by small pillows, the weight of the bedclothes taken by a cradle and great care taken not to pull at the catheter during bedmaking. Pressure areas need careful attention and the bowels should be watched as constipation is common and causes additional discomfort. Extra visiting and plenty of occupation will help to take the child's mind off his condition.

Undescended Testicle

The testes undergo migration in fœtal life from a position high up in the abdomen through the inguinal canal and into the scrotal sac. They usually reach this final position by the time of birth. In some cases, however, migration is incomplete on one or both sides. On examination it is usually possible to determine the exact position of the testicle and the length of the spermatic cord. In many cases the testicle lies subcutaneously near the opening of the inguinal canal and can be brought down without difficulty. Although it may retract again it can be expected to descend by the time puberty has been reached. In other cases it has to be brought down by operation and stitched into the scrotal sac. There may be an associated hernia, which can be repaired at the same time.

Postoperatively a few days' bed rest is necessary but other nursing care presents no problems. If bilateral and if left untreated, undescended testes cause sterility and in later life malignant changes may develop. Sometimes hormone therapy replaces operation but not all cases are suitable for this method of treatment.

Hydrocele

A hydrocele is a swelling of the scrotum caused by fluid which accumulates in the scrotal sac. It may be unilateral or bilateral. The cause of the condition is unknown and so is the reason for its spontaneous disappearance, often after a period of several months. Because the hydrocele may cure itself, operation is sometimes delayed unless swelling is sufficiently large to cause discomfort or embarrassment. Aspiration of the fluid is useless and the sac is usually incised and evacuated. The operation is a simple one which causes little discomfort and few problems in the after care. The child may be treated as an out-patient or as a day case.

Exomphalos with or without Ectopia Vesicæ

If the anterior abdominal wall is absent or if fusion of the abdominal muscles is incomplete, the abdominal and pelvic organs may be exposed or even lie on the surface at the time of birth. Malformation of this kind may be associated with malformations of the penis or the vagina and with absence of the urethra or bladder wall or eversion of the bladder. If this is the case, the ureteric openings can be plainly seen and there is a constant trickle of urine. Ammonia dermatitis and excoriation of the surrounding skin develop and may lead to an ascending infection of the renal tract. Until operation can be undertaken the skin should be protected by sterile ointments and barrier creams. Sterile pads are applied to absorb the urine. These should be changed at frequent intervals.

If possible the skin and bladder wall are sutured but it is

often necessary to leave the repair of muscle to a later date. If there is a normally functioning urethra, repair is comparatively successful but often urethra and sphincter control are defective or absent and transplantation of the ureters into the sigmoid colon, ileum or rectum is necessary. The abnormal bladder is then removed at the same time.

Transplantation of Ureters

The operation of transplantation of ureters is done in cases in which there is either an abnormal or diseased bladder or an absence of sphincter control. This is frequently associated with malformation of the vagina such as a rectovaginal fistula.

A course of phthalylsulphathiazole and oral neomycin is given to sterilize the bowel pre-operatively and the operation is often done on one ureter at a time. The operation is a difficult and extensive one and post-operative shock may be considerable.

Complications. These include œdema at the site of repair causing obstruction of the urinary flow and resulting uræmia. The fluid intake and output have to be measured carefully in order to detect this complication at an early stage and drainage of the kidney by a temporary nephrostomy may become necessary. Occasionally there is reabsorption of urinary chloride ions through the bowel wall, causing hyperchloræmia and acidosis. In order to prevent these complications and to allow the ureters, kidneys and bowels to get used to their new function, a drainage catheter may be left in the rectum for approximately 10 days following operation, but even so inflammation of the bowel lining is common and this may not clear up for some time. Gradually, however, the bowel becomes used to holding urine and with sympathetic training the child learns to control the urge to go to the toilet and can achieve control of micturition compatible with ordinary life.

Until continence has been achieved the care of the perineum is important. Baths should be given twice daily and a barrier cream applied to both perineum and buttocks. Absorbent pads (sphagnum moss pads are very useful) are worn and changed frequently. At night exposure under a bed cradle may help to keep the skin intact. A urinary antiseptic is often given and may have to be continued over a period of years as there is always a danger of infection travelling up the renal tract from the bowel.

Recently successful operations have been performed in which the ureters are brought out onto the abdominal wall.

Each ureter then empties into a plastic colostomy bag. Alternatively a loop of ileum is cut off from the alimentary canal and utilized as a bladder, an opening made onto the surface and urine drained into a colostomy bag; this lessens the risk of infection.

Nephrostomy

Drainage of the kidney proper is called nephrostomy. It is performed when some obstruction in the urinary tract has caused long-standing back pressure and dilatation of the ureters and renal pelvis (hydro-ureter and hydronephrosis) or when œdema following operation on the ureters obstructs the normal urinary flow. A Foley's catheter is introduced into the pelvis of the kidney and stitched in position, while a piece of corrugated rubber serves to drain the tissues around the kidney. The nephrostomy tube is kept *in situ* until all urinary leakage has stopped and the ureters regain their normal function. Occasionally irrigation may be necessary. The importance of an accurate record of fluid intake and output morning and evening is obvious. The general care of a patient with a nephrostomy is similar to that of nephrectomy. The skin around the wound should be carefully cleansed and protected against excoriation by the application of a barrier cream. Extra lengths of drainage tube are often used to allow for free movement without pulling on the tube, when this kind of drainage is used in children.

Nephrectomy

The removal of a kidney is never considered unless full investigations have shown that the other kidney is healthy and capable of taking over the total renal function. The tests carried out include intravenous pyelography, retrograde pyelography and excretion tests. It is also usual to ensure that the remaining kidney will not be at risk from the presence of infection elsewhere in the body. Throat swabs and Mantoux tests are carried out and tonsillectomy may be considered.

Reasons for undertaking nephrectomy include congenital abnormalities of the ureters or kidney, hydronephrosis and Wilms's tumour. Tuberculosis of the kidney is rare in childhood. The child is usually admitted several days prior to operation to allow him to get used to the ward. Fluid intake and output are carefully measured for comparison with the post-operative fluid balance. A urinary antiseptic such as a course of sulphonamides may be ordered. In the case of Wilms's tumour, operation may be considered urgent and no time may be allowed for any special preparation unless a course of deep X-ray therapy is given.

Pre-operative Preparation. This includes blood grouping, hæmoglobin estimation and urine culture. Some surgeons like an aperient to be given two nights before operation. Skin preparation varies according to the wishes of the surgeon but a bath or a thorough wash with soap and water, paying special attention to axillæ, groins and umbilicus should be given shortly before operation.

The Operation. The incision is usually a long one running roughly parallel with the margin of the ribs. After the kidney has been wholly or partly removed, the ureter is tied off and the wound closed. A corrugated rubber drain or small rubber tube is stitched in position to drain the kidney bed. Post-operative primary and secondary bleeding is a fairly common complication and the drain serves the dual purpose of showing any such bleeding and draining the area around the kidney of serum and blood. The pad of cotton wool which covers the area should be frequently inspected. The drain is usually shortened after 24 hours and removed after 48 hours.

Return to Consciousness. When this occurs the patient is made comfortable with several pillows. He is tilted slightly to the affected side to allow for better drainage and should be moved from side to side at intervals as this reduces abdominal distension and further assists with drainage and prevents chest complications.

Nursing Care. The pillows should be protected with plastic covers and so arranged as to allow a hollow for the drainage tube. A small pillow placed between the knees avoids pressure and gives added comfort.

Adequate fluid intake is important and the nurse may have to spend a good deal of time persuading the reluctant patient to drink. A variety of fruit juices, tea and proprietary drinks should be given to make drinking more interesting and the young patient can be encouraged by keeping up his own fluid chart, collecting stars or making little drawings (see page 88). Pain may prevent deep breathing and so predispose to chest complications. The patient is nursed on the affected side or in the supine position to allow for good ventilation of both lungs. Breathing exercises and games which encourage deep breathing should be started as soon as possible. Regular bowel action is important.

The urinary output may at first be low and the urine blood stained, but output should be normal and the urine regain its normal colour approximately 24 hours after operation.

In the majority of cases, nephrectomy should not present many problems. Occasionally uræmia develops, either because fluid intake has been inadequate or because the remaining kidney has not proved equal to the additional work (for uræmia see page 280). The patient is usually allowed up on the second or third day and discharged on the tenth or twelfth day. Nephrectomy should not disable the patient markedly and should not be a bar to vigorous activities or pregnancy.

Wilms's Tumour (Nephroblastoma)

Wilms's tumour, which arises from the kidney, is the most commonly occurring malignant growth of childhood.

Signs and Symptoms. Frequently the first signs noticed are an enlargement of the abdomen. Pain, hæmaturia and suppression of urine together with general malaise, anæmia and failure to thrive occur rather later and these children do in fact remain surprisingly well for a long time despite the great malignancy of the condition and its tendency to form metastases in other parts of the body, particularly the lungs. The tumour is as a rule unilateral.

Treatment. This should be started without delay. A minimum of palpation for diagnostic purposes is allowed as there is a danger of dispersing the tumour cells into the lymphatic system and so encouraging spread. An intravenous pyelogram will reveal distortion of the renal pelvis and displacement of the kidney. The treatment consists of deep X-ray therapy given at the same time as injections of actinomycin D intended to reduce the size of the tumour prior to nephrectomy. A further course is given after operation to minimize the tendency to metastases. Unfortunately secondaries often arise within a year and there is a very high mortality rate.

Nursing Care of Patients on Radium or Deep X-ray Therapy. Patients on radiotherapy are usually given a card with instructions telling them about the treatment, of local or generalized reaction or signs of intolerance to its treatment. In the case of children the mother will be given these instructions before the child is discharged home. Points of particular importance are:

Care of the Skin. No part of the skin which has been exposed to radiation should be touched by water or washed for 1 month after treatment has been stopped. If reddened or sore a good talcum powder should be dusted over the area and if there is any reddening of the skin lanolin or Hibitane cream may be applied and is usually very soothing. The skin should not be exposed to any heat or to the sun and clothing should be very light, loose and of a smooth texture.

Generalized Reactions. These include general malaise, weariness and vomiting. Sympathy, gentleness and all nursing care to give maximum rest and comfort are all that can be done for the first two reactions. Vomiting may be reduced by the administration of drugs such as chlorpromazine (Largactil). Some surgeons order pyridoxine and iron as a routine. Fluids should be given in small, frequent amounts to prevent dehydration but occasionally an intravenous infusion is necessary. The diet should be light and predigested. Milk drinks such as Bengers are often well tolerated. Extra glucose should be given with all drinks and many children enjoy sucking barley sugar and plain boiled sweets.

The care of patients following nephrectomy and of terminal, malignant illnesses is discussed elsewhere and all that has been said applies to these unfortunate children. It is often possible to discharge the patient home after the course of deep X-ray has been completed even though readmission after some months must be expected. In that case every effort is made to admit the child to the same ward so that he is familiar with the surroundings and at least some members of the staff.

17

DISEASES OF THE NERVOUS SYSTEM

Basically, examination of a child's nervous system is the same as for an adult and it requires the same equipment. A child, however, is unable to describe his symptoms accurately and he will often be irritable and uncooperative. It will always help if a nurse whom the child knows and trusts can be present to assist the physician. It is important to undress the child completely and to allow plenty of time for him to settle in the unfamiliar surroundings.

Most of the history will be obtained from the mother and it is taken back to include information about pregnancy and delivery. It is important to know whether there were signs of cyanosis or asphyxia at birth and whether the baby was premature or born at term. The doctor will also want to know whether there is any family history of epilepsy, mental deficiency or any other illness, which might have a bearing on the present condition.

Examination. The physician will note any abnormality of the skull such as bossing, asymmetry and the size of the fontanelle. In certain cases, such as suspected cerebral lesions or intracranial tumours, it may be important to notice the way in which the child holds his head. Facial palsy may cause him to dribble saliva from one corner of the mouth or cause only the unaffected side of the mouth to be drawn up when laughing or smiling.

The child may be unable to reach accurately for objects held out to him or he may have tremor of the hand. In certain diseases, the way in which the child raises himself from the floor to the standing position is in itself diagnostic. Sometimes the absence or presence of normal skills give the best guide towards assessment and diagnosis.

The reflexes, as tested with the aid of a jerk hammer, are important. Reflexes in the very young infant are unusually brisk and the plantar reflex is still extensor and only becomes flexor, as in the adult, when the child starts to walk.

Measuring the Head Circumference. The rate of growth of a child's head is often significant. In order to get accurate and comparable readings, the same person should always take the measurements if possible. The tape measure is taken round the head over the middle of the forehead and the most prominent part of the occiput.

Shaving a Child's Head. Considerable skill is needed to shave the skull of a young child as he cannot be expected to keep still for any length of time. Two nurses should always work together, one holding the child firmly to avoid any accidents. It is usually best to wrap the child securely in a blanket with his hands well out of the way and to lay him across the cot. One nurse stands at his feet and bends over the child with one hand placed either side of his face, while the other gets on with the shaving. In this way the nurse has complete control but at the same time can talk to the child, all equipment being kept well out of his sight.

Signs of Raised Intracranial Pressure

While diagnosis must always be the doctor's province, early observations and accurate reporting on the part of the nurse may be invaluable in securing early and effective treatment. The signs to watch for include:

Vomiting unrelated to meals and without previous warning.
Headache, which is sometimes eased when the head is raised.
A tense, bulging anterior fontanelle.*
Distension of the scalp veins.*
Separation of sutures.*
Increase in the circumference of the head.*
Papillœdema.
Slowing of pulse rate.
Convulsions.
Meningeal cry.
Head retraction.
Arching of the back.
Internal strabismus.
Irritability.
Resentment at being touched.
Drowsiness.

*Symptoms marked * apply to infants only.*

Some Neurological Procedures

Lumbar Puncture

Lumbar puncture is the same for children as for adults and is done for the same reasons. It is, however, important to have complete control of the child when holding him and only an experienced person should attempt to do this. Very young children are often best lifted on to a table or a well-padded locker. Really adequate control is as a rule best achieved by the following means. The child is made comfortable on the pillow or mattress and the back flexed as much as possible in order to separate the spinous processes of the vertebræ. The nurse then hooks one arm round the neck, the other round the crook of the flexed knees and allows her hands to meet in front of the patient, so forming a complete circle with her hands and arms and the child's body. Although safely restrained the child can breathe adequately and the nurse does not tire easily as pull on her own hands gives her strength and support. The child should be absolutely still, neither struggling nor crying while the pressure is being read, lest false readings be obtained.

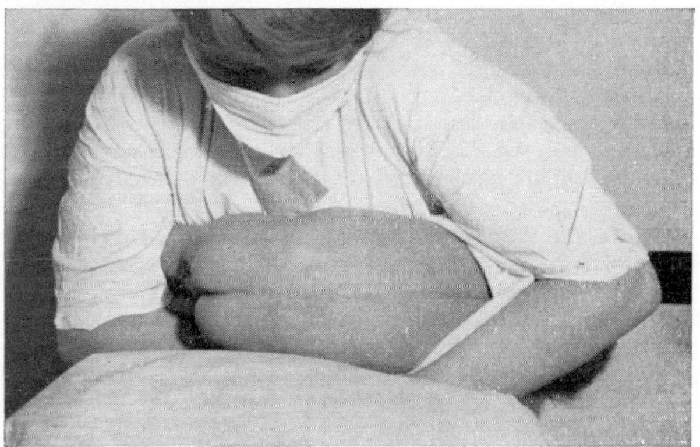

Fig. 52. Lumbar Puncture Performed on a Young Child.
Note the way neck and flexure of the knees are made to fit into the crook of the nurse's elbows.

Whenever it is thought that lumbar puncture may have to be done repeatedly, a sedative should be given so as to minimize possible fear and psychological trauma.

In children headaches rarely follow lumbar puncture and the routine of keeping the patient flat and the foot of the bed raised is not necessary unless air has been injected as for the purpose of an air encephalogram.

Cisternal Puncture

When a block between the *cisterna magna* and the distal end of the spinal canal obstructs the free circulation of cerebrospinal fluid, cisternal puncture may be done instead of a lumbar puncture. A small area of hair is shaved at the nape of the neck and a special cisternal puncture needle is used. This is inserted at a point where an imaginary line, drawn from one tip of the mastoid process to the other, crosses the spine, while the head is held in complete flexion. In all other respects the procedure is the same as for lumbar puncture.

Other, more extensive procedures may be both frightening and very uncomfortable and they are therefore done under a light general, or a basal anæsthetic. It is also easier to obtain the necessary positions with the anæsthetized patient than with an uncooperative one.

In conditions in which congenital abnormalities or hydrocephalus are suspected it may be necessary to outline the ventricles of the brain. This can be done by filling them with air or pure oxygen before taking X-ray pictures. Irregular outline, displacement or defects in filling may show up and these findings are valuable in coming to a diagnosis and in deciding on treatment. There are two methods in common use.

Pneumo-encephalogram. A lumbar puncture is performed in the usual way and several millilitres of cerebrospinal fluid are withdrawn. The fluid is replaced by filtered air or pure oxygen, injected through a syringe attached to the lumbar puncture needle. This process is repeated several times until about 40 millilitres have been exchanged. When the child is sat up, the air rises within the cerebrospinal canal, like an air bubble rising in water. If there is no abnormality present the ventricles of the brain will fill with air and their outline and position can be clearly seen on X-ray. Air encephalogram is never carried out in cases of suspected space occupying lesions as these cause raised intracranial pressure and the withdrawal of cerebrospinal fluid may lead to "coning" of the brain-stem through the foramen magnum into the spinal canal, resulting in sudden death from pressure on this vital part of the nervous system.

Ventriculography. For ventriculography the head has to be shaved, as the blunt cannula is introduced through the scalp, directly into the ventricles. In young infants this can be done through the still-open fontanelle or the still-ununited sutures.

In older patients it is necessary to make burr holes in the skull. Approximately 40 millilitres of filtered air or pure oxygen are then injected after withdrawing a similar quantity of cerebrospinal fluid.

In either case, X-ray pictures are taken immediately after the air has been injected. By placing the patient in different positions the movement of the air through the ventricular system and the shape, size and position of the ventricles can be clearly seen. Alternatively a filling defect of any part of the cerebrospinal or ventricular system will be a valuable aid to diagnosis. Ventriculography is used when a brain abscess or intracranial tumour is suspected.

Radio-opaque Methods

Angiography is used when it is desirable to outline blood vessels of the brain. An injection of a radio-opaque dye is made into the main carotid artery in the neck. As the dye circulates through the arteries their outline can be seen on the X-ray screen or film. Pictures are taken in rapid succession. In this way abnormalities such as angiomata of the brain can be clearly seen and accurately located. Angiography is a valuable diagnostic aid, particularly prior to certain operations on the brain (see Sturge-Weber Syndrome, page 307).

In cases of suspected non-communicating hydrocephalus (see page 313) radio-opaque media may be injected into the ventricle through the anterior fontanelle or through burr holes, and the site of a hold-up may be seen in the radiograph. Radio-opaque substances may also be injected into the spinal cord to discover the site of a spinal tumour.

The procedures described above are not without hazard and shock may be considerable. Children do not complain of headache but on return to the ward their colour may be poor and they may be restless or irritable. As soon as their condition permits, extra fluids should be given as this seems to ease their discomfort and helps in their recovery.

Electro-encephalogram

It is known that rhythmical electric charges of a certain pattern and frequency are exhibited in the human brain and that both pattern and frequency change in disease. Recordings can be made by means of electrical leads placed on the patient's scalp. The graphs obtained are typical of certain diseases or abnormalities and are a valuable aid to diagnosis. It is desirable to have a fully cooperative patient, capable of obeying instructions (for example to open or close his eyes) and this is often achieved by arranging for the mother or for the child's own nurse to be present. Frequently, however, a sedative has to be given.

Disturbances and Diseases of the Nervous System

Convulsions

Convulsions are very common in childhood and should be considered as a symptom of disease rather than as a disease in themselves. Some young children have a convulsion with every pyrexial illness and they can be expected to grow out of this tendency as they grow older. In others the convulsions are caused by brain damage or illnesses such as meningitis.

Treatment and prognosis will obviously depend on the cause of the convulsions. Intellectually, many of these children develop quite normally though sometimes interrupted schooling or misguided over-protection by the parents makes them compare unfavourably with their contemporaries.

Children whose fits are due to true epilepsy with frequent attacks need special protective measures and may have to attend special schools, but their chances of employment and their psychological adjustment can be greatly improved by attendance at ordinary schools, and understanding teachers often make this possible without any detriment to the other pupils. As normal a life as possible should be encouraged, though regular routine with regard to meals, sleep, work and recreation can often help to keep attacks down to a minimum. Convulsions seem to occur less frequently in the well-occupied child who has plenty to interest him than in those who never know what to do with themselves. Occasionally, risks have to be taken and are likely to be less serious than the effects of over-protection and constant restrictions, though common sense precautions such as fireguards and adequate cot-sides should be provided. The parents may well be deeply affected by their child's misfortune and nurses should never forget that they deserve both sympathy and understanding.

Petit Mal

Attacks of minor epilepsy may be so mild that they are only noticed by those who are in constant contact with the patient. The loss of consciousness may be so fleeting that, after a momentary pause, the patient immediately resumes his activities as if nothing had happened. The eyes may take on a momentary dazed look or there may be a feeling of giddiness or a loss of postural control. In hospital it is at times necessary for a nurse to "special" a patient in order to see one of these attacks.

Major Epilepsy

The stages of a major epileptic attack are the same in children as in adults, but children frequently become irritable or cling to their mothers as if seeking comfort during the period of aura. Occasionally there is no loss of consciousness nor are there true convulsive movements but the child shows considerable behaviour disturbances or temporary loss of memory and, in some cases, unexplained headaches or abdominal pain are thought to be of epileptic origin.

Except where children admitted during a convulsion are known to be epileptics of long-standing, investigations including lumbar puncture are carried out to exclude any acute illness. Later a full neurological examination and an electroencephalogram are usually undertaken.

A great variety of drugs are used to control convulsion, including phenobarbitone, Mysolin, Epanutin, paraldehyde or various combinations of anticonvulsant drugs. Some of these drugs have serious side-effects and the nurse should be well informed about these, and make careful observations. Mustard baths are still occasionally given but it is not likely that the hospital nurse in this country will be asked to use this method of treatment.

In dealing with a child in a convulsion, the principal concern is to keep him from harming himself. If he has been up and about, the nurse should lie him on a bed or on the floor away from any harmful object. The child's head should be turned to the side to allow saliva to drain freely and so prevent inhalation. Tight clothing should be loosened and the patient kept warm. If the attack occurs in bed, pillows are best removed and, if possible, a mackintosh and anæsthetic cloth should be placed underneath the head to protect the bed. A soft, firm wedge or bandage should be inserted between the teeth to prevent the patient from biting his tongue. Restraint is best avoided. If the attack occurs in the ward, screens should be placed around him and he should be kept as quiet as possible.

As the patient regains consciousness he is likely to be bewildered and reassurance and comfort should be given. A warm drink may help to send him into a restful sleep.

In hospital, a tray containing recovery instruments and swabs is usually kept near the beds of known epileptic children but this should be covered and out of sight of both child and visitors. Occasionally oxygen has to be given and paraldehyde may be ordered. This may be given by intramuscular injection or per rectum.

While looking after the patient the nurse should make careful observations and chart these as soon as she is free. The points to watch for are suggested in the following list.

Observations. How did the fit start? Was there an aura, noise in the ears, flash of light? Were there any movements? Where did they begin? Where did they spread to? Were the movements tonic or clonic? Was there a tremor and eye movements?

Did the patient lose consciousness? Were the eyes open or closed? If closed, could they be opened? Towards which side were they turned? If lightly touched, did the eyes blink? Was there incontinence, cyanosis, breath holding? Did the patient bite his tongue? What was the duration of the fit? Was the patient drowsy after the fit or was he confused? Did the patient show abnormal or unusual behaviour after the fit? What could the patient remember about the fit?

Temperature, pulse and respirations should be taken and recorded as soon as the convulsion is over.

Points of Interest. Although intelligence in epileptics is average in most instances and may even be above normal, mental subnormality occurs more commonly in epileptics than in other children, and the inevitable use of drugs often slows the mental processes in these children.

Pink Disease
(Erythroedema, Acrodynia, Polyneuritis)

Incidence. Pink disease affects children of both sexes from earliest infancy to about five years and while very common in some parts of the world (e.g. in Australia) is almost unknown in others (e.g. in Israel).

Cause. Since mercury has been removed from teething powders, the disease has markedly diminished, so that it is thought that the cause was probably hypersensitivity to mercury.

Signs and Symptoms. These may vary from moderate irritability, attributed to teething, a prolonged cold or mismanagement, to a picture of the most intense misery. The child with pink disease presents typical features in varying degrees of severity.

In a severe case it is the picture of a deeply miserable,

negative child. As the name suggests, there is pinkness of certain parts, mainly distributed over the nose and forehead and on the extremities in a "glove sock" distribution. The skin feels moist and cold and flaky peeling is caused by the child rubbing hands and feet together. The extremities are often swollen though the tissues do not pit on pressure.

Photophobia is marked and as the child lies in the knee elbow position burying his face in his pillows the nose and forehead are rubbed and this adds to their red appearance. All muscles are flabby and relaxed causing the lips to hang loosely and giving a "duckbill" expression with a constant dribble of saliva. The toddler who has been walking no longer stands or sits up and often adopts unusual positions made possible by the general hypotonia. Rectal prolapse is a common feature. Skin infections develop readily and whitlow is almost the rule.

In severe cases it is difficult to prevent stomatitis. The gums are swollen and spongy, and teeth may fall out prematurely. This adds to the already severe anorexia. Trophic changes cause gangrene of the fingers and toes. The hair becomes dull and sparse and as the child plucks at it, in his attempt to allay irritation, bald patches develop. Older children report severe burning and itching as if the extremities had been immersed in boiling water. The constant restlessness and the marked anorexia cause serious wasting and loss of weight. Sleeplessness is extreme and sedatives have little effect.

The blood pressure is raised to approximately 120 to 140 millimetres of mercury but the erythrocyte sedimentation rate remains normal.

Investigations. These merely serve research purposes as the typical symptoms and signs make a clinical diagnosis easy. Specimens of urine are usually examined for the presence of mercury.

Treatment. As little is known about the disease, treatment remains symptomatic and experimental. In cases where sweating is severe and much salt is lost, extra salt is given and belladonna preparations may be ordered to help dry up secretions. Penicillamine or calcium disodium versenate given intravenously are used, in the same way as for the treatment of lead poisoning (see page 308). Experiments with vasodilator drugs and ganglion blocking agents have given occasional encouragement to research workers. Sedatives such as chloral hydrate and phenobarbitone have to be given to secure rest and sleep.

Prognosis. The illness is a long one and may continue for 6 to 9 months with several periods of remission. Intercurrent infections may prove serious and must be carefully guarded against, but in uncomplicated cases recovery is complete.

Nursing Care. Children suffering from pink disease should ideally be nursed at home where the risk of intercurrent infections is small. Frequently, however, the mother becomes exhausted by the constant care of a child who, suffering from severe insomnia and anorexia, needs constant comforting and attention for several months. Unless considerable help can be given in the home, admission to hospital may become unavoidable to allow for a period of rest for the mother, although she should be allowed to visit freely and help with the care of her child lest she develops a sense of failure.

Cubicle nursing is essential. The nursing care is exacting and chiefly aims at relieving the symptoms as far as is possible and at supplying an adequate food intake. For the skin irritation and sweating, light clothing of cotton, aertex or silk should be worn and this should be washed frequently. Sponging and alkaline baths such as sodium bicarbonate 1 drachm to 1 pint and application of a calamine with 2 per cent. phenol lotion may help to allay irritation. The skin should be kept dry and cool and this is best achieved by the use of a good dusting powder. Cotton gloves and socks may stop the rubbing of hands and feet. Recently the use of Tubegauz in place of socks and gloves has proved most satisfactory.

The cot should be screened from light on account of the photophobia but the room should be well ventilated and of an even, cool temperature. If elbow splints are applied they should be of the lightest type and the usual padding modified as overheating would add to the already distressing irritation. A bed cradle is useful to take the weight of the bedclothes and to allow air to circulate and at the same time to give shade to the eyes.

Feeding presents serious problems and may call for great patience and ingenuity. Small, frequent amounts should be given whenever the child is likely to take them and bottle feeding may have to be continued much longer than is usual. Pretty crockery and carefully arranged, colourful food may stimulate the appetite in the older child. The diet should be nourishing and well balanced with plenty of fresh fruit and vitamins. Whenever stomatitis is present food should be soft or semi-solid. Occasionally tube feeding becomes necessary and it may be useful to pass a tube at night and give fortified milk by the drip method while the child is asleep.

Mentally these children remain normal and alert but often regression in training habits is marked.

Great patience and understanding and the best nursing attention only, will manage to keep these entirely negative little patients from abysmal distress and no amount of nursing and comforting should be considered as spoiling or as a waste of time.

Meningitis

Meningitis is more common in children than in adults but the causative organisms are the same as in adults with the exception of *Escherichia* (*Bacterium*) *coli* which occasionally causes meningitis in new-born infants. Generally speaking, the acute types present a common picture and basically investigations, treatment and nursing care are the same. Infections which present special problems are mentioned under the appropriate headings; for example, tuberculous meningitis under the heading tuberculosis.

Signs and Symptoms. Most commonly the onset is sudden, with headaches, vomiting, high fever, neck stiffness and photophobia. The pulse varies and may be either increased or slower than usual. From time to time the child gives a shrill, high-pitched scream known as the meningeal cry. He is irritable at first and resents being touched. Soon, however, he becomes drowsy, the eyes take on a staring expression and the pupils may be unequal and sluggish in their reaction to light. A squint may also develop. Occasionally convulsions occur and as a rule these must be regarded as a serious sign. As the irritation of the spinal meninges increases and the muscles of the neck become involved, head retraction and backward arching of the back result: this is known as *opisthotonos*. Cheyne-Stokes type of breathing may develop and delirium, stupor and coma supervene.

As the illness progresses, generalized septicæmia may set in and in these cases the skin takes on a grey colour, and feels cold and clammy. The pulse rate rises and the volume becomes poor. The blood pressure falls. Constipation and retention of urine are common.

Examination. This shows the infant to have a tense, bulging fontanelle and older children will have papillœdema, sure signs of increased intracranial pressure. Lumbar puncture will confirm the diagnosis and determine the causative organism and its sensitivity to drugs.

Treatment. This consists in giving the appropriate drug orally or by intramuscular or intrathecal injection. Occasionally a block forms in the channel of the cerebrospinal fluid with the result that the drugs do not reach the focus of the infection. In such cases lumbar puncture may be replaced by cisternal or ventricular puncture and surgical intervention may become necessary to assist drainage and prevent permanent damage. Sometimes fluid collects in the subdural space, causing the fever to persist and the head circumference to increase. Daily subdural taps will be necessary until no further fluid is obtained.

Prognosis. In most instances complete recovery may be expected, but much depends on early diagnosis and prompt, effective treatment. The outlook is most serious in very young infants and in all cases the illness is a long and serious one and the prognosis should always be somewhat guarded.

Complications. These include neurological disturbances, hydrocephalus, mental deficiency, paralysis and convulsions. A special point worth remembering is that, in young infants, meningitis may occur in a subacute form. There may be little or no fever; diarrhœa and vomiting may lead to dehydration and sunken eyes and fontanelle. Together with these misleading symptoms neurological examination is difficult and often atypical in babies and only lumbar puncture can confirm the diagnosis of meningitis.

Meningococcal Meningitis

Meningococcal meningitis presents some special features which are particularly important as this type of meningitis is often seen in children's wards. The patient often comes from overcrowded surroundings, and the infection which is spread by droplets invades the nasopharynx and blood stream. The course of the illness may be fulminant and, if coupled with septicæmia, may rapidly lead to collapse and death. Complications such as petechial hæmorrhages, temporary blindness, opisthotonos, peripheral circulatory failure, *taches cérébrales* and convulsions are common if treatment is delayed. In cases where there are signs of hæmorrhage into the skin, cortisone or prednisone are given, either by intravenous or intramuscular injection. In the less acute types, the patient is severely ill for two or three weeks.

A great danger is that an exudate may form at the base of the brain. Surgery can sometimes be carried out to remove the fibrous membrane formed but if it is not successful, blocking of the fourth ventricle, hydrocephalus, spasticity, loss of vision and hearing and mental defect may develop. With modern diagnostic methods and drug therapy, these severe cases and complications are fortunately rare in this country.

It should be remembered that meningococcal meningitis is a notifiable disease. The incubation period is 4 to 5 days only and carriers are common.

Hæmophilus influenzæ Meningitis

Hæmophilus infection causing meningitis occurs mostly during the pre-school age. Once invariably fatal, the outlook is now much more hopeful due to treatment with drugs such as chloramphenicol combined with a sulphonamide and possibly also polymixin, given by intramuscular or intravenous injection. There remains a danger of nerve damage, causing complications such as deafness or paralysis.

Nursing Care in All Cases of Meningitis

A quiet, well-ventilated room should be chosen, and certain types of meningitis will have to be nursed with full barrier precautions. Careful observations, coupled with sound knowledge of the possible complications, are of prime importance and the observations should be carried out continuously and conscientiously.

The child's position in bed may point to increasing intracranial pressure, for example turning away from the light or hiding under the bedclothes.

Pressure areas need careful attention on account of the severe wasting which is often present, and because of restlessness and incontinence. Water beds or sorbo mattresses are a great help. The skin should be kept healthy by careful sponging and this may at the same time serve to reduce the hyperpyrexia and help in the elimination of toxins. In all cases of bacterial meningitis broad spectrum antibiotics such as chloramphenicol are prescribed and must be given conscientiously, although the child may be very unco-operative about taking these drugs.

The bowels and bladder need watching as constipation and retention of urine are common. The urine should be tested for abnormal constituents, such as albumen, blood or acetone bodies.

Good ventilation and an electric fan may help in reducing high fever, and nursing aids such as bed cradles, ring pads for the heels and head, and soft bandages for the knees, should be used whenever necessary. Mouth toilet should be done frequently and the lips kept soft by applying petroleum jelly to prevent sores, particularly if the child is unconscious and unable to take fluids by mouth. A wedge and mouth gag should be kept at hand in case a convulsion should occur.

In the acute stages temperature, pulse and respirations are taken and charted 4-hourly and blood pressure readings may have to be taken frequently. Fluid intake and output should be measured and the charts kept up to date.

Diet. This should be light and nutritious, and fluids should be given in adequate amounts. Artificial feeding by nasal tube may become necessary. The problem of feeding may be aggravated by persistent vomiting. It often pays to allow the mother to bring a favourite dish from home and to give in to the child's whims where the diet is concerned, in order to maintain adequate nutrition.

Continuous and expert nursing care, using every available nursing aid and enlisting the help of occupational therapist, remedial physiotherapist and extra visiting, may help to bring these seriously ill children back to normal health, once they have passed the acute stage of the illness.

Cerebral Abscess

Cerebral abscess is often difficult to diagnose as the onset is insidious and neurological investigations in children a difficult task. For this reason such cases are often seen in medical wards, though the condition is essentially a surgical one.

Causes. These, in children, are the same as in adults, except that children with congenital heart disease are occasionally the victims of cerebral abscess caused when a small embolus reaches the brain and becomes infected.

In the early stage of the illness the symptoms resemble those of meningitis but, as the infection becomes localized, convulsions, visual disturbances, toxæmia, drowsiness and facial palsy may develop. At this point the temperature may be only slightly raised. The diagnosis is confirmed by ventriculography, immediately prior to surgical intervention.

Treatment. Antibiotics are given in large doses and, as soon as the abscess is sufficiently localized, an operation for drainage is carried out. The subsequent treatment is purely surgical.

Although this is a long and serious illness the prognosis is by no means hopeless, though children who have recovered in all other respects may be left with convulsions.

The *nursing care* includes all points observed when looking after seriously ill or even unconscious patients suffering from a prolonged illness, as well as the care for the underlying condition, for example endocarditis or otitis media. These patients may become very restless and difficult to manage, and need careful and constant nursing attention.

Intracranial Tumour

Intracranial, space-occupying lesions are fairly common, particularly in children of five to ten years old. Treatment is surgical or by deep X-ray therapy. According to their situation the lesions cause complications by pressure, for instance pressure on the pituitary gland, causing *diabetes insipidus*. Some of these tumours are malignant and inoperable but in many cases there is reasonable hope of successful treatment. The commonest site is the cerebellum and the pressure here causes the patient to suffer from vomiting which is difficult to control. Papillœdema is usually present and the child is grossly ataxic.

During the period in which investigations are carried out it is important to keep these children happy and generally fit. Whenever possible they should be up and about and gentle physiotherapy helps to keep their muscles in trim. But as these patients are often unstable on their feet this places extra responsibility on the nursing staff to avoid accidents. When deep X-ray therapy is given, vomiting and anorexia may become a problem and ingenuity is needed in keeping up the patient's nutrition. Avomine and other drugs may be prescribed to stop vomiting.

Sturge-Weber Syndrome

Some children have a facial nævus and a nævus of the meninges on one side, associated with hemiplegia of the opposite side and fits which may affect only the opposite side or be general. This is known as Sturge-Weber syndrome. The nævus on the meninges consists of dilated capillaries of a web-like appearance (telangiectasis) which calcify after a time. The associated convulsions may be so severe as ultimately to affect the child's mental development.

Treatment consists in trying to control the convulsions by drugs but frequently surgical treatment becomes necessary. In this case either the affected area or the entire hemisphere has to be removed (hemispherectomy).

Acute Encephalitis

Acute encephalitis may be caused by virus or bacterial infection, specific fevers or influenza.

Signs and Symptoms. The onset of the disease is very acute, with high fever, severe headache, vomiting, visual disturbances and sometimes convulsions and loss of consciousness. Patients may be so confused as to become irrational and violent to an extent which necessitates restraint.

A high lymphocyte count in the cerebrospinal fluid confirms the diagnosis. The illness is a short one and has a high mortality rate. Brain damage may be permanent in those children who recover from the acute illness.

Treatment. This is symptomatic and principally aims at reducing the intracranial pressure by repeated lumbar punctures. The nursing care is exacting as the patient cannot be expected to cooperate. Restlessness creates problems regarding pressure areas. Artificial feeding may become necessary during the confused stage and constant vigilance is essential to keep up a high standard of care and prevent accidents.

Rare types of encephalitis include encephalitis lethargica, which is now hardly ever seen in this country, post-vaccination encephalitis and toxoplasmosis.

Toxoplasmosis

Toxoplasmosis is a rare form of infection caused by a protozoon.

The child is affected *in utero* and the symptoms are present at birth. The infant fails to thrive, vomiting and diarrhœa, convulsions and changes in the retina develop and, as the lesions rapidly become calcified, they cause blindness, mental deficiency and hydrocephalus. The outlook is bad but not hopeless.

The presence of the disease is confirmed by serological tests. Early treatment with pyrimethalamine (Daraprim) has been found to result in some improvement, but prolonged use of the drug may cause megaloblastic anæmia, due to folic acid deficiency.

Lead Encephalitis

Lead encephalitis is mentioned mainly because it should be possible to avoid its occurrence altogether. It is wholly due to the use of paint containing lead which, in one way or another, has come within reach of young children. Toddlers, who carry everything to their mouths or who rub their sore gums on the cool bars of their cots when teething, are particularly exposed to this danger. By law, lead paint may not be used where such risks arise, but sometimes fathers may brighten up the child's furniture or toys with a little paint left over from an outside painting job, and so become the unwitting cause of the illness. By health teaching nurses can do much to prevent such accidents.

The symptoms include convulsions, anæmia, symptoms of intracranial pressure and neuritis.

Penicillamine or calcium disodium versenate given by the intravenous route are used to treat lead poisoning. The intravenous infusion must be given slowly as there may be a rapid fall in blood pressure if this is not done.

Cerebral Palsy

Cerebral palsy is caused by damage to the brain affecting the upper motor neurones and liable to occur any time before, during or after birth. Muscular control may be so little impaired that it is barely noticeable, or all muscle groups of the body may be involved, completely incapacitating the victim.

Some of the sufferers appear mentally defective as they are unable to control their facial expressions, but in reality half are mentally normal or of superior intelligence. Inability to enunciate may add to the impression that there is mental impairment.

Premature babies in particular seem likely to be affected, but there are many other causes, including ill health during pregnancy and an abnormal delivery.

The earlier these children can be treated, the greater the hope of teaching them sufficient muscular relaxation and control to make their lives tolerable to themselves, their parents and the community in general.

Nurses have special opportunities for spotting these cerebral palsy babies who are sometimes admitted to the children's ward under another diagnosis. These may include babies who suck and swallow badly, babies who are abnormally quiet or always restless, babies who start up with a jerk at a sudden noise, babies who never cry and those who let their heads drop back when they are picked up or always hold them turned towards one side. Babies who suffer from hæmolytic disease of the newborn (see page 57) are potential cerebral palsy sufferers and should be kept under careful supervision, so that treatment, if necessary, may be started at the earliest moment.

These babies should be brought to the notice of a doctor without delay so that they can be watched, and physiotherapy started as soon as possible. Where there is doubt, the nurse should compare her patient's progress with the milestones set out in Chapter 1 and try to judge whether her young charge's achievements fall within the normal limits of development. Mothers are often reluctant to admit, even to themselves, that their own child's progress compares unfavourably with others, and tact and careful observation may be needed if treatment is to be started at the best time.

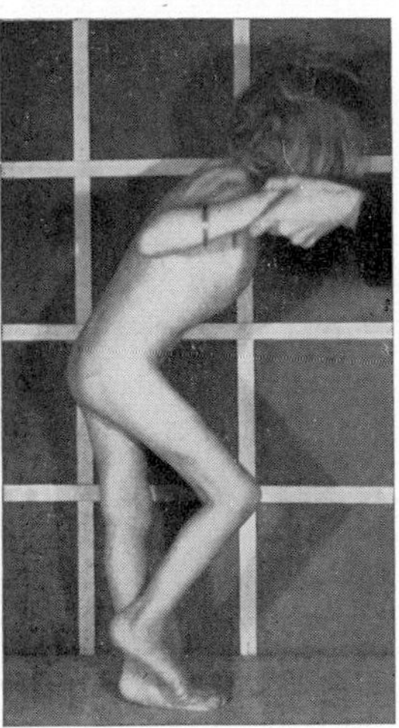

Fig. 53. Cerebral Palsy.
Note the typical stumbling gait.

Children suffering from cerebral palsy have difficulty in carrying out coordinated movements. The adductor muscles of the thigh in particular go into spasm (the scissor attitude). The gait is unsteady or clumsy, and is often reminiscent of a drunken man, charging forward, dragging a foot and stumbling about (Fig. 53), or the movements may be slow and writhing. Speech is difficult if the lip, tongue and laryngeal muscles are affected and the child may grimace in an attempt at forming words. What speech is possible is often explosive and the abnormal functioning of the respiratory muscles causes the child to make uncontrolled, animal-like noises. This may intensify the impression that the child is mentally abnormal. In addition he has difficulty in swallowing and he may have a constant dribble of saliva down his chin. Poor mastication causes dental decay, anæmia and malnutrition.

Many spastic children have a squint caused by muscle spasm, and visual disturbances such as double vision are common. Hearing defects are often associated with cerebral palsy, and these and the visual defects are often partly responsible for the delay in acquiring speech and learning to read.

Some of these children have particularly lovable ways, but others suffer from temper tantrums brought on by frustration and by a tendency to convulsions. Doctors and nurses can help to enlighten the general public about cerebral palsy sufferers and thus get them accepted with constructive sympathy.

Investigations should be carried out by a specialist and should be very extensive. The aim is to make a full assessment and then set to work on those muscle groups and abilities which give hope of response and seem capable of development. Teamwork is the essence in the treatment of cerebral palsy. An educational psychologist is asked to assess the child's mental ability, a very difficult task as poor muscular control and sensory defects, such as deafness or double vision, may make the use of the usual testing material impossible.

It is often possible to correct or alleviate some of the associated defects, by giving the child glasses, a hearing aid and walking calipers. The general health should be regularly supervised. As these children have difficulty in masticating due to bad muscular coordination, malnutrition is common and the teeth may be bad or ill developed. Septic tonsils are frequently another cause of general ill health. Deformities of various kinds may develop, caused by the unequal pull of muscles on the bony structures. The pædiatrician will therefore often enlist the help of orthopædic, dental, ear, nose and throat and ophthalmic surgeons who may be able to correct or ameliorate existing defects.

From the earliest moment the use of splints, small pillows, specially constructed chairs, gentle, passive movements and massage should be encouraged and teaching of conscious relaxation started.

The brunt of treatment will fall on the parents, teachers and physiotherapist. These children can attend nursery schools and schools for the physically handicapped, where physiotherapy is available and where they can be shown how the powers left to them can be used to the best advantage. Often this means tedious exercises in relaxation and only when this has been mastered will it be possible to teach voluntary movements with success. Progress will be slow and such aids as mirrors, walking skis and rails at suitable levels may give the much-needed encouragement. Tape recorders, on which progress in speech can be followed, are an invaluable stimulus both to the children and to their parents and teachers.

Films taken of the patient at various stages may also be used to remind all concerned of the initial difficulties and so make them appreciate better what has been achieved. Building up the handles of eating utensils, adjusting lavatory seats and other ingenious adaptations may be learnt at special centres and schools or thought of by intelligent, enterprising parents.

Parents of spastic children have in fact come together and founded a society through which they work for better treatment and education for their children as well as encouraging each other and exchanging useful ideas on their children's upbringing.

Later in life, no trouble should be spared to integrate these young people into the life of the community, and it will be found that given suitable help and employment a large majority can earn their living and fend for themselves.

The problem, though great, is one where there is no need for despair, and the reader will be rewarded if she makes a more thorough study of this condition about which only a little can be said within the scope of a small text-book.

Friedreich's Ataxia

Friedreich's ataxia is a fairly uncommon condition and the reader is referred to larger text-books for greater detail. The disease is familial, and usually becomes established at the age of five to ten years; it is caused by degenerative changes in the spinal cord and cerebellum. The child develops uncoordinated movements, ataxia, difficulty with speech and swallowing, generalized weakness and mental deterioration.

There is no known cure for this disease and nursing and medical care are confined to symptomatic treatment and prevention of deformities.

Progressive Spinal Muscular Atrophy

In this condition the motor cells in the spinal cord fail to develop properly and in consequence the muscles of the limbs and trunk are very feeble and flaccid. In one form, *amyotonia congenita*, most of the damage occurs before birth and the infant can merely lie flat. Some slight improvement may occur and permits life to continue for years, but sooner or later, respiratory infection causes death, for the child is unable to clear the respiratory passages by coughing.

In another form, *Werdnig-Hoffman's disease*, the condition is less severe at birth but weakness increases and death occurs at an early age. Nursing care concentrates on preventing inhalation of food and infection and in moving the child and changing his position and caring for the skin. Diagnosis in both instances is confirmed by electromyogram and muscular biopsy.

Hydrocephalus and Spina Bifida

Although both these conditions are frequently seen in medical children's wards and in maternity units, treatment is mainly on surgical lines and the reader is advised to consult a surgical text-book for detailed information. The nursing problem is, however, a considerable one and often confronts general pædiatric nurses while the baby is awaiting transfer.

Hydrocephalus

Hydrocephalus is the name given to an excessive accumulation of cerebrospinal fluid within the skull. The resulting pressure causes the skull bones to separate, the skull circumference to increase, the ventricles to become distended and the substance of the brain to be compressed.

The excess accumulation is produced by obstruction of the flow or absorption of the fluid, due to congenital malformation, birth injury, inflammatory processes or pressure from a tumour.

Nurses will hear the doctors mention a communicating and a non-communicating type of hydrocephalus and investigations will aim at establishing which of the two varieties affects the child.

In the *communicating type* there is a block within the subarachnoid space although there is free communication between the ventricular system and the spinal theca.

In the *non-communicating type*, the outflow from within the brain to the subarachnoid space is blocked; in either case various methods of drainage have been tried with some success. Lately the use of the *Spitz-Holter valve* has given good results in a proportion of cases. Details of the nursing care of these patients should be sought in specialized text-books.

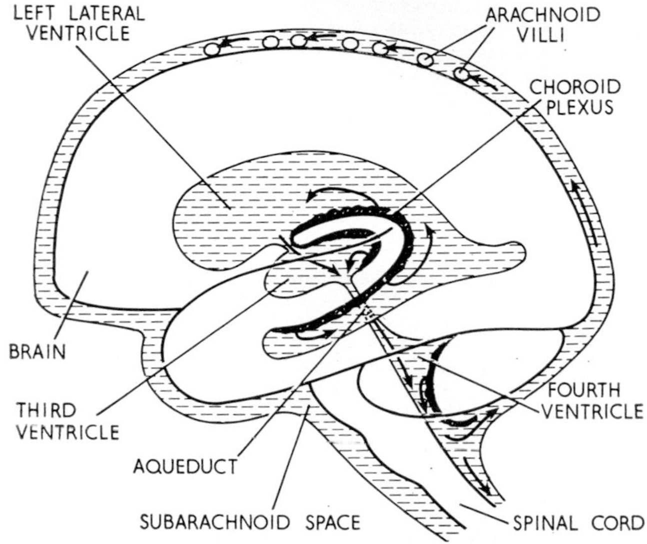

Fig. 54. DIAGRAM OF SKULL AND BRAIN, SHOWING THE VENTRICLES AND THE CIRCULATION OF CEREBROSPINAL FLUID.

The *nursing care* of hydrocephalic children is chiefly concerned with the prevention of pressure sores and of hypostatic pneumonia. Owing to the considerable weight of the head, these patients are unable to move themselves freely and they have to be turned carefully every few hours. The weight of the head also causes great pressure on the scalp and ingenuity is needed if pressure sores are to be avoided. Soft pillows are unsuitable for young children but foam rubber pads covered with some washable material give the necessary softness. Sometimes an extra ring of foam rubber can be used to give added protection to any prominence on the skull.

When lifting the infant from his cot the head must be picked up first and given adequate support before the rest of the baby is lifted out. It is unnecessary and unkind to deprive these infants of the usual "cuddle" for fear of "breaking the neck" and skill and the help of a soft pillow, on which to support the head while feeding, makes it perfectly possible to pick them up in the usual way.

Babies with hydrocephalus often have pretty faces which

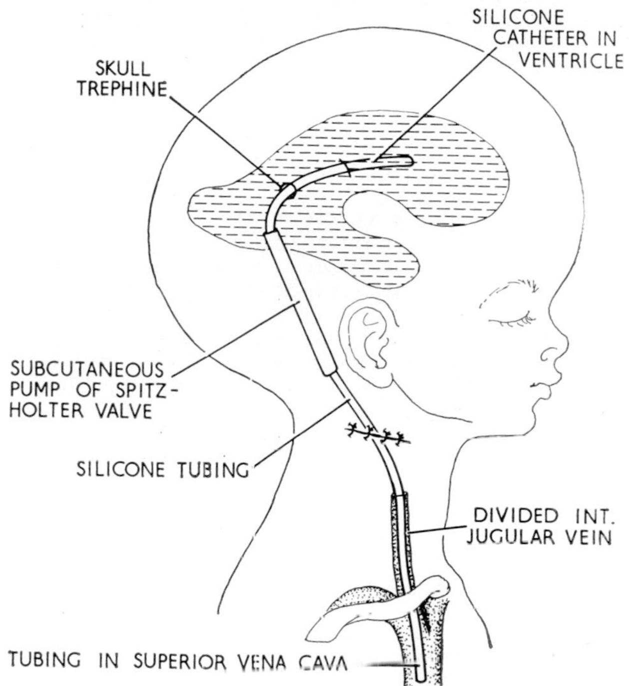

Fig. 55. Diagram of a Child with Hydrocephalus Treated by Drainage with the Aid of a Spitz-Holter Valve.

seem doubly dainty compared with the large vault of the skull. The forehead is usually drawn up tightly and it is not always possible for these infants to close their eyelids. Castor oil or Albucid 1 per cent drops should be instilled every four hours to keep the cornea moist and free from infection and injury.

Some hydrocephalic babies are troubled by persistent vomiting. In these cases the feeds should be small and frequent, and diluted or Bengerized milk is sometimes well tolerated even though the vomiting is of cerebral and not of digestive origin. Special care must be taken to avoid inhalation of vomitus. Convulsions and screaming attacks are common, and should be dealt with in the usual way.

In many instances the condition is not amenable to treatment and the infant survives for a year or more and may present a grave problem within a family. Many are alert and intelligent in spite of their deformity. They should never be allowed to vegetate, but their cots should be raised so that they can look around, and they should be given extra attention whenever possible to keep them happy and help them to develop.

If these children are nursed in general pædiatric wards, nurses should always remember that they may seem frightening or repulsive to other children and to lay personnel. Their beds should therefore be appropriately placed and their heads covered by a shawl or a pretty bonnet.

In some children the condition is arrested spontaneously. If this happens before there is damage to the brain, they may be able to lead a near-normal life, attending ordinary school and attaining average standards of education.

Spina Bifida

Spina bifida is a congenital abnormality due to a defect in the formation of the skeletal arch enclosing the spinal cord. It occurs most frequently in the lumbar region but may be present anywhere along the spinal column or even on the skull.

There are various degrees of this abnormality. In the mildest there is nothing beyond the bony defect. Next in severity is the *meningocele* in which case the spinal meninges herniate and the sac contains cerebrospinal fluid. If the sac contains nerve tissue as well as fluid the lesion is called *meningomyelocele.* Motor and sensory loss are often associated with this type of deformity; early operation may lessen the danger of these becoming worse, as the risk of infection is thus removed. The most severe type is not compatible with life, as the central canal is exposed on the surface of the body and the sac is filled with nerve tissue.

Occasionally it is possible to excise the sac with good results, but often the patient develops a hydrocephalus following the operation and, when nerve tissue is involved, paralysis may result. In many instances operation cannot be attempted and treatment is confined to supplying a more adequate covering for the sac and so preventing infection. This can be done by means of a skin graft or with the aid of some device such as a polythene or rubber case. Rings, made of foam rubber, are often a good means of support and protection.

Figs. 56–57. Myelocele Protection used in Connection with Tulle gras or a Dry Dressing.

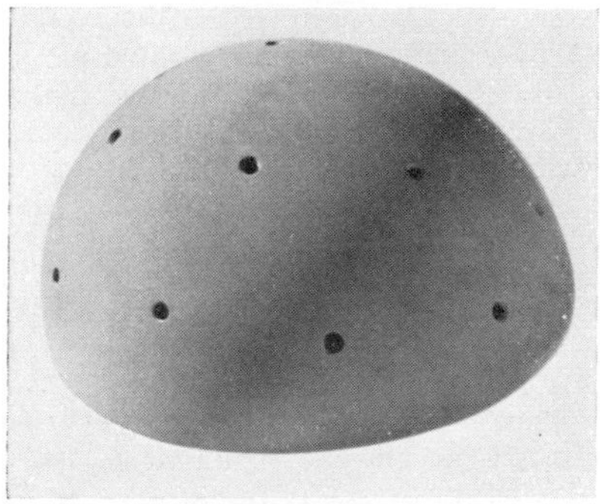

Fig. 56 (*above*) Semi-rigid perforated rubber cap made from an ordinary rubber ball.

Fig. 57. (*below*) Protection made from an ordinary kitchen sieve. The handle can be sawn off and tapes attached to the stump and the two hooks. This device allows for free circulation of air.

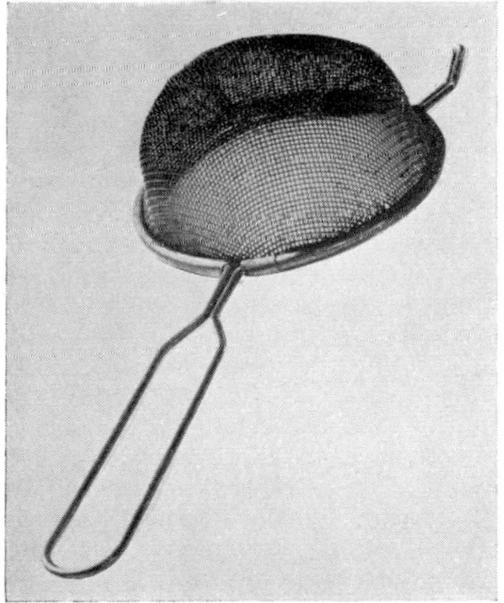

The *nursing care* mainly aims at keeping the area dry and clean, not always an easy task with a young baby. The protruding sac must also be kept free of friction, and injury and abrasions prevented. The skin is best covered with a soft sterile dressing or tulle gras and a protective barrier should be devised between the buttocks and the meningocele. It is often most satisfactory to nurse these infants in the prone position by means of building up pillows and sand bags. The chief difficulty is to leave the face free and to give an adequate air way. Special care should be taken to prevent trophic ulceration and to keep these babies warm, bearing in mind the fact that many are paralysed and lack sensory appreciation. A bed cradle can be used but this should be covered with soft bandages to prevent the baby injuring himself on the frame of the cradle. Warmth can be supplied by hot-water bottles secured around and outside the structure of the cradle.

The prognosis is poor as removal of the sac frequently leads to complications which leave the patient no better off; and in any case there is no hope of improving the sensory or motor disturbances already present. Many of the lesions break down, become infected and set up a meningitis from which the infant rarely recovers.

Some Behaviour Problems

Enuresis

A child who repeatedly passes urine involuntarily at an age when he can normally be expected to be toilet-trained is said to be suffering from enuresis. He may either never have been dry, or may have relapsed after a period of normal control of micturition. Wetting may occur several times a night, very occasionally, or perhaps once or twice per month.

Causes include renal infections, nephrosis, diabetes, psychological disturbances, congenital abnormalities of the urinary tract, spina bifida, neurological lesions, mental subnormality, chronic constipation, and intestinal worms. A frequent cause is behaviour disturbance following the birth of a new baby, a change to a new school, a severe illness or other experience causing a loss of security.

Full investigations of the renal tract are usually done to exclude organic disease, and if these are negative, psychological treatment may be advised. This will include full enquiry into home background, and the parents will be interviewed as well as the child. They may be advised to restrict fluid intake during the evening, to rouse the child and offer a pot before they themselves go to bed and to leave a small light burning. Punishment and scolding are as a rule out of place, although an overworked exasperated mother may well be forgiven if she loses patience with the child. Constant wet sheets may be a great trial in a small town flat and the criticism of neighbours is not easy to bear.

Every small improvement should be hailed as a hopeful sign and encouragement and praise given whenever possible. Sometimes drugs are given which dry up secretions or relax the bladder. Others are prescribed to lighten sleep so that the stimulus of a full bladder can waken the child (e.g. Dexedrine). A "conditioned reflex" can be created in older children by using a specially designed buzzer which goes off and rouses the child as he starts to void urine. Properly used these may score successes in 75 per cent. of cases treated.

Fæcal Incontinence (*Encopresis*)

Fæcal incontinence, i.e., soiling at an age when a child may reasonably be expected to be toilet-trained, may be due to a number of reasons. A common cause is constipation with overflow, and reasons for this situation range from "pot refusal" due to painful anal fissure in toddlers, to emotional disturbances, congenital abnormalities and bad housing conditions. Another example is the child who notes his mother's distress if he does not have his bowels open regularly and uses bowel function to attract attention, "please" or "punish". Sometimes the lavatory itself is to blame: it may be situated on a dark landing in an old tenement building or in the garden, or it may be so high that the child dreads using it for fear of falling in.

The cause of fæcal incontinence should therefore be investigated very carefully and patiently. Good teamwork between parents, pædiatrician, Child Guidance Clinic and Health Visitor will usually cure the condition, but sometimes repeated enemata or such medicines as Isogel or Senokot may be prescribed.

Although chronic constipation very frequently has a psychological background, it is also a common complication in mentally subnormal children and in those suffering from such conditions as spina bifida and neuromuscular diseases. If due to psychological reasons, the condition usually starts after the child has been successfully toilet-trained. Strange habits such as passing a stool "secretly" and "hiding" it in strange places may develop. Only skilled psychiatric treatment can successfully cure such children.

18

DISEASES OF THE SKIN

Infantile Eczema

Infantile eczema mostly affects very young children. It is rarely seen before the age of three months and with the exception of localized patches may be expected to clear up by the age of 2 to 3 years. A definite family history of eczema, asthma or hay fever is typical and some children who suffer from eczema in infancy develop asthma later in life.

Boys are more frequently affected than girls and the babies are often blue-eyed, fair-haired and frequently delightful patients to look after. Allergy to certain foods such as eggs, fish, cow's milk and certain pollen or household dust can sometimes be found, either by taking a careful history or by performing intradermal tests.

Signs and Symptoms. The rash is commonly first noticed over the forehead, cheeks and scalp but the areas around the mouth stay clear. As the eczema spreads the flexures of the elbows and knees and the folds behind the ears become affected and patchy areas may occur in any part of the body. Initially the skin is red, hot and scaly but soon papules and vesicles appear and as they break down clear serum exudes from the lesion. This is known as weeping eczema and at this stage the skin easily becomes infected. Irritation is intense and it may be almost impossible to stop the infant from scratching. As the exudate dries up thick crusts are formed. In spite of the extensive lesions, eczema leaves no scars.

Treatment. This often includes a full investigation of the possible exciting causes. Intradermal tests with certain proteins, pollen or dust may show a positive reaction to a certain agent which can then be eliminated from the diet or the child's environment. Psychological disturbances may be present and both parents and patient need guidance and psychotherapy. Dietary idiosyncrasies must be corrected and certain foods may have to be excluded from the diet. Starchy foods should be given in moderation, but extra protein in the form of Casilan or Complan are useful during the acute, weeping stage. Occasionally there is an intolerance of cow's milk and this can be substituted by soya-bean "milk". Special dried milks such as Allergilac (Cow & Gate) are on the market.

Local Treatment. This includes the use of coal tar preparations, calamine lotion with or without an oily base and the addition of a mild antiseptic. More recently creams containing hydrocortisone have been used with good effect though improvement is often not maintained when treatment is discontinued. Irritation may be allayed by giving medicated baths, and bath time is often the only happy time in a baby's day. A 1 per cent. solution of common salt may be used, or sodium sulphate to make a 1 per cent. solution to which is added unguentum emulsificans, a soothing preparation which is used instead of soap and also aids the separation of crusts. A soft towel should be used for drying and the skin gently dabbed and never rubbed.

The Applications. These vary according to the stage of the rash. When dry and scaly, creams or liniments may be ordered. They are either applied direct to the skin and left exposed or thinly spread on to old linen and bandaged to the affected area. Infected areas may be treated with some kind of antiseptic lotion or cream such as, for instance, proflavine or an antibiotic. When weeping eczema has caused crusts to form, starch poultices may be used to soften the scabs. It is usual to leave a starch poultice on for 6 to 12 hours and on no account should the starch be allowed to dry up. When the poultice is due to be removed, a small dressing tray is taken to the bedside. After removing the poultice the remaining scabs are gently loosened with the help of olive swabs and dressing forceps and any lotion or cream applied as ordered. Bandages should always be of the open woven type as they are cooler and more economical than other types. Tubegauz is very useful as it is easy to keep in position, porous and light. The skin of convalescent children can be suitably protected by Tubegauz "sleeves, stockings and mittens". When elbow splints are applied, they should be made of spatulæ or cardboard (see page 92) and a minimum of padding used to avoid overheating the skin. Any knots should be tied on the posterior aspect of the splint so that the child cannot rub his face on them.

Nursing Care. The brunt of the treatment will fall on the mother or nursing staff. Irritation is intense and the infant manages to scratch by every possible means. Even when the extremities are effectively restrained he manages to wriggle his little body and roll his head and if inadvertently released, a newly healed area may be scratched to bleeding point in next to no time. Mittens made of Tubegauz (see page 92) may have to be left on during a bath to prevent scratching and the hands always dried first and clean mittens applied after a bath.

The infant should be kept cool and well occupied. During the acute stages it is necessary in many cases to secure rest and sleep by sedation. Special smooth sheets should be used. With small children it has been found useful to nurse them on a large sheet of X-ray film or acetate sheets which are smooth and cool and can easily be cleaned. Tied to the mattress this can be a most effective means to comfort. Clothes must be light and cool and should be of thin cotton or silk. The patients are often happiest if left entirely without clothes. They are best done up in the front as buttons or tapes down the back give the baby an opportunity for scratching by moving his body. Mittens and socks can be used to keep the extremities warm but they should be of cool light cotton or Tubegauz. The bedclothes are best cradled and an electric fan may be used to keep the air circulating and cool. Sedatives such as chloral hydrate in large doses, Benadryl, Phenergan and Disprin may be ordered. It is usual to admit these infants into cubicles to minimize the danger of cross infection but this consideration must be carefully weighed against the need for company and diversion. Extra visiting and attention from the mother are desirable not only because she can divert the infant but also because she can learn to handle her child and assist with the care of his skin while under expert supervision. Thus she will gain confidence and the child will learn to accept treatment from her. A good ward sister may also be able to observe any psychological conflicts which may exist between mother and child.

Children suffering from eczema are prone to bronchitis and gastro-intestinal upsets. The latter may cause alarming losses of weight and apparent wasting due to the loss of abnormal fluid present in the tissues. Both these complications may prove serious and babies with infantile eczema should be nursed with special care. Exposure to infection is minimized by admission to a cubicle or a "clean" ward. Barrier gowns are worn and anyone suffering from a cold should keep away from these babies. Exacerbations during teething are common.

Care has to be taken to avoid indiscretions in the diet where an allergy is known to exist. Not infrequently there is a definite psychological background, as in many allergic conditions. This point must never be ignored and a child guidance expert may be able to help and advise. A happy emotional background is of great importance. The mother-child relationship should always be carefully examined, but even if the mother is entirely adequate, exhaustion from nursing the child and constant disturbed nights may be so great that a period of rest is imperative and the infant's admission to hospital unavoidable. A calm but non-restrictive atmosphere in the home is of prime importance.

Immunization and Vaccination. Children with eczema can be treated as any others with regard to immunization. Vaccination against smallpox may, however, be highly dangerous and the child should never be allowed to go near another child recently vaccinated. There is a great risk of generalized vaccinia together with severe toxic symptoms. This very serious condition is known as Kaposi's varicelliform dermatitis. Kaposi's dermatitis is, however, more often due to infection by the virus of herpes simplex.

Making a Starch Poultice. One tablespoon of starch powder, half a teaspoon of boracic powder and boiling water are needed. The starch and boracic powder are mixed with a little cold water to form a smooth paste. Boiling water is then poured on to the paste while stirring rapidly until the starch has turned from a white paste to an opaque mucilage. When this has been allowed to cool it is spread on to old linen of an appropriate size and shape and applied. The skin is sometimes previously softened by a medicated bath. The poultice is left on for 6 to 12 hours but should never be allowed to become dry.

NOTE. Unless the water is really boiling the starch cannot be expected to set. The mixing bowl should be taken to the boiling kettle in the same manner as one would take the teapot to the kettle, and not vice versa.

Impetigo Contagiosa

Impetigo is a skin infection caused by the streptococcus or staphylococcus. It is very common in children of school age and spreads easily, particularly in overcrowded homes with poor hygiene. The organism enters the skin through a crack or a scratch and for that reason is often associated with an infested head.

At first small vesicles appear and as they break the lesion becomes red and weeping and as the exudate dries up thick crusts form. Typical sites are on the scalp, the chin and around the lips. The crusts have the appearance of being "stuck on".

Local Treatment. This consists in softening the crusts with olive oil, warm saline bathings or a solution of potassium permanganate 1 in 4,000. A starch poultice may be applied (see page 321). The skin may be painted with an antiseptic preparation such as boracic cream, gentian violet 1 per cent. aqueous solution or an antibiotic cream. Occasionally antibiotics may be ordered by mouth if the infection is severe or fails to respond to local treatment. If the hair is crusted, a small area may have to be shaved after obtaining medical and parental consent.

The child suffering from impetigo is likely to infect others and if admitted to hospital should be nursed with barrier precautions. Crockery and cutlery should be sterilized until the last lesion has healed. Scratching is prevented by splinting in the same way as in the case of infantile eczema (see page 320).

The condition may clear within a few days and rarely leaves any scars. Recurrence should be prevented by giving the mother guidance with regard to personal hygiene and building up the child's general resistance, by good diet, exercise in the fresh air and an adequate vitamin intake.

Scabies

Scabies is a skin infestation caused by a minute parasite. The female mite burrows into the skin where she lays her eggs, and it is usually possible to see the burrows with the help of a magnifying glass. As the eggs hatch, the larvæ move to the hair follicles. Intense irritation results and this is particularly marked when the skin becomes warm at night. In young babies the soft skin allows for access in any part and lesions are found anywhere on the body. In babies who have not started walking, lesions may even occur on the soft skin of the soles of the feet. Secondary infections are common as a result of scratching.

Treatment. This aims at softening the skin and opening the burrows prior to the application of benzyl benzoate (25 per cent. solution). The patient is given a warm bath after which the skin is dabbed dry and the whole body painted with benzyl benzoate and allowed to dry. On the second day the body is again painted all over and on the third day a final bath is given. After that, both personal clothing and bed linen are changed. The infected clothing and linen are sterilized by boiling or by pressing with a hot iron.

Benzyl benzoate may sting on application, particularly if

there are open scratch-wounds. Care must be taken not to apply the lotion too near the eyes. For small infants Eurax 10 per cent. ointment may be used instead of the benzyl benzoate. This is applied in the same manner as benzyl benzoate.

19

DISEASES OF MUSCLE, BONES AND JOINTS

Muscular Dystrophies (Myopathies)

A number of variants of the myopathies exist which all have the characteristics of progressive, degenerative changes in the muscle fibres, leading to wasting and weakness. The nerves are not affected in this group and there are neither sensory changes nor paralysis. The diseases are often hereditary and familial and usually lead to early death due to intercurrent infections such as pneumonia. A proportion of children with muscular dystrophy are mentally handicapped but the majority are of normal intelligence.

The various types of myopathies affect different muscle groups in particular, causing degenerative changes in the muscle fibres and their replacement by connective tissue and fat. Whole groups of muscles may thus be weakened and although the process may be a very slow one, it is always progressive and the patient eventually becomes completely incapacitated and crippled.

Diagnosis. This is confirmed by electromyography by which means the changes can be differentiated from those in other diseases of muscles. The destruction of muscle causes excretion of creatinine in the urine.

Pseudo-hypertrophic Muscular Dystrophy

The most common of the myopathies in childhood is pseudo-hypertrophic muscular dystrophy so called because of the enlargement of certain muscles in this condition.

Signs and Symptoms. The child may be normal up to school age but gradually it is noticed that he tires easily, that he prefers to sit about rather than play with other children, and finds it difficult to walk up stairs without the help of the banister. The gait becomes unstable and he is easily pushed over in play. The muscles of the shoulder girdle may become so weak that the child cannot raise his arms above his head and when the doctor places his hands underneath the arms to lift the patient, the child literally slips through his hands.

Weakness of the muscles of the pelvic girdle and the spine lead to kyphosis and lordosis. The gait is waddling at first and later walking becomes impossible. When the child tries to raise himself from the lying position, he first has to roll on to his front and then raise himself on to his hands and knees; by gradually moving one hand after the other up his legs and above his knees he eventually succeeds in raising himself to the upright position. This manœuvre is very characteristic of the disease.

As the muscular weakness progresses the child becomes bedridden and deformities through contractions develop.

Treatment. This aims at preventing crippling and wasting by massage and exercises. Movement should be encouraged as disuse leads to more rapid wasting. Pneumonia usually causes death after a few years.

Other Types of the Myopathies. These affect specific muscle groups in particular. The rate of progress may vary greatly and in spite of crippling the patient may survive into middle age. The more common varieties are the facio-scapulo-humeral type and myotonia-congenita. As the name implies, the muscles affected in the facio-scapulo-humeral type, are those of the face, arms and shoulder girdle. The first signs may be difficulty in sucking and in closing the eyes completely. The handicap is as a rule slight and a fairly normal existence is possible. Myotonia congenita causes voluntary muscles to go into protracted contractions followed by slow relaxation. Muscle biopsy shows enlargement and thickening of muscle fibres. Muscle biopsy and electromyography are usually carried out to confirm diagnosis as the changes in the electrical activity in the muscle and those in the structure of the muscles are characteristic of the various types of the disease.

Torticollis (Wry Neck)

Torticollis may be present from birth or arise later in life caused by diseases such as inflamed glands of the neck, tuberculosis of the cervical spine and paralysis. Occasionally the cause is psychological.

The postural changes are characteristic and include rotation of the head to one side with head flexion and a raising of the shoulder on the other. If allowed to persist, the angle at which the head is constantly held causes visual disturbances.

Treatment. This depends on the child's age and on the underlying cause. In infants stretching and passive exercises should be carried out several times daily and correct posture maintained by means of sandbags and possibly a cap and light harness made of 1-inch webbing. Collars made of corrugated paper covered with a piece of soft material, Perspex splints and supports and collars made from plaster of Paris are used to keep the head in an over-corrected position. In resistant cases, subcutaneous or open tenotomy may have to be carried out to lengthen the sternomastoid muscle. Post-operative over-correction is maintained for some time by one of the methods given above.

Sternomastoid Tumour

Difficult labour associated with excessive rotation and lateral extension of the neck and head are occasionally the cause of a sternomastoid tumour. The tumour is rarely noticed before the baby is about two weeks old. It is painless and firm and the size varies from a small lump the size of a pea to that of a walnut. The condition is harmless and resolves spontaneously after some weeks. Passive movement and massage are given to help recovery and minimize any risk of permanent torticollis from habitually wrong posture.

Perthes' Disease

Although the cause is rarely known, Perthes' disease is probably caused by injury to the hip joint. The disease almost always affects boys of 3 to 8 years but occasionally Perthes' disease follows correction of a congenital dislocation of the hip joint in girls. Pain may be absent or referred to the thigh and knee, the general health is unaffected, the erythrocyte sedimentation rate is normal and a limp is often the first sign of the disease.

Examination. This reveals that the range of movement is limited in all directions. Changes may not show up on X-ray for some time. During the initial stages of the disease there are degenerative changes in the head of the femur and rarefaction of the epiphysis leading to flattening of the femoral head. This is called mushrooming. After several months' rest the area recalcifies. At this stage X-ray appearance is mottled like a snow storm. Healing may not be complete for one or two years.

Treatment. This concentrates on preventing deformity of the femoral head by relieving pressure on it and by immobilization. This is done by traction and splinting until there is evidence of regeneration. After that, walking with a non-weight-bearing caliper may be started. There are various methods of immobilizing the hip joint and some splints allow for a great deal of freedom and general mobility while achieving traction and local immobilization. Alternatively trochanteric osteotomy is performed. This may shorten the course of treatment considerably. The reason for this is at present unexplained.

Nursing Care. This includes daily removal of the bandages and care of the skin and release of the groin strap and corset for toilet purposes. The groin strap is undone twice daily and the groin washed and carefully dried. Powder, zinc and castor oil cream (with or without the addition of a little compound tincture of benzoin sufficient to colour the cream a light brown) and padding with a layer of lint are various ways by which any initial soreness can be prevented. The patient usually gets used to the strap after a short time.

General muscle tone should be maintained by giving daily massage and exercises. As the stay in hospital may extend over many months, schooling and occupational therapy should be made available and whenever possible little treats such as outings or a week-end visit home can be arranged.

Prognosis. This is excellent provided adequate, early treatment is given but late cases may develop severe arthritis when they grow older.

Congenital Dislocation of the Hip Joint

Congenital dislocation of the hip joint occurs mostly in fair-haired, blue-eyed girls; the condition runs in families and although usually present at birth it is often not noticed until the child begins to walk.

Signs and Symptoms. When the baby is examined lying on her back, the thighs are flexed at the hips and the knees rotated outwards at right angles. If there is a dislocation, movement is limited, particularly on abduction, and sometimes a definite click can be felt on rotation. The perineum is wider than usual and sometimes a telescoping movement of the leg is possible. One leg may be shorter than the other. When the child is lying prone, the gluteal crease on the affected side is higher than that on the good side, and the buttocks may be flattened.

Children with congenital dislocation of the hip joint have an abnormally shallow acetabulum which causes the femoral head to be displaced upwards and backwards when the child begins to put weight upon the limb. The neck of the femur may be shortened and the capsule becomes stretched. Sometimes the femoral head lies outside the acetabulum at the time of birth. As the child walks she dips on the affected side or has a waddling gait if the dislocation is a bilateral one. Because the pelvis is tipped forward, lordosis develops.

Treatment

This should be started as soon as the condition has been recognized as its duration and success depend on the age of the child. In very young babies a special webbing harness may be used. Older children may be placed on a special abduction frame and skin traction is applied to bring the head of the

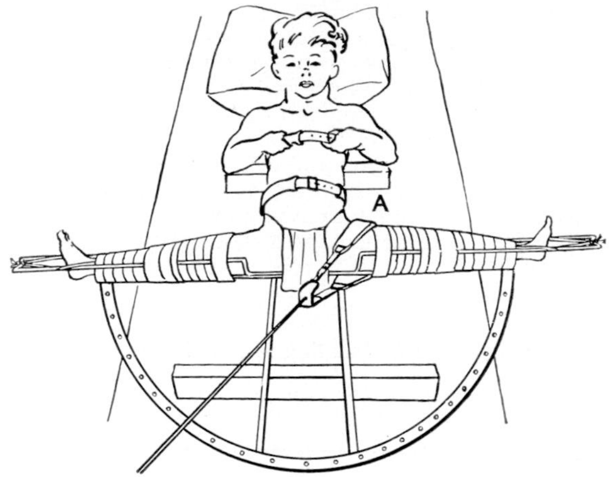

Fig. 58. Complete Abduction of Both Legs.
A. indicates cross pull over felt to get the head of the femur into the acetabulum.

femur into position opposite the acetabulum. The legs are gradually abducted, one leg at a time, at intervals of 2 or 3 days to allow for gradual stretching of the muscles. When both legs have been abducted to right angles to the trunk, the child is taken to the theatre (Fig. 58).

Two different methods of treatment are commonly used, depending on the age of the child, X-ray appearance and the surgeon's wishes:

1. The dislocation is reduced and the legs rotated to bring the femoral head into the acetabulum. The legs are fixed externally rotated and in full abduction with the knees flexed at right angles to the femora. A so-called *"frog plaster"* is applied, which reaches from the nipple line to the ankles.

2. The dislocation is reduced, the femora internally rotated and the legs fully abducted from the knees downward. A plaster, reaching from the groins to the ankles enables the child to move freely in the hip joint while maintaining flexion and extension. A wooden cross-bar is incorporated into the plaster from one knee across to the other: this is called a *Batchelor plaster* (Fig. 59). After a time the child learns to move about and even to "walk" on her knees.

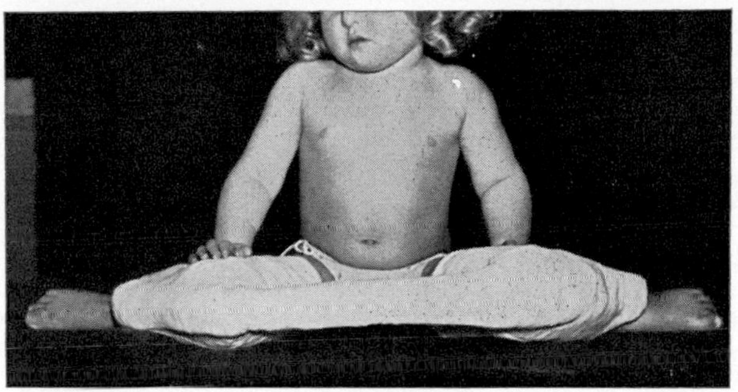

Fig. 59. Batchelor Plaster.

In either case treatment has to be continued for a year to 18 months and during that time the child may be discharged home and brought back for changes of plaster at intervals of approximately 3 months. Occasionally neither of these methods is successful and open reduction and rotation osteotomy to correct the angle of the femur on the hip may be necessary. In very persistent cases shelf operation, acetabuloplasty, is performed to deepen the acetabulum, and a hip spica applied.

Nursing Care

During the stage of abduction the child suffers considerable discomfort and frustration due to the immobility and her position on the frame. Firm sympathy, a great deal of individual attention and occupation and free visiting all help to comfort the child and in the initial stages sedatives should be given generously. The nurse will have to use much patience and imagination to get the child to take fluids and food in this position and to teach her to pass urine and fæces without unduly soiling the padding of the frame. The bandages are taken off the legs daily and the skin inspected for reaction to strapping. They are washed and powdered before re-applying the bandages. The frame padding or plaster can be protected by thin plastic sheeting or waterproof adhesive tape.

After manipulation and application of the plaster the new position will again cause distress for some days and sleep may be very light and disturbed. Individual small pillows to support arms, shoulders and feet should be available. Even though the plaster is left exposed to allow for drying, the chest and extremities should be covered with little blankets, bootees and mittens. The toes should be carefully watched. They should be warm and rosy and should flush quickly with blood on release of digital pressure. The patient is turned 4-hourly to ensure drying of the plaster on the back as well as the front.

As soon as the plaster has set, the child should be turned on to her side and front at intervals for change of position and to reduce abdominal distension as far as possible and give a different outlook. A special watch should be kept for possible plaster sores. The young child is unable to express her pain and discomfort but restlessness, itching, fretfulness and a slight rise in temperature should all be considered carefully as possible signs of trouble. It must always be remembered that, once the sore deepens, all pain disappears. A foul smell and staining of the plaster are later, more obvious signs that a sore has developed. As the child digs her elbows into the bed in an attempt at raising herself to look round, the elbows are particularly liable to get sore. Heels and ankles should also have attention and be kept off the bed by support with small pillows or heel rings while lying down. Various adjustable frames (Figs. 60–61) with a detachable tray can be used to support the child in the upright position and some children can even manage to "walk" in a frog plaster.

Treatment has to continue over a period of 1 to 2 years depending in part on the age of the child, as the longer the condition has been left untreated the more difficult is successful treatment. When the plaster is eventually omitted, the child is at first allowed the freedom of the bed. Daily physiotherapy is given and after about 3 weeks, if X-ray appearance is satis-

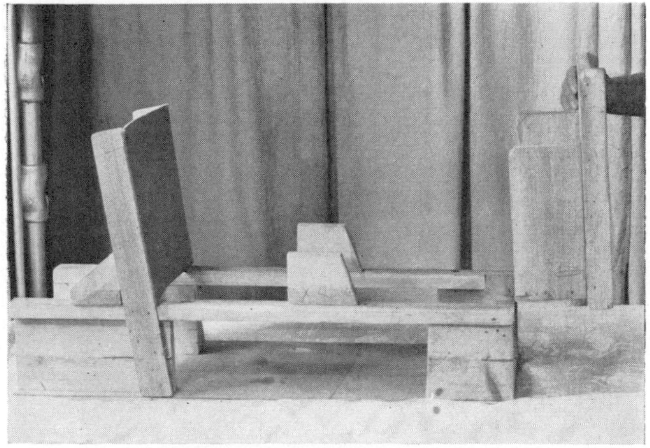

Figs. 60–61. Wooden Frame for Children with Congenital Dislocation of the Hip Joint, Treated in Frog Plaster.

A detachable tray placed on top of the frame makes a good table for toys and at meal times. For toilet purposes, a "pottie" or bedpan can be inserted underneath the opening in the seat.

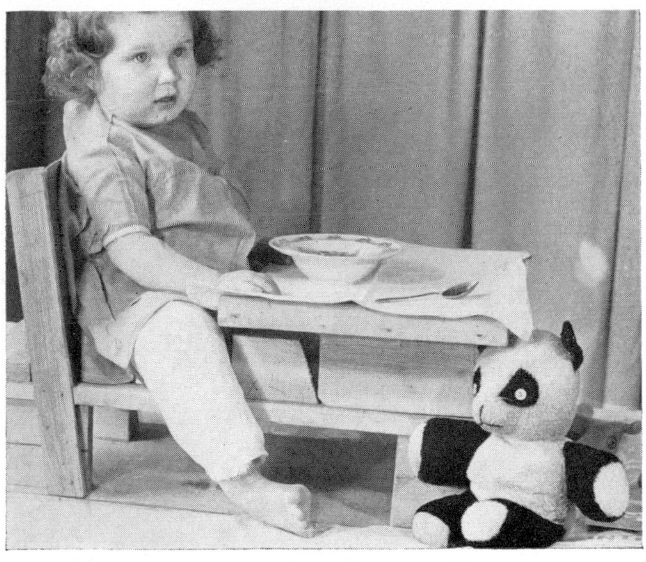

factory, is allowed to start weight-bearing. In early, successful cases, walking should be normal and a complete, permanent cure can be expected.

If home conditions are good, the child is usually sent home and only readmitted for change of plaster and reassessment at intervals of two to three months. The mother can be taught how to keep the plaster clean and special little supports and chairs can be made at low cost to facilitate sitting up and for toilet purposes. If the child has to remain in hospital, everything should be done to keep up contact with the home by allowing free visiting and if possible week-end visits home. Suitable occupation and little outings to the hospital grounds or even the surrounding streets are important if the young child is to be given a chance of developing the experiences appropriate to her age. If these points are neglected it may well happen that as a result of treatment the hip joint is normal at the expense of serious psychological disturbance in the young patient.

Talipes (Club Foot)

Talipes may occur on one or both sides and is often associated with other congenital abnormalities such as spina bifida. There are four types, and any may be seen in varying degrees of severity.

1. *Talipes equinovarus.* The deformity consists of inversion (turning in) of the forefoot, internal rotation of the tibia and plantar flexion of the ankle joint.
2. *Talipes calcaneovalgus.* The deformity consists of eversion (turning out) of the foot and dorsiflexion at the ankle joint. The tendo Achillis is lengthened. This deformity is less severe and yields more easily to treatment than the equinovarus deformity.
3. *Talipes equinovalgus.* In this deformity there is eversion and plantar flexion.
4. *Talipes calcaneovarus.* In this deformity there is inversion and dorsiflexion.

The two last mentioned types are rare.

Treatment

This should be started within 36 hours of birth and its success depends greatly on the promptness with which it is started. The foot is manipulated manually until the little toe touches the peroneal surface of the leg. The over-corrected position is maintained by adhesive strapping, splints, plaster of Paris or special Denis Browne boots. Manipulation is repeated weekly at first. Kicking and standing on the splints when the child is old enough are encouraged as this helps to develop the leg muscles.

Manipulation often causes reactionary swelling and as treatment is often given in the out-patient department full instructions to bring her baby back if there is reason for concern, should be given to the mother, in the same way as would be done in cases of fractures treated by plaster of Paris. If the baby is treated while in the maternity ward, the weight of the bedclothes is taken off by using a cradle and the feet are inspected frequently to make sure that swelling is not excessive and that there is no serious constriction to the blood supply. As it would seriously interfere with treatment if the splints were to be left off, even for short periods, it is necessary to persevere regardless of strapping reactions or even blistering of the skin. If treated from birth correction may be complete by the age of 6 months or a year, but a special night boot is usually worn for another year or two. Occasionally the outside of the shoe heel is raised or an inside iron with a "T" strap fixed to the shoes when the baby starts to walk. Cases treated less promptly, may need many years of treatment and cure may not be permanent. Parents are usually very pleased with the initial improvement and it may be difficult to impress on them the importance of continuing treatment for a number of years. Sometimes manipulation, stretching and splinting fail and operation becomes necessary. This may be either open or closed tenotomy, Steindler's operation or triple arthrodesis. Supervision by the orthopædic surgeon is as a rule maintained until growth is complete.

Osteomyelitis

Osteomyelitis used to be one of the most severe illnesses of childhood usually affecting children whose general health was poor and who came from overcrowded homes. With the advent of modern drug therapy the outlook has greatly improved, but the patient may still be seriously ill and relapses are common.

The disease usually attacks children between the ages of 5 and 10 years. The femur, humerus and clavicle are common sites of infection and there may be evidence of a recent knock or injury. There is frequently a history of infected tonsils, boils or septic spots and the causative organism is then in many cases a staphylococcus, although in recent years other organisms, e.g. *E. coli*, have caused osteomyelitis. The condition in the latter case is not so acute, but the site has to be drained more often before the infection is overcome.

Signs and Symptoms. The onset may be acute with hyperpyrexia, tachycardia, headaches, rigor, toxæmia or septicæmia, but at times it may be quite insidious. Infants appear to have little pain, but the general disturbances include vomiting and diarrhœa, causing dehydration. In older children pain can be very severe until tension subsides following the discharge or release of pus or decrease of infection following treatment with antibiotics. The limb is held immobilized in a relaxed position and occasionally the condition may be mistaken for some form of paralysis. Any handling is deeply resented. The skin over the affected area may be found to be red, shiny and hot, although it may take a day or two for the inflammation to become obvious. The white cell count is high (mainly polymorphonuclear cells) and blood culture is sometimes positive. X-ray appearance is rarely abnormal before the second or third week.

Treatment. Large doses of antibiotics together with immobilization, may bring about a cure, but sometimes the patient does not respond well.

Nursing Care. As there may be exquisite pain, jarring of the bed must be avoided and for that reason the bed should be situated in a corner of the ward in the acute stage. Temperature, pulse and respirations are taken every 4 hours and fluid intake and output charts kept up to date. Abundant fluids are given and as the child is often negative and reluctant to drink, it is important to vary the drinks by using different flavours and by alternating hot and cold drinks. Savoury fluids, such as Bovril or Marmite are at times taken when sweet drinks are refused. They serve the additional purpose of causing thirst because of their high salt content. Once the fever has subsided, a nourishing, high protein diet is given to build up the child's general health. Small pillows, sandbags and air rings should be used to ensure a comfortable position and rest for the affected part. As the illness may be a long one, the child should be wheeled into the fresh air whenever this is possible and schooling, occupational therapy and extra visiting are important if general morale and happiness are to be maintained.

Achondroplasia

Achondroplasia is a congenital abnormality which runs in families and is characterized by a shortness of the limbs and a large head with marked frontal bossing. The long bones are short, thick and curved and the overlying subcutaneous tissues and skin are in folds as if there were more of them than fits the length of the limb. The hands are broad and the child is unable to extend the elbow joint fully. The ligaments are relaxed and this produces a waddling gait. Growth is slow and this fact, together with the shortness of the long bones causes dwarfism. The patient has a peculiar ability to rise from the sitting position on the ground to the standing position without using his hands. Adults with achondroplasia often earn their living as clowns in a circus. So far there is no known treatment.

Syndactyly

Syndactyly or webbing of the digits of the hands and feet may be partial or complete. The underlying bones and joints may be normal, or sections may be missing or fused. The plastic surgeon may be able to separate the digits and to give the hand an æsthetically good appearance, without much difficulty. Or it may be necessary to utilize one of the fingers as a thumb by transplanting muscles in such a way as to bring one digit into apposition to the others to make gripping possible. Frequently skin grafting is undertaken to supply skin for the surfaces between the divided digits.

In looking after these patients postoperatively it is important to watch for signs of impaired circulation, sometimes a difficult task as the entire hand or foot may be covered in a tight crêpe bandage. Fine judgment may be needed in assessing any complaints of discomfort the child may make. As a rule children are very adaptable and manage to lead a normal life in spite of their handicap and up to the age of approximately 10 years they rarely seem aware of, or disturbed by their appearance.

Osteogenesis Imperfecta (Fragilitas Ossium)

As the name suggests the bones in fragilitas ossium are fragile and fractures occur on the least provocation. There are two main types of the disease. In the antenatal variety most of the bones of the fœtal skull and skeleton have sustained fractures before birth. Callus formation causes the bones to be thickened and deformed. Babies with this complaint have markedly blue sclerotics. The condition is familial and severe cases become seriously handicapped, while others die at birth due to fractures occurring during labour.

In the second variety the fractures occur mostly after the first year of life. The bones are porous and the teeth translucent. Although the fractures heal rapidly, deformities inevitably result and these children lead sheltered lives with schooling frequently interrupted by treatment or admissions to hospital. Occasionally the condition improves at puberty. Neither the cause nor any effective treatment are known.

Correction of Deformities caused by Paralysis

The abnormal and imbalanced pull of certain muscle groups against others weakened by paralysis can cause severe and progressive deformities in the growing child. Surgical treatment is often necessary to prevent deformity and to stabilize joints and so to improve function. The results of infantile paralysis, congenital abnormalities of the spine (e.g. myelomeningocele) and cerebral palsy are examples.

Corrective operations include transplantation of tendons in the leg or foot. This transplantation aims at counteracting an abnormal pull from a group of healthy muscles which would lead to deformity. Transplantation of the tendons of the hamstring muscles, for instance to the back of the femur, may enable a child with spastic paralysis to straighten his knees and to walk almost normally.

Tenotomy may be performed to lengthen certain tendons, a contracted tendo Achillis is a typical example. Paralysis of one leg only, may cause the healthy leg to grow and develop more rapidly than the affected one. The growth of the sound leg can be slowed down by inserting staples into the epiphysis and in this way both legs will be equal and the need for a surgical boot become unnecessary.

The nursing care of these patients is the same as for any child in plaster or extension and should not present any special problems.

20

TUBERCULOSIS IN CHILDHOOD

Tuberculosis is not hereditary but it is thought that a susceptibility to tuberculous disease may be inherited. Coloured races seem to be more vulnerable than white. This is probably due to the fact that poverty and malnutrition are widespread amongst such people and that, unless they have been in contact with European or other white peoples, they have little or no natural immunity. Other predisposing causes include bad living conditions, overcrowding, malnutrition and such illnesses as measles and whooping cough.

In Great Britain tuberculosis is a notifiable disease but neither treatment nor segregation of people suffering from it is compulsory.

Immunity

Acquired immunity may develop through infection by repeated small doses of tubercle bacilli. Children living in large cities can become immune in this way, even though the symptoms of infection may be so slight as to go unnoticed. Artificial immunity may be conferred by inoculation with B.C.G. vaccine.

Bacille Calmette-Guérin (*B.C.G.*)

Calmette and Guérin developed non-virulent tubercle bacilli and used them for inoculation. This raises the body resistance to tuberculosis and so immunity is conferred. In some countries all children are immunized, with the result that the incidence of tuberculosis has decreased to negligible proportions. In Great Britain B.C.G. is reserved for those who are exposed to special risks on account of their work, for infants where there is a close relative suffering from tuberculosis and for children about to leave school. In the case of infants the inoculation is done within the first two or three weeks of life and the child tested after approximately 8 weeks, when conversion is likely to have taken place.

Tests

Various tests are used to check whether individuals have

been exposed to tuberculous infection or are infected at the time of exposure. A positive reaction shows that the person has developed immunity after having been infected with tuberculosis or is developing it. These tests include the Mantoux test, the tuberculin jelly or patch test and the Heaf test.

Mantoux Test. In the Mantoux test 0·1 ml. of a 1 in 10,000 solution of Old Tuberculin is injected intradermally into the forearm, sufficient to raise a small bleb. Sometimes additional injections of stronger solutions, up to 1 in 100, are used as well. Some solutions used must not be older than one week. The test is read after 48 and 72 hours respectively and an area of induration of not less than 6 millimetres in diameter is considered to be positive, that is to say the patient has either been exposed to tuberculosis at some time and developed immunity, or is at the present moment suffering from active tuberculous disease.

This test is most valuable under the age of 5 years as a positive Mantoux reaction at that age should put the doctor on the alert in his watch for active tuberculous infection. After the age of 5 years, a positive Mantoux test is not necessarily a reason for concern. Indeed, if the tests are still negative, B.C.G. vaccination will most probably be given in order to protect the child from tuberculosis.

Purified Protein Derivative (P.P.D.) is sometimes used for this test.

Tuberculin Jelly Test. In doing the jelly test the skin between the scapulæ is prepared by cleaning it with acetone to rid it of all grease and, in children more than 5 years old, by rubbing lightly with fine flour paper. Jelly containing Old Tuberculin is applied in "T" form and a piece of adhesive tape applied directly over it. A control test with plain jelly is done at the same time in the form of a "C". The mother is instructed to keep the area dry and to remove the strapping after 48 hours. Small vesicle formation shows the test to be positive. The test is comparable to a Mantoux test in a dilution of 1 in 1,000 and has the advantage of avoiding an injection.

Heaf Test. For Heaf's test a specially designed instrument is used. A solution of Purified Protein Derivative (P.P.D.) is applied to the area. Small punctures are made in the skin by pressure on the plunger of the instrument whose sharp points penetrate the skin. The P.P.D. is absorbed through the punctures. The reaction is similar to that of the Mantoux test and the results are read in the same way and at the same time intervals.

General Nursing Care of Tuberculosis

Since the introduction of modern surgery and drug therapy tuberculosis has lost much of its terror and the vast majority of patients may be expected to make a complete recovery. But the illness is usually a protracted one and general nursing care presents special considerations and problems.

Observations. Primary lesions of tuberculous infection do not always remain confined and it is important that a nurse should at all times be on the alert, for any changes in her patient which might indicate a spread of the disease, so that treatment may be started at the earliest moment. Changes in the pattern of the temperature chart are important. A rising pulse or respiratory rate may point to an aggravation of the toxic state or involvement of a vital part of the respiratory system. Changes in the patient's temperament are often significant. An otherwise cheerful and contented child, who suddenly loses interest or becomes fractious or demanding may for instance be showing early signs of meningitis. Stiffness or reluctance to use a limb should be reported as this may prove to be an early sign of tuberculous disease of a joint or of abscess formation. The excreta should be watched, as pale or relaxed stools, more frequent than usual, may be the first indication that the alimentary tract is becoming involved. Constipation is among the early symptoms of tuberculous meningitis. Frequency of micturition and blood in the urine may be early signs of tuberculosis of the urinary tract.

General Care. Bed rest, fresh air and a diet rich in vitamins and providing adequate calories are the important basic principles in the treatment of all types of tuberculosis.

The child's bed should be in a light place in the ward and preferably near a door or window which can be left open day and night. A french window leading to a garden or balcony is a great asset. Direct exposure to sun should as a rule be avoided but in sanatoria graduated exposure under strict supervision is often part of the treatment. All nursing aids such as bedrests, comfortable pillows, air rings and a good mattress help to make the patient comfortable and more willing to rest quietly.

Barrier nursing is considered unnecessary by the majority of pædiatricians as the type of tuberculous infection from which children suffer is in most cases not harmful to others.

Occasionally, however, the child may be suffering from miliary tuberculosis or there may be positive cerebrospinal fluid, infected discharge or even a productive cough with positive sputum. Strict precautions must then be observed. In addition, any sputum or gastric washings should be adequately disinfected before putting them down the sluice. Sputum containers should if possible be of destructible material. It is best to use paper handkerchiefs as they can be placed in a paper bag and burned after use. Any food left over is wrapped in newspaper and taken to the incinerator instead of the pig bin.

Diet. The basic diet should be augmented by extra milk and cream, and a little butter can be added to all vegetables and potatoes. Special dishes prepared by the patient's own nurse or a particular "treat" brought in by the mother may help to vary the monotony of hospital meals. When anorexia is marked, 5 to 10 millilitres (1½ to 3 drachms) of sherry, given half an hour before meals in a little water and sweetened to taste, is often very helpful and usually enjoyed. Vitamins should be given in liberal amounts, and cod-liver oil is particularly valuable.

Occupation. Adequate occupational facilities for the child are of prime importance and toys and books should be easily accessible to the young patient. Many of these children are well enough to attend hospital school or occupational therapy and during convalescence visits to a nearby park or shop may be possible and will do much towards keeping the child interested and happy.

Routine Tests

During treatment a weekly weight chart is kept and the height of the patient is measured on admission and at monthly intervals.

The erythrocyte sedimentation rate is taken weekly and this is one of the best guides to progress. The amount of exercise permitted as well as permission to get up are usually based on this test. A return to normal, that is to say approximately 10 millimetres sedimentation in the first hour, is as a rule the signal for getting the patient up and for allowing increased activity.

X-ray pictures of the affected part are taken every month and in cases of tuberculous meningitis check-up lumbar punctures are performed for many weeks after clinical recovery.

Gastric Washings

As young children are not as a rule able to cooperate in producing specimens of sputum and as they frequently have an entirely unproductive cough, it may be necessary to do gastric washings in order to obtain a specimen.

Method. Unless the milk supply is known to be absolutely safe from tubercle, dried milk is given for 3 days prior to the washings. Immediately after waking and before anything has been given by mouth, a gastric tube is passed and any resting juice withdrawn. This is placed in a sterile bottle and labelled. A few millilitres of sterile saline are then introduced through the tube and withdrawn. This specimen, which usually contains a fair quantity of mucus, is placed in a second bottle and again appropriately labelled. The specimen is sent to the laboratory. Gastric washings are repeated on three successive mornings. The nurse will have to use much tact and sympathy when carrying out this unpleasant procedure, but if approached in the right way children are as a rule wonderfully co-operative and easily managed.

Urine Tests. In order to eliminate any danger of overlooking an infection of the renal tract weekly tests are done to exclude blood, albumen and pus cells in the patient's urine.

Drugs Used in the Treatment of Tuberculosis

The main drugs used in the treatment of tuberculosis are:

1. *Streptomycin.* (a) By intramuscular injection (44 milligrams per kilogram body weight per day). Side effects: rashes, nausea, vomiting, giddiness, and deafness.

   (b) By the intrathecal route: 50 to 100 milligrams daily.

2. *Para-aminosalicylic acid* (PAS) given orally as tablets, syrup or enteric-coated granules 250 milligrams per kilogram weight daily in divided doses.

   Side effects: nausea, vomiting anorexia, rashes and jaundice. Patients usually get used to the drug rapidly and tolerate it well after the early difficulties.

3. *Isonicotinic acid hydrazide* (INAH). 2 to 8 milligrams per kilogram body weight is given as a mixture and is usually well tolerated.

   Side effects: rashes, purpura, dizziness, convulsions and neuritis.

As a rule two of these drugs are given at a time and their combination varied during the course of several months' treatment. The giving of more than one of these drugs appears to make each more efficacious and prevents the tubercle bacilli from becoming resistant to either of them.

Other Drugs. Sedatives may occasionally be necessary, particularly in some cases of tuberculous meningitis. Aperients, potassium citrate in the case of urinary complications, iron and vitamins are among the other medications frequently prescribed as need arises.

Convalescence

After all types of illnesses caused by tuberculosis infection, prolonged convalescence under good conditions and in country surroundings is essential. This is often difficult to arrange, as many convalescent homes do not accept these patients, but the help of a relative living in the country can sometimes be enlisted.

On return home, the patient should remain under regular supervision and care must be taken that all other members of the household are healthy or being adequately treated should this be necessary. A nurse's duty does not therefore end with the discharge of her patient, but must include much thought and organization for the future.

Taking a History

In cases of tuberculous infection it is particularly important to get a complete and reliable history of the patient and his family. The child has probably become infected by an adult in his close surroundings, possibly a member of the family. Contacts should therefore be X-rayed and generally watched so that treatment can be given at the earliest moment should need arise. The local chest clinic will usually provide the necessary care.

Most people are still reluctant to admit that there is any tuberculous infection in the family, so that patient, repeated history-taking may be necessary to elicit the source of the infection. By giving the parents confidence the nursing staff are often able to do more in this respect than the doctor.

Mass X-ray is doing much towards enlightening the population and detects early cases before they become a danger to themselves or their families. Universal pasteurization of milk and encouragement to farmers to keep attested herds will also improve public health. In spite of this all milk given to children under the age of about three years should be boiled.

Primary Tuberculosis of Childhood

In childhood, infection with the tubercle bacillus follows a fairly set and typical pattern.

As a rule the tubercle bacillus reaches the lungs by inhalation and produces a local lesion which is frequently so slight that it goes unnoticed. The infected area is drained by the local lymph glands and eventually becomes encapsulated by fibrous tissue and calcium deposits. Such a calcified area in the lung may be the size of a split pea. It is known as a *Ghon focus.* As a result of the tuberculous infection the glands at the roots of the lung become enlarged and on X-ray reports reference is made to enlarged hilar glands or mediastinal lymph nodes.

The Ghon focus and enlarged hilar glands form what is known as the *primary complex*, and this may now develop in any of the following ways:

1. The primary focus becomes arrested and heals by calcification, that is to say the patient is cured.
2. The primary focus becomes arrested but is reactivated later in life.
3. The pressure of the tuberculous glands causes collapse of a part of the lung, in which case the lung may eventually re-expand spontaneously or the gland may rupture into the bronchus and cause tuberculous bronchopneumonia, which will show as a wedge-shaped shadow on X-ray.
4. The infection spreads via the blood stream and may cause miliary tuberculosis, tuberculous meningitis or any other tuberculous infection of the bones, the urinary tract or alimentary canal.

The Primary Complex

Signs and Symptoms. The child is usually quite well and frequently the infection is only detected when contacts of tuberculous adults are X-rayed. Occasionally, however, the child may be less active than usual, demand more attention, lose interest in his food and so fail to gain weight. There may be slight anæmia. The mother may give a history of a recent chill after which the child has failed to return to normal.

The temperature and pulse rate may be slightly raised and a mild, dry cough, often paroxysmal in nature, arouses the mother's concern. The erythrocyte sedimentation rate is increased to about 20 to 40 millimetres in the first hour.

When an infected gland presses on a bronchus the cough may be very irritating and have a brassy tone. Dyspnœa may develop and become quite alarming at night. Bronchiectasis may result as a complication.

Treatment. Bed rest, fresh air, good food and a very gradual return to normal activities is often all that is needed. In more severe cases one or several of the modern drugs for the treatment of tuberculosis are used. Progress is guided by the improvement in the erythrocyte sedimentation rate, a gain in weight, the return to normal of temperature and pulse rate and signs of calcification on X-ray. X-ray pictures and general follow up should be continued for several years. The outlook with modern treatment is as a rule excellent.

Nursing Points. What has been written about the general care of tuberculous children applies fully in these cases. The nurse should, in addition, remember that prolonged bed rest and restricted activities over a period of several months may be very irksome for a child who is feeling perfectly well. More perhaps than in any other condition she will have to devote a good deal of her time to playing with the child, supplying him with suitable play material and toys and giving help with his education according to his age and ability. Television, pets and frequent visiting may allay some of the boredom, and visits to the hospital grounds or local parks may be possible during the later stages of convalescence. The diet should be varied and served as attractively as possible. This type of tuberculous infection is not contagious and children having treatment for primary tuberculosis can be nursed in general wards without protective precautions for their neighbours or the staff.

Complications. Given unfavourable conditions such as malnutrition, debility or sudden excessive development at puberty, a dormant and apparently cured childhood infection may become reactivated.

Pressure by an inflamed lymph gland may cause collapse of a lobe or segment of the lung by blockage of a bronchus. The right middle lobe and a segment of the upper lobe are most frequently affected. Occlusion of the lumen of a bronchus by tuberculous granulations may also cause collapse as described above. The symptoms are similar.

Treatment of Collapse of Part of the Lung. Treatment is once again on the general lines described. In suitable, quiescent cases postural drainage and physiotherapy are given. When tuberculous granulations occlude the bronchus, bronchoscopy may be carried out.

Granulations, caseated material and stagnant secretions are often sucked out through the bronchoscope, with excellent results. More rarely an infected gland may rupture into the pleural cavity causing tuberculous pleurisy or alternatively into the bronchus causing tuberculous bronchopneumonia.

Prognosis. This, in the majority of cases, is good. The lung may expand spontaneously as the lesion heals, though this may take many weeks.

Tuberculous Pleurisy

Pleurisy is not an uncommon complication of tuberculosis in older children and usually occurs within 2 years of the original infection.

Signs and Symptoms. Either no symptoms are present and the condition is detected on routine investigations, or the onset is very sudden. In the latter case the child complains of severe pain which may be either in the side of the chest or in the abdomen. The pain may be referred through the intercostal nerves to the lower abdomen and may simulate acute appendicitis, or via the phrenic nerve into the shoulder, on the affected side. It is a sharp, knife-like pain and may cause great distress in breathing.

Chest movements are restricted to avoid pain, but pleural fluid forms rapidly and as the two surfaces of the parietal and visceral pleura become separated, the pain subsides. Large amounts of pleural effusion may cause difficulty in respiration and may displace the heart and trachea. In these cases a paracentesis thoracis is carried out to relieve the symptoms. The fluid which is withdrawn is straw coloured, pale and clear or slightly milky in appearance. On pathological examination the tubercle bacillus may be found.

Sometimes the pleural effusion becomes purulent instead of resolving and causes an empyema. This condition is fortunately uncommon in children. (The management of empyema is described later in this chapter.) Adhesions may form but they are rarely of much importance.

Nursing Care. General good care, fresh air, nourishing light diet with extra milk and vitamins, and prolonged bed rest are needed.

Pressure areas require attention during the acute stages of the illness and a good bedrest and comfortable pillows will do much to relieve the child's restlessness and discomfort. Very frequently the child will place himself on the affected side thus instinctively limiting the movement of the chest wall on the affected side. Alternatively the severe pain may be relieved by applying heat in the form of a light poultice, warm cotton wool or a well protected hot-water bottle (N.B. this need only be filled at the hot tap and boiling water should never be used). Poultices should be used only on medical advice as their weight may lead to further embarrassment of respiration.

Abundant fluids should be given and the diet should be light but nutritious and attractively served.

The weight is checked every week and the usual blood tests carried out. All considerations for the general care of tuberculous patients mentioned at the beginning of this chapter apply when nursing these children.

Drugs. In addition to the usual drugs used in the treatment of tuberculosis some pain relieving drugs will be required, and nurses should remember that pain from an early pleurisy is among the severest pains that can be experienced.

In many countries counter-irritants such as mustard plasters, painting with 10 per cent. iodine or cupping are still used. Occasionally a small artificial pneumothorax is induced to keep the pleural layers apart and so reduce the painful friction of the two inflamed surfaces rubbing on each other.

Phlyctenular Conjunctivitis

Phlyctenular conjunctivitis appears to be a hypersensitivity reaction to tuberculin and it is most frequently seen in debilitated children of early school age.

Signs and Symptoms. The conjunctivæ and occasionally the cornea are infiltrated by small, raised nodules, grey in colour but surrounded by an area of inflammation. Photophobia is marked and the child may refuse to open his eyes which he keeps very tightly shut. Irritation and excessive lacrimation may cause the child to rub his eyes. Occasionally a discharge is present.

Treatment. A swab for culture should always be taken and the sensitivity of any organisms established. There may be a superimposed infection which will require separate treatment.

Treatment is general, on the usual lines for tuberculosis, as well as local. The eyes should be gently bathed with warm saline or boracic lotion. Hydrocortisone eye drops instilled thrice daily usually clear the local condition quite rapidly. Pad and bandage should not be applied but relief may be obtained from the use of dark glasses or alternatively the room in which the child is being nursed should be kept darkened during the acute stage. Antibiotics are given by mouth or by injection. They include streptomycin, PAS (para-aminosalicylic acid) and INAH (isonicotinic acid hydrazide).

Prognosis. Complications, such as a prolonged course of the infection or corneal ulceration, are now rarely seen.

Erythema Nodosum

Erythema nodosum appears to be another allergic reaction to tuberculin which arises within 2 to 3 months after the incubation period. The rash is most frequently seen over the shins or occasionally over the forearms, the elbows or the malar bones on the face. The rash is tender to touch, red and slightly raised. After 2 to 3 weeks it disappears spontaneously often leaving brown or purple markings which persist for some time.

Treatment. No treatment is needed but discomfort may be relieved by local application of calamine lotion or lead lotion or by administration of aspirin. Both phlyctenular conjunctivitis and erythema nodosum can be regarded as warning signs of active tubercle infection or simply of a recent infection now overcome, for which careful observation of the patient, rest and dietetic treatment are still necessary.

Miliary Tuberculosis

Miliary tuberculosis results from a dissemination of tubercle bacilli via the blood stream and usually occurs between the ages of 1 to 3 years and approximately 3 months after the primary tuberculous infection. Lesions may arise in any part of the body such as the lungs, the peritoneum, the urinary tract, the central nervous system or the eyes. The deposits are about the size of a millet seed, hence the name miliary tuberculosis.

Signs and Symptoms. The onset is frequently an insidious one. The child is a little fretful and listless, often lies down during play, refuses his food and loses his usual good colouring and weight. Much later a raised, swinging temperature, a rapid pulse rate and persistent cough may be noticed. The respirations are rapid, due to the toxic state and often quite out of keeping with the severity of the infection in the lungs.

Gradually the whole appearance of the child becomes toxic, he shows signs of having a headache and may become drowsy. On examination the spleen is found to be enlarged. An X-ray picture of the lungs will show disseminated lesions which give the appearance of a snow storm.

Investigations. Chest X-ray, erythrocyte sedimentation rate and blood tests are done. As children rarely bring up any sputum, gastric washings are sent for culture. After dilating the pupils with a mydriatic the eyes are examined to exclude papillœdema and choroidal tuberculomata. Mantoux tests are carried out. Specimens of urine are sent for culture to exclude tuberculosis of the urinary tract.

Lumbar puncture is always carried out in the early stages and repeated weekly at first in order to exclude and detect any invasion of the meninges at the earliest moment.

Treatment. This follows the general lines described for tuberculous infections, with special treatment and care of specific infections which may arise. The usual drugs used in the treatment of tuberculosis are given over a prolonged period of time.

Prognosis. Though prognosis used to be hopeless, a very high rate of complete recovery may be expected with early, modern treatment by streptomycin, para-aminosalicylic acid and isoniazid.

Tuberculous Meningitis

Tuberculous meningitis is fortunately far less often seen in the United Kingdom than it used to be. With adequate treatment the course of the illness may not be unduly serious and, although treatment will in most cases continue for approximately 6 months, the young patient begins to feel and look well after a comparatively short while. He will start to play happily, eat well and gain weight. Treatment may be possible at home. However, severe cases are still seen, and for that reason such a case is here fully described. The intelligent nurse will at all times adjust management to the situation on hand.

Although tuberculous meningitis may occur at any age, it is most commonly seen between the ages of 2 to 10 years. It is never a primary lesion and is frequently associated with miliary tuberculosis.

Signs and Symptoms

The onset of the disease is slow and insidious. The normally lively child gradually becomes quiet, prefers sitting in his chair to getting about, sleeps more than usual, vomits occasionally and the vomit is quite unrelated to meals. He eventually becomes irritable and demanding and finally drowsy.

When lying down he curls up and, as there is photophobia, either turns away from the light or pulls his sheet over his head. Constipation is a typical symptom: older children may complain of having a headache. Neck rigidity and a positive

Kernig's sign develop. As anorexia becomes established there is failure to gain weight. Wasting rapidly sets in and soon causes the typical scaphoid, indrawn appearance of the abdomen. The skin is dry and inelastic. The temperature rises, the pulse rate slows down and respirations are irregular. In spite of underlying pallor the child looks flushed and typical red spots known as taches cérébrales may be noticed. Convulsions are a frequent complication.

In very young children the fontanelle is tense and bulging and in older ones there may be papillœdema and squints and the pupils are dilated and unequal. On examination of the eyes tuberculomata may be seen on the fundus and the choroid. Nystagmus is also often seen. The child frequently has a typical, high-pitched, meningeal cry which may present a very real problem in an open ward.

The child's attitude in bed is of interest. He is frequently restless and picks continually at his bed clothes and often also at his nose; many of these patients are inclined to masturbate. Opisthotonos may be extreme (see page 303). Teeth grinding is common and can be a distressing feature. As the disease progresses food may be altogether refused, the mouth becomes dry and dirty despite all nursing efforts, and severe wasting occurs. The limbs may be held in spasm and a squint is very often present.

A block may develop in the cerebrospinal system causing hydrocephalus. This may have to be treated surgically.

Investigation

Early recognition of the disease is of vital importance if treatment is to be successful, the most conclusive and reliable investigation being lumbar puncture.

The Cerebrospinal Fluid. On lumbar puncture pressure is often found to be raised (over 200 millimetres of water). The cell count is higher than usual (50 to 200 cells per cubic millimetre). The protein rises to 45 to 80 milligrams per cent. while the sugar shows a marked drop to 15 to 30 milligrams per cent. Acid fast bacilli may be found on staining or by inoculation into a guinea pig. The chlorides fall well below 700 milligrams per cent. As the disease progresses, the abnormalities in the above figures become grossly exaggerated. To the naked eye the fluid may appear clear but on standing a fine spider web clot of fibrinogen may form.

Urine and Stools. These may be sent for culture for acid fast bacilli.

The Mantoux Test. This is as a rule positive in a dilution of 1:10,000 though it may become negative in the later stages of the disease.

Gastric Washings. These are usually performed to prove the presence of the tubercle bacillus.

Examination of the Eyes. After dilating the pupils with 1 per cent. atropine drops, or ointment, the fundi of the eyes are examined for papillœdema and for the possible presence of tuberculomata.

A full examination of the central nervous system is done at regular intervals.

X-ray of the chest is a monthly routine.

Weight. The child is weighed weekly.

Treatment

Treatment is mainly based on drug therapy. Although the frequency and period of time over which streptomycin and the other anti-tuberculosis drugs are given varies from one hospital to another the basic principles remain the same.

In the early stages daily lumbar punctures may be performed and streptomycin given by the intrathecal route. In that case steroids are also given to prevent the resultant inflammatory changes in the meninges which might otherwise cause permanent complications. In many instances combined drug therapy may be expected to give excellent results and intrathecal injections over a prolonged period are now rarely necessary. In either case the child is given streptomycin by intramuscular injection twice a day, isonicotinic acid hydrazide (INAH) orally three times a day and para-aminosalicylic acid (PAS) 4-hourly. The combination of any two of these drugs reduces the danger of the tubercle becoming resistant to streptomycin. Isoniazid also has the added advantage of easily reaching the theca and the meninges while streptomycin does not diffuse well into the thecal spaces.

Antihistamine drugs may be prescribed if giddiness and vomiting are troublesome. Vitamins, iron therapy and sedative drugs are frequently necessary. If the child is either very young or very ill, steroids (e.g. prednisolone) may also be given in the initial stages.

Nursing Care

It is obvious that the most careful and expert nursing will be needed for children so seriously ill for a matter of months.

The bed should be in a quiet part of the ward and easily screened for the purpose of treatments and special visiting. The distressing meningeal cry may well disturb other patients and this too should be considered when choosing a bed. A blind to darken the ward is an asset.

Sorbo mattresses are invaluable and water beds give much comfort though they are less firm and may present difficulties when lumbar punctures are performed on the patient's bed. The bedclothes should be light and warm and their weight should be taken off the feet and limbs by using bed cradles. These patients are as a rule best nursed with one pillow only, but care must be taken to turn them at frequent intervals so as to prevent hypostatic pneumonia. For unconscious patients the foot end of the bed may be raised in order to facilitate drainage.

As these children are often doubly incontinent for many weeks every precaution should be taken to prevent the skin from breaking and pressure sores from developing. After the routine treatment it is useful to massage some cod-liver oil into the area. This serves the dual purpose of keeping the skin supple and of supplying vitamins. Silicone barrier cream may help to keep the skin intact.

The patients are often restless and this fact together with the extreme wasting makes frequent nursing care essential. Bony prominences should be placed on small pillows or pads of wool and ankles, knees and elbows bandaged with protective cotton wool.

The infection of the cerebrospinal system may cause serious disturbances in the heat regulating centre of the body.

Oral toilet needs constant attention. Carious teeth so often seen in these children should be removed as tooth grinding is apt to break them and the broken-off bits may be inhaled.

Constipation may be obstinate. Fruit juice and abundant fluids should be given whenever possible, but glycerin suppositories and small enemata are often necessary. The nurse should remember that constipation is one of the causes of restlessness. Urinary incontinence is common and much trouble can be avoided by fixing up some means of collecting the urine. Paul's tubing leading to a urinal or even a urinal left *in situ* may help in this matter in the case of boys.

Convulsions are likely to occur and a covered tray containing a mouth gag, spatulæ, wooden peg and tongue holding forceps should be kept at the bedside.

Spastic contractions are common. Splinting with light plaster of Paris splints and relief of spasm by application of warmth and frequent massage should be instituted at the earliest moment. Passive movements and physiotherapy are invaluable and should be carried out by the nursing staff in the absence of a physiotherapist. In the convalescent stage re-education in walking and maintaining of balance may prove a time-consuming effort.

Painful areas caused by the intramuscular injections can be treated by the application of warmth. It is useful to keep a record of the site into which the last injection was given so as to ensure that nurses alternate the injections between the thighs and deltoid muscles regularly when giving them. Occasionally an abscess forms where injections have been given. Visual disturbances such as double vision, nystagmus and even blindness are among the complications which may occur.

Drugs

Drug therapy has already been mentioned. Iron therapy and para-aminosalicylic acid are inclined to cause anorexia and toxic symptoms and these must be dealt with in an imaginative way as they arise.

Diet

The resourcefulness and patience of the nurse will be taxed to the full. It may well take half an hour to persuade the child to take two to three spoonfuls of nourishment. Food should be as varied as possible and contain a very high calorie value. Quite big children may regress to baby stage and feed from a bottle, others may develop fads (such as demanding jellied eels) or refuse all food except that brought by the mother from home. It is well worth while giving in to any of these whims during the critical stage in order to maintain the child's state of nutrition.

Artificial feeding often becomes necessary and even patients who can take a certain amount by mouth may need a continuous tube feed over night in order to get the necessary calories. A length of polythene or Plexitron tubing passed nasally can often be left in position for three or more weeks without causing any trouble. Through this, a high calorie mixture can be given and not infrequently it is the best way in which to give oral drugs. A suitable high calorie mixture may be made by adding one or two eggs, a teaspoon of Casilan and 1 ounce of glucose to a pint of milk. If the patient has difficulty in retaining such a mixture the feed may be diluted or given by continuous drip method over a period of time.

Special Complications

Occasionally the subarachnoid spaces and areas round the midbrain become blocked by constrictive exudate. The drugs given will not in these cases reach the meninges and streptomycin may have to be given by cisternal or ventricular puncture. Burr holes may have to be made in the skull and drugs injected through these either by puncture or by indwelling catheter. Drainage too may be established in this manner where there is danger of hydrocephalus developing. When the analyses of the lumbar and ventricular cerebrospinal fluids are entirely different and the flow of cerebrospinal fluid diminishes, it is a warning that these complications are arising.

Prognosis

Before the advent of streptomycin therapy coupled with isonicotinic acid hydrazide and para-aminosalicylic acid, tuberculous meningitis used to be a 100 per cent. fatal disease. Nowadays, however, those patients who are conscious on admission, and who receive adequate treatment with the combined drug therapy, may be expected to make a complete recovery. Others, less fortunate, may be left with permanent disabilities such as partial or total deafness, visual defects, recurrent epileptiform attacks, cranial nerve palsy and mental deterioration and retardation.

A great deal depends on early diagnosis and expert treatment.

Duration of the Illness

A hospital stay of many months is likely to be necessary and even after discharge patients require a long period of convalescence and rehabilitation during which time regular visits to hospital for the purpose of check-up lumbar punctures will be necessary.

Convalescence

Convalescence is slow and tedious, the total stay in hospital often being 9 to 12 months. Occupation according to age and stage of convalescence is most important and distractions such as television and wireless in the ward may be a great help in relieving boredom.

The Relatives

Much time may have to be spent in keeping up the courage and hope of parents who will be deeply distressed to see their child so seriously ill and so changed. Their patience will be taxed to the extreme by the fact that for weeks it may not be possible to give anything but noncommittal and guarded information because of the uncertainty of complete recovery.

Abdominal Tuberculosis

Tuberculous ulceration of the bowel, tuberculous peritonitis and tabes mesenterica are the most usual manifestations of abdominal tuberculosis in childhood, though even these are only rarely seen in this country. The infection is frequently of the bovine type or is carried from other foci via the blood stream. The onset is, as a rule, slow and insidious.

Tuberculosis of the Bowel. In tuberculosis of the bowel the tubercle bacillus invades the bowel mucosa and may either perforate into the peritoneal cavity setting up peritonitis, or heal by scarring which often causes narrowing of the lumen of the bowel. The infection is as a rule a secondary one arising from the swallowing of tuberculous sputum.

Signs and Symptoms. Loose offensive stools containing mucus and blood are characteristic. The child is often fairly fit but in more severe cases wasting and toxic manifestations may be very marked.

Treatment. This is on general lines and symptoms such as pain, high fever or severe diarrhœa are treated as they arise.

Tabes Mesenterica. Involvement of the glands of the abdomen is frequently met with in children. It may cause little general or local disturbance. Occasionally however there is general malaise, lassitude, rise in temperature and failure to gain weight. Intermittent, vague abdominal pain and occasional vomiting are often misleading symptoms and acute appendicitis may be wrongly suspected. Cases are known in which the glands are so situated as to cause obstruction of the bowel.

Prognosis. Calcification occurs eventually but the glands may remain palpable for many years even though general recovery has been complete.

Tuberculous Peritonitis. The signs and symptoms of tuberculous peritonitis differ little from those of other types of peritonitis (see page 224) but are less acute. When much free fluid is present in the abdominal cavity paracentesis may have to be performed, but there is great likelihood of adhesions forming after the release of the fluid. If the fluid is left, it gradually becomes absorbed leaving fibrinous deposits which organize into a soft, doughy mass involving the omentum as well as loops of bowel. Obstruction and perforation may result.

Prognosis. In spite of the severity and long duration of the illness, recovery may be expected and is often complete.

Tuberculosis of the Kidney. Tuberculous infections of the kidney are rarely seen in children unless associated with miliary tuberculosis.

Signs and Symptoms. The child is debilitated and complains of frequency of micturition. Hæmaturia may occur. Cystoscopy may show tuberculous ulcers of the urinary tract and inoculation of a guinea pig with infected urine will confirm the diagnosis.

Treatment. In cases where one kidney only is affected nephrectomy can be performed; in others treatment is the same as for miliary tuberculosis (see page 349).

Tuberculous Cervical Adenitis

Tuberculous infection may reach the lymph glands of the neck from the tonsils or adenoids or via the blood stream from any primary focus. Children under the age of three are rarely affected.

Signs and Symptoms. The onset is insidious and the child seems well in himself. A hard lump can be felt in the neck which gradually increases in size. It is painless but may cause stiffness of the neck and torticollis. The Mantoux test is positive.

If left untreated the infected gland may calcify or it may caseate and form a cold abscess which breaks through the skin and forms a discharging sinus.

Treatment. This includes the general care given to children with any type of tuberculous infection. In addition, the head is immobilized between sand bags or in a plaster of Paris or Perspex collar. Aspiration with a large bore needle and syringe, curettage or dissection of the gland may be necessary. If the condition is treated early, the after-care presents no problems and the prognosis is good provided cross-infection is avoided. If it is neglected and the abscess breaks through the skin, a permanent sinus may result from added septic infection.

Tuberculosis of Bones and Joints

Tuberculous infections of bones and joints are sometimes of the bovine type, alternatively the infection is blood borne and carried from a primary focus. Rest of the affected part by means of splints, plaster of Paris and general treatment for tuberculosis are given concurrently. Full drug therapy is employed and the chest should be examined to exclude tuberculosis of the lungs. The prognosis is good if treatment is given early and if it is adequate. The details of nursing and orthopædic care are the same as in adults although special problems arise on account of the long duration of the treatment. These problems have already been mentioned in the chapter on diseases of the bones and joints.

21

INFECTIOUS FEVERS

The tables on pages 363–367 give a summary of the acute infectious fevers which may be encountered in a children's ward. Further details of each condition can be found in specific text-books. Brief notes on other conditions that may be met follow, but larger text-books should also be consulted.

Coxsackie and Echo Virus Group

The Coxsackie and Echo viruses cause a variety of conditions, and include those listed below.

Benign Lymphocytic Meningitis, with fever, headache, nausea, neck stiffness and raised cells in the cerebrospinal fluid (predominantly lymphocytes).

Epidemic Myalgia (Bornholm's Disease) (Coxsackie). Acute, severe pain of the intercostal muscles, painful, rapid shallow respirations, pleural rub, low grade fever, possibly lymphocytosis. Lasts 7 to 10 days. Symptomatic treatment.

Herpangina (Coxsackie Group A). Mild febrile illness of infancy. Vesicular and ulcerative lesions on soft palate and in fauces.

Epidemic Diarrhœa (Echo)

Aseptic Meningitis (Echo)

Without paralysis or sequelæ.

Adenovirus

Acute upper respiratory tract infection or severe influenza-like fever. Sore throat. Cough. Conjunctivitis. Painful enlargement of lymph glands. Sometimes causes pneumonic consolidation.

Catscratch Fever

Probably a virus infection. Cat apparently healthy. A few days after scratch, ulcer or sore. A week or two later—regional lymph nodes very enlarged, some fever. Nodes may suppurate or adenitis persist for some months. Pus sterile, white cell count normal. Treated with broad-spectrum antibiotic to prevent suppuration.

Post-infective Encephalitis and Encephalomyelitis

May follow measles, whooping cough, mumps, chickenpox, German measles, scarlet and glandular fever, and vaccination and immunization. Tends to occur in small epidemics, within 2 weeks of initial condition. Varying severity-headache, drowsiness, irritability, vomiting, fits, coma, pareisis, signs of meningitis, cranial nerve palsies, transient lower motor neuron weakness in limbs. 10 to 50 per cent. mortality. Possibly residual hemiplegia, cranial nerve palsies, mental deficiency or Parkinsonian syndrome.

Tetanus (Lockjaw)

Caused by *Clostridium tetani* found on cultivated land. Anærobic bacillus—danger in deep penetrating wounds which do not bleed much. Exotoxin forms, which attacks muscle, motor nerves, central nervous system.

Incubation period variable. The shorter the time, the worse the prognosis. Non infectious.

Signs and Symptoms. Local muscle weakness, trismus, spasm of face muscles (risus sardonicus), tonic spasm-opisthotonos, rigid abdomen. Fever common. Paroxysmal state, precipitated by any disturbance such as feeding, noise, examination, painful spasm, arching back, extension of limbs, clenching teeth. Lasts seconds or minutes. If severe or increasing frequency—death from exhaustion.

Treatment. Intravenous antitoxin after subcutaneous test dose initially (need to be prepared for anaphylactic shock) followed by intramuscular injections of antitoxin daily. One hour after antitoxin—surgical débridement under light anæsthetic. Muscle relaxants to control spasm. Penicillin prophylaxis. If respirations cease—oxygen from anæsthetic machine, tracheal intubation as soon as relaxed, tracheostomy later, elevate foot of bed, sucker, intragastric feeds at first, intravenous fluids and electrolyte balance.

Prophylaxis (Prevention). Active immunization—tetanus toxoid by triple immunization or separately (see page 13). Booster dose at 4 to 5 years, and every 5 years, and 0·5 millilitre if the patient has an accident involving penetrating wound or possible infection.

Passive Immunization—anti-tetanus serum at time of accident. Not as efficient and more danger of anaphylactic reactions.

Poliomyelitis

Virus infection of nasopharynx or alimentary tract.

Incubation period. 7 to 14 days or 21 days depending on type. Isolate for 6 weeks.

Signs and Symptoms. Coryza, fever, malaise, headache, vomiting, neck and back stiffness or rigidity, drowsiness or irritability; pain in limbs when patient sits up—back rigid and hands placed behind "tripod sign", to support the body; Kernig's sign may be positive. Cerebrospinal fluid under increased pressure, 10 to 200 cells/cubic millimetre, at first polymorphonuclear, later lymphocytes, protein sometimes increased, this increases with paralysis, raised globulin; sugar and chlorides normal.

Virus affects anterior horn cells and motor nuclei of brainstem. The poliomyelitis may be abortive, or progress to a flaccid paralysis of legs, arms, trunk, tongue, pharynx, larynx, face, diaphragm and intercostal muscles, or respiratory centre in the medulla. There is no sensory loss and the paralysis develops rapidly, but may advance for 3 to 5 days, during which time fever subsides. There may be retention of fæces and urine, and reflexes are absent or decreased, although in pre-paralytic stage they may be increased.

Treatment—symptomatic. In *pre-paralytic stage*—rest, analgesics (exertion increases likelihood of paralysis and respiratory difficulty). Isolation. Reassurance.

If paralyzed—gentle, frequent passive movements to weak limbs, hot packs to painful muscles, cradle, footrest, prevent shortening, expression of bladder to prevent retention of urine, enemata, adequate airway and oxygen, tracheostomy if necessary, probably with cuff and intermittent positive pressure or artificial respirator.

After acute stage—early and vigorous activity, schooling, rehabilitation, active physiotherapy. Paralysis usually diminishes over two or more weeks, or improvement may continue for several months; deformity can be minimized by adequate splinting where indicated, and if necessary tenotomy or arthrodesis can be performed at a later date.

Bulbar Involvement. Early difficulty in swallowing and speaking. Patient nursed in respirator to prevent mucus and vomit going into lungs, with head tilted down for drainage. Alternatively respirator with tracheostomy and suction or positive pressure respirator with tracheostomy and suction. *Never* put patient with bulbar paralysis in ordinary respirator without prior tipping, or secretions are immediately sucked into lungs.

Prophylaxis. Prevents disease and epidemics (see page 13). Gamma globulin can be given for passive immunity to close contacts who have not been immunized.

NOTE. Immunization against diptheria and pertussis should be avoided if there is a poliomyelitis epidemic, as the injected limb is more liable to paralysis if the child develops poliomyelitis. A child who develops poliomyelitis after a recent tonsillectomy is prone to develop bulbar paralysis.

PRINCIPAL INFECTIOUS DISEASES

DISEASE	INCUBATION PERIOD	ORGANISM AND MODE OF SPREAD	SIGNS AND SYMPTOMS	TREATMENT AND COMPLICATIONS	OTHER REMARKS
Measles (Morbilli or rubeola)	10–14 days	Virus. Droplet.	Running eyes and nose. Dry, irritating cough. Conjunctivitis. Photophobia. Pyrexia. Transient prodromal rash. Koplik spots—white on red base on buccal mucous membrane. 3rd day: temperature subsides. 4th day: rash appears—dusky red macular rash behind ears→face, trunk, limbs. Temperature again elevated. Rash becomes large irregular blotchy areas of darker red.	Bed. Symptomatic. Antibiotic for secondary infections. Otitis media. Blepharitis. Corneal ulcerations. Bronchopneumonia. Collapsed lobe of lung. Bronchiectasis and Lung abscess (if collapse insufficiently treated). Tuberculosis. Encephalitis and Encephalomyelitis. (Gastro-enteritis in infancy.)	Notifiable. Segregate until rash fades. Passive immunity for three months after birth (if mother has not had measles). Older or sick children are given convalescent serum 5–10 mls. or adult serum or gamma globulin for protection. *Gamma globulin* 250 mg. prevents attack under one year, attenuates attack at all ages. Later 750 mg. should prevent attack. Second dose after six weeks.
German Measles (Rubella)	14–21 days	Virus. Droplet.	Mild malaise and pyrexia day before rash. Generalized tender lymphadenitis especially posterior cervical and occipital. Rash: pink macules and papules at first discrete then confluent.	Very little necessary—symptomatic. Occasionally: Encephalitis. Arthritis.	Danger to fœtus during first 14 weeks *in utero* if mother affected. Baby may be born deaf, with cataract, glaucoma, or heart disease (also risk of abortion). Mother should be given gamma globulin.
Scarlet Fever (Scarlatina)	1–7 days	Hæmolytic streptococci (Lancefield Group A) Droplet, fomites, milk.	Headache, vomiting, pyrexia. Sore throat—soft yellow exudate. "Strawberry tongue". Polymorphonuclear leucocytosis. Raised antistreptolysin titre. Cervical lymphadenitis. Rash—punctate erythema, bright scarlet, behind ears and sides of neck→whole body except circumoral pallor. Desquamation after 1 week.	(Septic and toxic forms very rare.) Bed. Penicillin and sulphonamides. Fluids. Mouth care. Pneumonia. Septicæmia. Otitis media. Acute nephritis and Rheumatism. Anaphylactoid purpura. Sinusitis. Encephalitis. Quinsy. Retropharyngeal abscess. Cervical adenitis and abscess.	Notifiable. Dick test for diagnosis—rarely used. Possibility of cardiac lesions from acute rheumatism. Scarlet fever antitoxin sometimes given.

DISEASE	INCUBATION PERIOD	ORGANISM AND MODE OF SPREAD	SIGNS AND SYMPTOMS	TREATMENT AND COMPLICATIONS	OTHER REMARKS
Whooping Cough (Pertussis)	7–14 days	*Bordetella* (*Hæmophilus*) *pertussis*. Droplet.	Cold→chest infection→cough which becomes paroxysmal with vomiting. Ulcer on frænum. Lymphocytosis. Low erythrocyte sedimentation rate. Baby vomits, cyanosed, limp, no paroxysms.	Feed after vomiting. Sedation. Chloramphenicol for pertussis—5-day course only; other broad spectrum antibiotic for secondary infections. Deal with debility—long convalescence, high-calorie diet. Otitis media. Bronchopneumonia. Pulmonary collapse. Bronchiectasis. Tuberculosis. Subconjunctival hæmorrhage. Cerebral anoxia or hæmorrhage. Convulsions. Rectal prolapse. Hernia. Spontaneous pneumothorax.	Notifiable. No passive immunity in babies. Mild abortive case in immunized child, but equally infectious. Child often "whoops" for months after attack—infectious. Routine Immunization—not to child with epilepsy or prone to convulsions—he may develop encephalopathy if immunized.
Chickenpox (Varicella)	14–21 days	Virus. Contact and droplet.	Minimal malaise and headache. Fever. Transient prodromal rash. Main rash appears in crops—mainly on face, head and trunk, (centripetal) oval, unilocular papules→vesicles→pustules→crusts. Irritating rash. Lymphocytosis.	Prevent from scratching to avoid scarring. Baths. Calamine. Keep cool. Short nails. Elbow splints if necessary. Antihistamines. Antibiotics for secondary infections—impetigo, boils, cellulitis, conjunctivitis, polyneuritis, encephalitis, transverse myelitis.	Notifiable only in smallpox epidemic. Herpes zoster closely allied. Severe or fatal if child has leukæmia or is on steroid therapy. Segregate until scabs dry.
Smallpox (Variola)	8–18 usually 10–12 days	Virus. Contact and droplet.	*Variola major* Sudden onset—headache, fever, shivering, severe pain in back and aching of limbs. Toxæmia. Prodromal rash—purpuric. True rash, 3rd day, 1 crop only. Thickest on peripheral parts of limbs (centrifugal), round, multilocular→confluent. Macule → papule → vesicle → pustule → crust → scab → scar.	Strict isolation until all scabs off. Care of mouth, eyes, skin, otherwise symptomatic. Antibiotics against secondary infections. Otitis media, conjunctivitis, corneal ulceration, nephritis, cardiac failure, septicæmia, bronchopneumonia, encephalitis.	Notifiable. *Variola major*—high mortality. Quarantine 16 days. Routine vaccination advised—except for children with eczema. Vaccination of contacts effective to modify the attack. Very high infectivity.

Smallpox (*cont.*)			Toxic, septicæmic, confusion state with pyrexia when pustules form. Slower developing rash than chickenpox. *Variola minor* Relatively trivial and difficult to distinguish from chickenpox.		
Mumps (Epidemic parotitis)	14–28 days	Virus. Droplet.	Fever, malaise, stiff jaw, swelling of salivary glands—parotid and submandibular. Unilateral or bilateral. Trismus. Pain on eating—especially sugars. Furred tongue, mouth dry—diminution of saliva. Moderate lymphocytosis.	Symptomatic. Mouth care—drink with straw. Avoid foods which are sweet and stimulate salivary glands. Mastitis, oophoritis, prostatitis, pancreatitis (all rare), meningitis, encephalitis (may lead to permanent deafness), facial paralysis. Orchitis—after puberty (give steroids to prevent sterility).	Complement fixation test reaction to confirm diagnosis—rarely necessary.
Influenza	1–2 days	Virus—A, B, and C strains. Droplet.	Sudden onset—fever, shivering, headache, upper respiratory tract infection. Profound malaise, severe aching in back and limbs. Remittent fever for up to 1 week—falls by lysis.	Analgesics when necessary. Antibiotics for secondary infections—pneumonia. Post-influenzal debility and depression.	Vaccines A and B strain—partial immunity for 6 months—used in epidemics.
Roseola Infantum (Exanthema subitum, Sixth Disease, Pseudo-rubella)	8–15 days	Virus. Droplet.	Fever, macular rash—appears immediately temperature fallen, fades on pressure. On trunk, neck, proximal part of limbs; *not* face. Lasts 1–3 days. Little malaise. Catarrhal pharyngitis, cervical lymphadenopathy. Neutrophil leucopenia with relative lymphocytosis.	NIL	

DISEASE	INCUBATION PERIOD	ORGANISM AND MODE OF SPREAD	SIGNS AND SYMPTOMS	TREATMENT AND COMPLICATIONS	OTHER REMARKS
Glandular Fever (Infectious mononucleosis)	6–14 days	Probably a virus. Droplet. Low infectivity.	Lassitude, anorexia, general malaise, pyrexia, headache, sore throat with tonsillar exudate which separates easily without bleeding. At times petechiæ on palate. Enlarged lymph nodes and spleen. Transient macular rash—chest, trunk, limbs and particularly dorsum of hands and feet. Leucocytosis with raised monocytes (atypical). Paul Bunnell test may be positive.	Symptomatic. Treat general debility and depression—prolonged convalescence. Treat secondary infections—hepatitis, meningitis, encephalitis, ruptured spleen, myocarditis.	Relapses common, but complete recovery eventually.
Diphtheria	2–7 days	*Corynebacterium diphtheriæ* (or Klebs-Loeffler bacillus) Droplet, Fomites, milk.	Malaise, headache, rapid, feeble pulse, some rise in temperature, toxic. Albuminuria, exhaustion. *Faucial:* Slight sore throat, continuous greyish membrane spreading to soft palate and pharynx, which bleeds when attempt made to remove. Glands of neck very enlarged.—"Bull neck", myocarditis. *Nasal:* Thin bloodstained nasal discharge with offensive smell. Crusting of external nares. *Laryngeal:* Croupy cough, laryngeal stridor, loss of voice, asphyxia.	Diphtheria antitoxin if any question of infection possible. Absolute bed rest, mouth care, tube feed if necessary. Tracheostomy before obstructed. Treat secondary infections. Respirator will be necessary if diaphragm paralysed. Physiotherapy after acute stage. Myocarditis, paralysis of limbs, palate, diaphragm, ciliary muscles and external rectus muscles, nephritis, peripheral neuritis.	Notifiable. Follow up contacts and possible carriers. Treat carriers with antibiotic and possibly tonsillectomy. Immunization advisable to prevent infection and epidemics. Schick test to assess immunity—negative if immune.

13+

Enteric Fever	2 weeks	Typhoid (*Salmonella typhi*) Paratyphoid A, B and C (*S. paratyphi* A, B and C) (non-lactose fermenters). Contamination of food or water by excreta from carriers or patients with the disease. Fomites, flies.	Headache, tiredness, aching limbs, cough, fever rising in "step-ladder" fashion, relative bradycardia, palpable spleen, abdominal discomfort, "rose spots" on abdomen or chest—constipated—later "pea soup" stools. Leucopenia if no secondary infection. Typhoid state—drowsy, confused, muttering, plucking at bedclothes, "coma vigil". Blood culture positive in first few days. Widal test—rising titre.	Symptomatic. High calorie, low roughage, diet. Care of mouth and skin. Watch for hæmorrhage from perforated Peyer's patches. Transfusion if necessary. Chloramphenicol for acute infection and relapses. Venous thrombosis, acute arthritis, cholecystitis, bone abscess and periostitis, peritonitis. Parotitis if inadequate mouth care.	Notifiable. Isolate until 2 negative stool cultures (consecutive). Immunize contacts. Treat carriers—if necessary with cholecystectomy.
Brucellosis (Undulant fever, Malta fever)	1–3 weeks	*Brucella abortus* (cattle) *Brucella melitensis* (goats) *Brucella suis* (pigs) Infected, unpasteurized milk, meat, dairy products. Infected hides and carcases.	Headache, malaise, anorexia, constipation, fever—settles by lysis in 10 days, but recurs. Cough, backache, profuse sweating, palpable spleen. Transient arthritis. *Abortus fever* (chronic brucellosis). Insidious, milder and more prolonged. Recurrent night sweats without serious general ill health. (*In both*) Blood culture may be positive. Rising agglutination titre. Leucopenia, mild anæmia.	Tetracycline, streptomycin, vitamin B. Symptomatic—treat debility with long convalescence Disinfect excreta—especially urine.	Notifiable. Recurring at short intervals for many months. Pasteurization of milk, clean water and destroying infected animals prevents disease.
Psittacosis (Ornithosis)	1–2 weeks	Virus from infected birds (who may not be ill). Most virulent strain from parrots. Droplet and contact with infected birds.	Gradual onset, cough, fever, relative bradycardia, headache, backache, general malaise, splenomegaly. Pneumonia spreading from hilum. White cell count low or normal. Diagnosis—complement fixation test.	Symptomatic. Tetracycline for 1 week. Convalescence slow and prolonged. Fulminating—high fever, delirium, rising pulse and respiration rate, poor prognosis.	

22

BURNS, SCALDS AND ACCIDENTS

Burns and scalds are among the most frequently occurring accidents in childhood—some thousand patients are admitted annually to the hospitals in the London area alone—and they are the more tragic, because so many of them are preventable.

Common Causes. The causes of such accidents are not only failure to use fire guards for open fires. In many households electric fires still remain unguarded, mirrors or pretty pictures hung above fireplaces attract children, saucepan handles are left within reach of toddlers, scalding hot water is left standing about in readiness for a bath, the weekly wash or for scrubbing the floor. Baths should never be filled with hot water before running in some cold, otherwise a small child may step into water which is hot enough to scald him, or the bottom of the bath may become hot enough to burn the soles of his feet.

Children admitted with burns are frequently little girls whose nightdresses have caught fire or who have stood in front of fires in flimsy party clothes in an attempt to keep warm. Young children of either sex should wear pyjamas or at least nightdresses made of flame-proof materials such as Proban.

Inadequate precautions are sometimes taken in the homes of mentally handicapped children and of those subject to epileptic fits. Table cloths should not be used in homes where there is danger of a toddler getting hold of the cloth and pulling the teapot over him. Older children run particular risks when playing with fireworks, partly empty oil cans or bonfires on demolition sites and rubbish dumps, and when playing games with matches.

First-aid Treatment. This should be confined to the following procedure. Very slight burns or scalds should be covered by a clean piece of linen soaked in normal saline or spread with a paste made of sodium bicarbonate and a little water. If available Anthisan cream may be applied, as this lessens pain and at the same time reduces blistering.

More severe burns and scalds should be covered with clean linen to exclude air. Burnt clothing—sterilized by the heat—

should be left untouched, but any wet clothing should be gently removed before covering the wound. Regardless of the possibility of an anæsthetic within a few hours, bland fluids such as sugar water or very weak tea should be given at once, as with children promptness in this respect may be the most important factor in saving life by reducing shock.

Classification of Burns and Scalds

Modern surgery refers to only two degrees of burns and scalds: superficial burns, and full thickness or deep burns. As a rule *superficial burns* may be expected to heal with little scarring, while *full thickness burns* are slow to heal and may cause scarring, crippling contractions and loss of function, and usually require skin grafting and prolonged and repeated treatment in hospital.

The extent of the burn is as important as the depth. For purposes of classification the "Waller Method" is frequently used. The body surface is divided into sections of 9 per cent. of the total and thus, with reference to a chart, it is easy to estimate the extent of the burn as being a multiple of 9 per cent. The seriousness of the burn or scald is often far more dependent on the extent of the affected area, than on the thickness. A child may lose his life with an 18 per cent. superficial burn but an older patient may be expected to survive deep burns covering 50 per cent. of the body surface.

The Lund and Browder method of estimating the extent of burns is given on the next page.

Treatment for Shock

No time should be lost in treating shock, even if the usual symptoms may at first not be evident because shock is delayed. Shock is always directly proportionate to the area involved as the loss of salts, protein and fluids into the tissue spaces and on to the body surface reduces the volume of circulating blood. The body reacts to this by a drop in blood pressure, subnormal temperature, pallor, thirst, restlessness and failure to secrete urine.

Intravenous Therapy

This is started in all cases in which the area involved exceeds 9 per cent. of the body surface. It is usual to take blood for grouping and hæmoglobin estimation before starting the infusion.

Plasma is the fluid of choice although fresh blood may be given according to the level of the hæmoglobin which should never be allowed to fall below 70 per cent.

The Lund and Browder Method of Estimating the Extent of Burns in Children

As in Waller's "Rule of Nines" method, the body is divided into areas each of which is given a percentage value, but the values of certain areas alter with age as the proportions of the child's body are changed by normal growth.

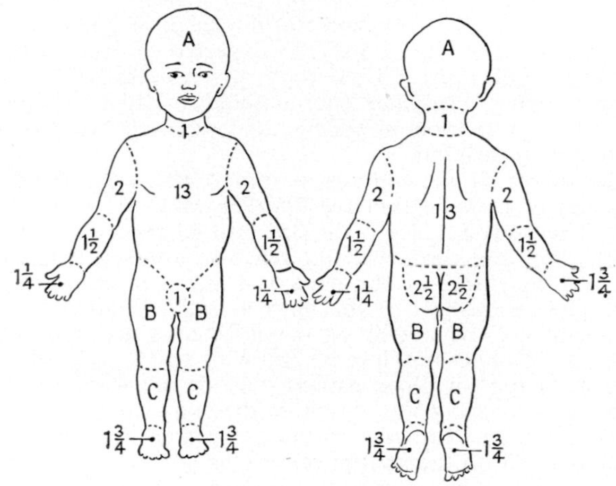

Fig. 62.

[From Lund, C. C., and Browder, N. C., *Surg. Gynec. Obstet.*]

Areas affected by Growth	*Age*				
	1 *month*	1 *year*	5 *years*	10 *years*	15 *years*
A = half of head	$9\frac{1}{2}$	$8\frac{1}{2}$	$6\frac{1}{2}$	$5\frac{1}{2}$	$4\frac{1}{2}$
B = half of one thigh	$2\frac{3}{4}$	$3\frac{1}{4}$	4	$4\frac{1}{4}$	$4\frac{1}{2}$
C = half of one lower leg	$2\frac{1}{2}$	$2\frac{1}{2}$	$2\frac{3}{4}$	3	$3\frac{1}{4}$

The rate of fluid loss is estimated by repeated hæmatocrit readings, the hæmoconcentration and the amount of urinary output. On the first day approximately two-thirds of the fluid loss is replaced in the first 8 hours after admission. After that, chemical tests of both blood and urine are done at least daily and the findings are taken as a guide for further intravenous therapy and blood transfusion. Blood replacement is of particular importance in preventing anoxia of the kidneys and liver. Transfusion is therefore given without delay as severe symptoms of toxæmia can so be prevented.

Fluids by Mouth

These are given liberally at the same time and a careful fluid balance record kept. For accuracy in measuring the output, patients with burns of 20 per cent. or over are often nursed with an indwelling catheter in the case of girls and Paul's tubing in the case of boys. The urine is measured and tested every hour until normal output has been restored. A catheter may be left *in situ* to ensure accurate collection and measurement of urine. Anuria which continues longer than 12 hours and hæmaturia both point to a bad prognosis.

Oxygen Therapy

Shock and the loss of red blood cells from the burnt surface may cause sufficient reduction in the oxygenating power of the blood to make oxygen therapy necessary. This is usually best given by nasal catheters as oxygen given by means of a tent interferes with local treatment and also influences bacterial growth.

Cubicle Nursing

Whenever possible the patient is admitted into a special cubicle which is kept as free from infection as possible by daily cleaning with plenty of soap and water, disinfectant solution, aerosol spray and special ventilation, and by employing barrier technique. The humidity is regulated according to need. At first a dry atmosphere (approximately 35 to 40 per cent. humidity) is maintained to allow for crust formation and to discourage bacterial growth, but humidity may be raised gradually to 50 or 60 per cent. particularly if chest complications are feared. The temperature of the cubicle is kept to 21° or 24° C. (70° or 75° F.), sufficient to keep the patient comfortable but not enough to encourage bacterial growth.

Local Treatment

Treatment of the burnt area may vary from one hospital to another and according to the wishes of the surgeon, and the nursing and laboratory facilities available. Prevention of infection and early grafting are accepted standards of treatment at the present time. Limbs are usually dressed and covered irrespective of age, but children are often best nursed by the exposure method, which has the advantage of inhibiting bacterial growth by keeping the area cool, dry and exposed to light, and eliminating painful dressings while promoting healing with a minimum of scarring. The patient can move around freely and observation of the progress is possible; both these considerations are of psychological and clinical importance. Few dressings under anæsthetic are necessary and this means, among other things, that nutrition is not constantly being interrupted.

The affected area and surrounding skin are usually cleansed with a solution of 1 per cent. centrimide or of Hibitane 1 in 2,000. Large, heavy blisters may be punctured and drained but small ones are left undisturbed and dead skin is not removed unless it is very dirty.

A hard, dry crust of plasma exudate usually forms within 24 to 36 hours and provides a sterile covering for the underlying surface. Air is allowed to circulate freely to aid the drying process and for that purpose special beds, extensions and slings may be used and the patient's position changed according to need. Pressure on the affected part must be avoided as a good blood supply is essential to healing.

Immediately on admission, and before cleansing the area, swabs are taken from various parts of the burnt area, the nose and throat and of one or two areas of normal skin. The swabs are dipped into sterile broth before use and they are sent to the laboratory for culture and sensitivity tests. In some centres human plasma is used to accelerate crust formation but in the majority of cases this is not considered necessary. In favourable cases the crusts begin to peel off after approximately 3 weeks when new epidermis has formed. Very thick crusts may be loosened by liquid paraffin soaks (gauze swabs saturated with paraffin) which are renewed every 4 hours. After approximately 12 hours much of the crust can be lifted off with the aid of sterile forceps. This should only be done if the treatment is entirely painless, i.e. if adequate healing underneath the crust has taken place.

Full thickness burns are treated in the same way initially,

but after 10 to 21 days the patient is taken to the theatre for thorough examination and wound toilet. By now it is possible to decide how much of the tissues are dead and consequently incapable of primary healing. As a rule partial thickness burns may be expected to heal in 3 to 4 weeks, but full thickness burns will require grafting and usually are associated with some degree of deformity. Any sloughs are removed and skin grafting is undertaken. This operation is called *escharectomy* (eschar=slough). Loss of blood may be considerable but by now the patient's general condition should be so much better that he can stand up to operation even though further blood transfusion may be necessary.

Following the grafting, both donor area and grafted area are bandaged and it is important that the nurse should watch any exposed and pendent parts for œdema and bleeding. The bandaging requires great skill as considerable pressure is required in order to prevent blood or exudate from lifting the graft off its bed. At the same time it is obviously dangerous to apply the crêpe bandages too tightly. Œdema may be severe and may cause the bandage to become tight and impede circulation with consequent death of the skin graft. Nursing methods, such as elevating the part, are attempted to reduce the swelling before interfering with the bandage as this is often applied with the intention of correcting deformities and contractions, as well as covering the operation area.

General Treatment

Drug Therapy

A broad spectrum antibiotic or a combination of one of these with penicillin is given prophylactically for the first 24 hours. The drug may then be changed according to the sensitivity report. Some surgeons change the drug routinely every time the patient has to be taken to the theatre in order to guard against his becoming resistant to any one drug.

Analgesic drugs are given freely for the first 48 hours but it is important to know that restlessness is often due to the need for more fluid rather than for more sedation. Heroin (0·6 mg. up to 3 years, 1·2 mg. from 3 to 7 years) given by injection and Nepenthe (0·06 ml. per year of age) given subcutaneously or by mouth are suitable drugs and can usually be repeated at 4-hourly intervals. After 48 hours pain subsides and drugs such as codeine or phenobarbitone are sufficient. Elixir Phenergan has a sedative effect and at the same time reduces tissue swelling. Sedatives at night may be necessary for some time and should never be withheld merely for fear of forming a habit. Iron in the form of Colliron 1–2 ml. ($\frac{1}{4}$–$\frac{1}{2}$ drachm) thrice daily is usually ordered.

Diet

Abundant fluids should be given from the start and the daily requirement is best divided into half-hourly amounts. A liberal addition of glucose (up to 1 pound a day) provides the necessary calories for the first day or two. Occasionally acidosis develops in young children and this can be treated by adding small quantities of sodium bicarbonate to the drinks, after seeking medical permission for doing so. On the second day diluted milk may be tried and after 48 hours gradually increased to full strength. A high calorie diet is introduced as soon as possible. It should be rich in vitamins, particularly vitamin C. Young children are often difficult in the initial stages but even at that point kind firmness is permissible as it may avoid much unhappiness and difficulty at a later stage.

Tube Feeding. If the burnt area exceeds 30 to 40 per cent. a tube is passed and left *in situ* and high calorie feeds given by the drip method. Excess of protein may cause liver and renal damage and for that reason adequate fat intake is important. An emulsion of arachis oil, glucose and Complan is suitable for tube feeding and satisfactory emulsions are best produced by using an electric mixer.

A suitable recipe which is almost identical to the one used for anuria (Bull's régime) is as follows:

Arachis oil	100 ml.	3,000 calories
Glucose	400 G.	
Gum acacia	25 G.	
Distilled water to	1 litre	

Complan can also be mixed into milk feeds and added to a variety of dishes. Abidec, a vitamin concentrate, may be given in conjunction with this feed.

As soon as the patient can tolerate it, a full diet is given which is augmented by eggs, milk, vitamins and foods which are rich in iron. Such foods are red meat, liver, kidney, sardines, dried fruits, green vegetables, tomatoes, cocoa, chocolate, black treacle, whole meal and rye bread and Bovril and Marmite. As most of these foods are both palatable and colourful, there should be little difficulty in arranging attractive meals. The food intake must be measured accurately and the amounts taken should be known and supplemented by tube feeding if necessary. Much patience and ingenuity may be needed to achieve the necessary fluid and calorie intake but as so much of the patient's treatment and progress depends on this factor, success brings its own reward.

Nursing Care

This includes recording of the oral or rectal temperature, blood pressure readings, accurate measurement of urinary output and calorie and fluid balance charts. If the foot end of the bed is at first raised to counteract shock it is necessary to watch for œdema of face and neck which may in turn spread to the brain and cause cerebral congestion. In this case the bed must be lowered at once and in more extreme cases the head end of the bed is elevated. Local œdema of the limbs and excess fluid loss from exudate is prevented by raising the affected extremity by means of extension. Sterilized foam rubber slings attached to a balkan beam or an intravenous stand and positioning with the help of foam rubber pillows is possible in most cases. Toddlers with burns of buttocks can sometimes be kept dry by using a gallows extension. Burns of the trunk may be nursed on a "Bradford frame" padded with sterilized polyurethane foam rubber, which is changed twice daily. The supporting nylon net is divided into sections and this facilitates the giving of bedpans without disturbance to the patient who lies, as it were, suspended over the gap. Intermittent pressure mattresses which move automatically in waves at about 10-minute intervals are suitable for older children. Foam rubber can be sterilized in the same way as rubber gloves and it is a good idea to use pads of different colours for the amusement of the child and so make a bit more tolerable the frequent change which may be a disturbing procedure to the patient.

Complications

Damage of liver and kidneys, pneumonia, reactions to blood transfusion, sepsis, uræmia and psychological disturbances are common. Treatment of any of these at the earliest stage is essential and in the majority of cases these complications can be avoided by adequate medical and nursing care. Local complications may arise from sloughs and crusts which by their position or extent may restrict chest movement or the blood supply to extremities, causing chest complications or thrombosis and gangrene of the parts. Burns and scalds of the eyelids are likely to cause contractions followed by exposure of the cornea, resulting in keratitis. Careful swabbing and instillation of lubricating eye drops every four hours may prevent complications but in some cases it is deemed best temporarily to stitch the upper and lower lid margins together or to excise them with a view to early grafting.

Burns of the hands and external genitalia present further problems which have to be dealt with as the individual case demands. Contractions of flexure surfaces are often prevented by plaster of Paris casts or Kramer-wire splinting. Lesions of groins, neck and armpits should be prevented from contracting by separating them or extending them fully with the aid of pillows or rolls of foam rubber. Steam scalds of face, neck and tongue may require tracheostomy and so add to the already difficult nursing problem.

Mental Welfare

However exacting the routine nursing care, no nurse must ever forget the mental welfare of these children. They are usually severely shocked and numbed in the first hours but after this initial stage they need a great deal of assurance, company and occupation. They are frightened by the accident and the sudden admission to hospital and often haunted by memories of the burst of flames and by feelings of guilt. Flame burns in particular cause severe nightmares after two or three days, and the children easily develop feelings of resentment and a bad relationship towards their parents.

Case assignment nursing and the presence of the mother for as much time as possible is of great psychological value. Any relatives or neighbours involved in the accident should be allowed to visit and speak to the child in order to reassure him. Sometimes it is possible to admit the mother with the child, provided she can spare the time from her other commitments. She can help to feed her child and play with him and sometimes may get him to sleep when he is wakeful or frightened. The idea that the mother can only be admitted or frequent visiting be arranged after the first days when the child is better, is completely mistaken. *It is in the first, initial stages that comfort from the mother is so important.* Although a physiotherapist will carry out daily treatment to prevent and correct contractions and bad posture, mothers can often be taught to assist, e.g. when games are played which encourage deep breathing and so help to prevent chest infections. As soon as possible full occupation is needed to keep these patients happy.

Boredom encourages scratching and picking at the crusts, both factors which may lead to infection, delayed healing and unnecessary scarring. Adequate occupation and company are far better means of preventing this than sedation or restraint. Toys and occupational material must at first be of the sterilizable kind. In situations of stress such as this, the child should not be deprived of a loved toy and if this cannot be sterilized even a teddy bear can be covered by a clean polythene bag.

It is interesting to note that children who sustain burns or scalds often appear to be of rather low intelligence and that they often come from homes with several other young brothers and sisters, so that the mother is overworked and unable to give much supervision. This also seems to be one of the reasons why many of these patients are still used to drinking from the bottle, well after the usual age. This possibility should always be kept in mind if there is difficulty in getting a young child to drink.

Children nursed by the exposure method often miss their usual coverings at first and if cold, can be covered by sterile towels and wear sterilized bootees and mittens. Little girls enjoy wearing pretty hair ribbons even if this is the only "clothing" they are allowed. The young patients soon get used to their nakedness and although they may at first feel cold when transferred to the open ward they then often dislike being dressed.

Consideration for the mental welfare of the parents is as important as for the child. Parents often blame themselves in some way for the accident and some time may have to be spent with anxious parents outlining the treatment, the probable outcome of the illness and the degree of scarring and length of hospitalization to be expected. Parents of newly admitted children should be encouraged to speak to those of convalescent patients as they may be able to give them comfort from their own experiences.

Convalescence

This may be prolonged in many cases and go on for months after the accident, until healing and repeated skin grafting are complete. Occupational therapy or schooling are essential during this period and short outings or a week-end at home should be arranged when possible. The skin is often kept supple by massaging with lanolin; this treatment together with exercising, helps to stretch newly forming skin and prevents contractions and should be carried out several times daily and not merely when the physiotherapist visits the ward.

ACCIDENTS

Dangers	How to guard against them
	FIRES
Electric Fires, Gas Fires, Coal Fires	Efficient guards fixed to fire surround. Fix on wall whenever possible. Wire netting fixed to fire.
	ELECTRICITY
Sockets	Locked sockets prevent children from poking fingers or pointed articles into the holes.
Flexes	Short flexes prevent accidents from tripping over them. Long flexes tempt children to pull on them, e.g. flex from electric iron.
	HOT WATER
Water Taps	Fix out of reach if possible. Detachable in bath room.
Baths	Run cold water in before the hot to prevent floor of bath from getting too hot.
Bath Water	Mix well, use thermometer, do not rely on sense of touch.
Hot-water Bottles	Use tap (not boiling) water. Cover completely with two protective layers. Never give hot water bottles to unconscious or paralysed patients.
	SCALDS
Teapots, Kettles	Point spout away from table or stove edge. Drinking from the spouts of teapots and kettles seems attractive to the very young child. Œdema of the mouth, larynx and œsophagus may necessitate tracheostomy. Keep well out of the way.
Table-cloths	Table-cloths should not be used or should at least not exceed the size of the table surface. If allowed to hang over table edge the toddler may tug on them when wanting to reach something on the table. Serious scalds may result, if there is a teapot on the table.
Saucepans	Saucepan handles should always be directed backwards or inwards. Safety rails for stoves are available. The child may reach for the handle in an attempt at "peeping inside" to see what is cooking.
Scrubbing Buckets	Buckets filled with scalding water should never be left standing on the floor unguarded. The young child may fall or plunge his hands into it.

ACCIDENTS—*contd.*

Dangers	How to guard against them
	SWALLOWING AND INHALING
Toys	Toys should be large enough to make it impossible for young children to swallow or inhale them. Beads, nails, and small marbles should not be given to very young toddlers. Toys should not have sharp edges—danger of cuts and abrasions. They should be coloured with vegetable—not lead—paint.
	SUFFOCATION
Pillows	Should not be used in cots before the age of 1 year or until the child can safely move himself. They are particularly dangerous if they are soft.
Plastic Bibs	Avoid. They may fall over the baby's face and interfere with breathing.
	GANGRENE
Mittens	These are best avoided. A thread of cotton or strand of wool hanging off the inside edge of the mitten has been known to wrap itself round the tip of a finger causing constriction and gangrene.
	FOREIGN BODIES
Small Objects	All body orifices offer opportunities for young children to push beads, peas, ball of paper, etc., into them. Sepsis and foul-smelling discharge will result. The observant and watchful mother or nurse should spot the toddler doing this sort of thing before the harm is done.
	SHARP THINGS
Knives, Saws, Axes, Scissors	All these should be kept out of harm's way. If left lying around they are likely to be misused and dangerous. Playing with them should be forbidden, while very young. When a little older their use should be supervised. The "first" scissors should have rounded ends and they should not be too sharp. A child who has "his own" will not want adult ones.
Safety Pins	If left lying around they should always be fastened. If in use they should be inaccessible to the child. On napkins they should be pinned horizontally.

ACCIDENTS—*contd.*

Dangers	How to guard against them
Pin Boxes and Needle Books	Should be kept well out of reach.
	FIRE AND BURNING
Matches	Children should be taught to respect matches as dangerous when used by very young people or indiscriminately.
Match-boxes,	Should not be left lying around the house.
Lighters	The same applies to them as to matches.
Fire-works, Bonfires	Children should know that both may be enjoyed only while supervised by adults.
Clothing	Pyjamas are preferable for girls as well as boys as their closer fit diminishes the danger of catching fire. Flame-proofed materials are obtainable, their advantages greatly outweigh the extra cost.
Mirrors	Should not be fixed over fireplaces. Clothes easily catch fire as one leans over the fireplace to look in the mirror.
	WINDOWS
Guards	Safety guards should be fixed on windows of any rooms in which young children may have to be left alone.
Chairs and Step Ladders	May invite the child to climb on to them and lean out of the window. If unguarded this may have serious results.
	STAIRS
Safety Gates	Where there is a toddler in the house stairs should be made safe by placing safety gates at the top and bottom of flights of stairs.
	LOTIONS
Disinfectants	Should be kept locked away or out of reach even if the toddler climbs to get at them. They should always be clearly labelled, but it must also be remembered that the child may not be able to read. Disinfectants should not be stored in old fruit-juice bottles which still have the original label on.
	POISONING
Marking Ink	Until it has been fixed by boiling, the aniline dye in marking ink (e.g. on baby napkins) may be absorbed via the skin and cause methaemoglobinaemia, a serious condition.

ACCIDENTS—*contd.*

Dangers	How to guard against them
	EATING HARMFUL THINGS
Pills	Pills should, if possible, be distinct in shape and colour. They should preferably be wrapped separately in tin foil or wax paper and put out of the child's reach. A national campaign to achieve this should be encouraged.
Berries	A firm warning against picking and eating berries must be given in early days.
Cosmetics	Cosmetics should be kept out of reach of toddlers.
	As the young child loves putting things in his mouth they should be inaccessible to him. Gaily coloured pills and berries are no exception. Pills often resemble familiar sweets and may be almost indistinguishable from them. Many cosmetics are harmful when taken internally.
	CLIMBING
Trees, Walls	Climbing is good exercise. The danger of climbing trees and walls is slight compared with the advantage of experience in adventure, balance and dexterity.
	WATER SAFETY
Paddling, Swimming	Young children should be taught to swim early in life. The child should be shown danger spots such as sudden drops in depth, dangerous currents and outlets from drains. When on holiday by lake, sea or river children should wear safety belts or jackets.
	Parents should insist on children paddling or swimming where other people are about.
	ROAD SAFETY
Road Injuries	The Safety Code should be taught untiringly by parents and in schools. In 1964, 823 children died in road accidents; 13,644 suffered serious injuries, and 45,090 minor injuries.
	GENERAL POINTS
	2,300 children lost their lives through accidents in 1962. Many more were seriously injured and are scarred or incapacitated for life. In addition to the more obvious results of accidents, psychological trauma resulting from shock, hospitalization handicaps and disfigurement must be of the greatest possible concern to all.

23

TERMINAL ILLNESS AND DEATH IN THE CHILDREN'S WARD

The care of children suffering from a hopeless disease calls for some of the nurse's finest qualities and there is probably no situation that taxes her emotions more severely, nor any other group of illnesses in which she would more sincerely wish to give of her best, both in the care of her patient and by offering mental and spiritual help to the parents.

Sometimes it is the nurse who is looking after the child, who, because she herself has a live faith and religious outlook, can give just the right kind of comfort by word or attitude. Even the parent who has not thought of religion and has got out of the habit of prayer may find solace in a prayer said together by the child's bedside. Some nurses feel that this aspect should be left to their seniors and to others more experienced in dealing with deep sorrow. But it is often in the unplanned and unexpected moment that the right word or action, however simple, brings greatest relief and assures the parents of the sympathetic sharing of their burden. The nurse closest to the child should at this time also be closest to the parents.

Once a hopeless diagnosis has been made, the parents will want to ask innumerable questions of every possible person, in the hope of getting some information which might give a ray of hope. It is best to allow only the smallest possible number of people to discuss prognosis and treatment, as doubts may arise even if merely different words are used to describe the same thing. Any information given should be consistent and it is often possible to lead up to the subject of a hopeless outcome in several separate conversations. Parents often sense what will have to be said and some will ask a direct question. An honest answer is probably the only right one in such a case but at the same time the parent can be assured that everything possible will be done to relieve pain and keep suffering to a minimum. Parents should be allowed to be with their hopelessly sick children as much as they wish, and should be allowed and encouraged to do those little things for the child which only a mother would know how to do. Both parents and child should be kept occupied and entertained as far as possible. As a rule it is kinder to keep the child in a general ward rather than in a side ward, unless the final weariness becomes too much for him.

Little treats, such as food brought from home, an unusual visit to another part of the hospital, or a week-end at home should all be allowed without fear of "spoiling the child". The visit of a granny, a beloved teacher or the family's vicar should always be permitted.

Children with malignant or terminal illnesses often develop curious fancies; one typical one is the desire to have "a special meal in the middle of the night". No nurse should be too busy or too rigid in her routine to grant such a request. There is always time to see to these children. There is little doubt that dying children sometimes realize what is about to happen. A compassionate nurse will be aware of this and often a little verse or story about Jesus who loves little children, or of happy children in God's blue heaven, is not mawkish and sentimental, but kindly and deeply comforting. No child should be allowed to die alone. Anticipation of impending death is one of a nurse's primary duties. If they desire it, parents should be allowed to sleep in the hospital and they should be called when the end approaches. When all is over, those nearest to the child should be left alone for a few moments by the bedside and then led away with quiet, sympathetic firmness. It is common-sense kindness to ensure some rest by giving the parents, with the permission of the attending house officer, one dose of sleeping tablets to be taken when they reach home.

Many hospitals have the services of a chaplain available. Whether normally religious or not, most people find it helpful to talk to him at this time and he should always be called. A sympathetic nurse will soon sense what kind of comfort will best help each individual parent. Often the parents have been so preoccupied with their dying child and their impending loss that they have for the time being hardly given a thought to their other children at home. The nurse can then remind them of the other children's needs and of their good fortune in having others who need their love. This is positive comfort and may be very helpful as it reminds the parents that their responsibilities have not come to an end and that there is much purpose left for them in life. The reminder that death is releasing their beloved little one from suffering or from an invalid life is comfort which may help in other cases

In all cases it is possible to remind parents that children probably lack the apprehension and fear an adult may feel and that their passing is thus made a great deal easier.

The parents' wishes as regards religious observances and orthodox rites should be ascertained and the necessary arrangements made in good time. It is every nurse's duty to be familiar with the practices of other denominations as well as her own, and all children should be christened, confirmed or given the last rites, as the case may be.

Last Offices

The general procedure of carrying out the last offices differs little from that customary for adults. Detail may, however, be adapted to suit the special cases. Unless the relatives have brought a little gown and socks, a plain white cotton gown or shroud is supplied by the hospital. This should be sufficiently long to cover the feet. If the jaw is inclined to drop, a one or one and a half inch bandage, still rolled up as supplied, can be used as a prop between chin and sternum and camouflaged by the gown. This is particularly easily done with infants whose necks are short. With young infants the knees may be drawn up, and they should be straightened by bandaging, some cotton wool being placed between the prominences of the knees to avoid marking the skin. The child's hands are placed together with the fingers interlaced, holding a little white flower. If the arms tend to sag, a roll of cotton wool or a rolled up napkin can be placed underneath the elbows beside the body to support their weight. The face is covered with a square of gauze or an embroidered handkerchief reserved for the purpose. After securing the body in a sheet, a pall is placed over it and it is carried to the mortuary. Fresh flowers should be placed in the chapel and a light is left burning until the body is removed for burial.

Personal belongings or toys are parcelled up in the usual way but occasionally the parents appreciate the suggestion that a beloved toy should be left with the child.

Answering the questions of other children in the ward about the sudden disappearance of a patient or the inevitable disturbance caused by a death may not be easy. Psychologists are not yet agreed as to what is the best way of dealing with the problem and no two children are likely to react in the same manner, though they will all sense that something unusual has taken place. In the majority of cases it is probably best to state the truth simply, as for instance "Johnny was so weak he fell asleep and will not wake up again because God has taken him to heaven". But the nurse should also add immediately—"this will not happen to you—you are not weak, are you", or words to that effect. As a rule children will be satisfied with this straightforward, honest statement. The few who may ponder or seem disturbed will soon be picked out by the ward sister, who can have a more personal talk with the individual child. The interest and variety of ward life will soon restore the usual, happy atmosphere.

Index

Principal references are in **bold type**

MADE AND PRINTED IN GREAT BRITAIN BY WILLIAM CLOWES AND SONS, LIMITED, LONDON AND BECCLES FOR BAILLIÈRE, TINDALL AND CASSELL, LIMITED

THE NURSES' AIDS SERIES

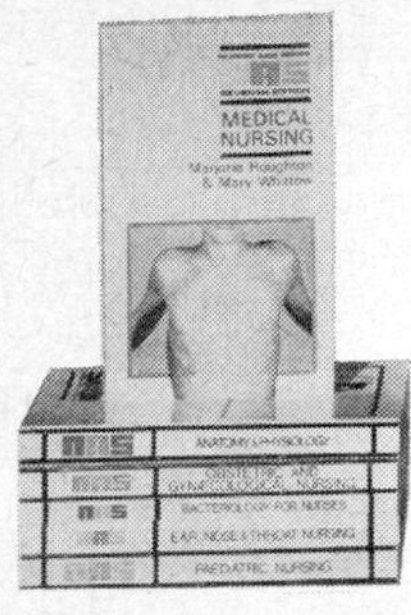

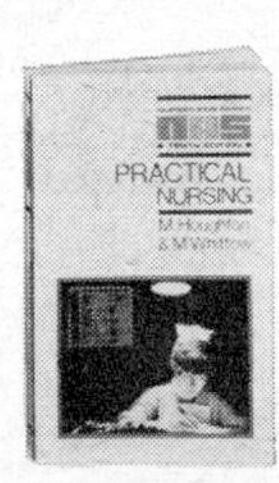

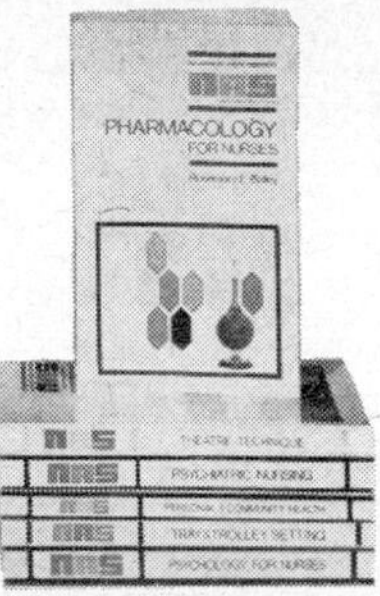

A series of complete illustrated textbooks covering the requirements of the G.N.C. Examination syllabus, each volume being written by an expert on the subject. New volumes or editions may have been added; up-to-date information will gladly be supplied on request.

ANATOMY AND PHYSIOLOGY

By **Katharine F. Armstrong,** S.R.N., S.C.M., D.N., formerly Sister Tutor, King's College Hospital, London.
7th edn. 12*s.* 6*d.*

ARITHMETIC IN NURSING

By **Wm. C. Fream,** S.R.N., B.T.A.CERT., Senior Tutor, Ballarat Base Hospital, Victoria, Australia. *3rd edn.* 12*s.* 6*d.*

EAR, NOSE AND THROAT NURSING

By **Susanna Marshall,** S.R.N., S.C.M., D.N., formerly Principal Tutor, Hitchin School of Nursing. *4th edn.* 12*s.* 6*d.*

MEDICAL NURSING

By **Marjorie Houghton,** O.B.E., S.R.N., S.C.M., D.N., formerly Sister Tutor, University College Hospital, London, and **Mary Whittow,** S.R.N., Ward Sister, Medical Unit, University College Hospital, London. *7th edn.* 15*s.*

BACTERIOLOGY FOR NURSES

By **E. Joan Bocock,** S.R.N., S.C.M., D.N., and **Katharine F. Armstrong,** S.R.N., S.C.M., D.N. *2nd edn.* 12*s.* 6*d.*

OBSTETRIC AND GYNÆCOLOGICAL NURSING

By **Joyce N. McNiven,** S.R.N., S.C.M., M.T.D., Midwifery Tutor, Guy's Hospital, London, and **Beryl Warne,** S.R.N., S.C.M., S.T.D., Nurse Tutor, Guy's Hospital, London. *7th edn.* 12*s.* 6*d.*

ORTHOPÆDICS FOR NURSES

By **Winifred Talog Davies,** S.R.N., S.C.M., formerly Sister Tutor, Royal Orthopædic Hospital, Birmingham.
3rd edn. 12*s.* 6*d.*

PAEDIATRIC NURSING

By **M. A. Duncombe,** S.R.N., R.S.C.N., S.C.M., Matron, Queen Victoria Hospital, East Grinstead.
2nd edn. 16*s.*

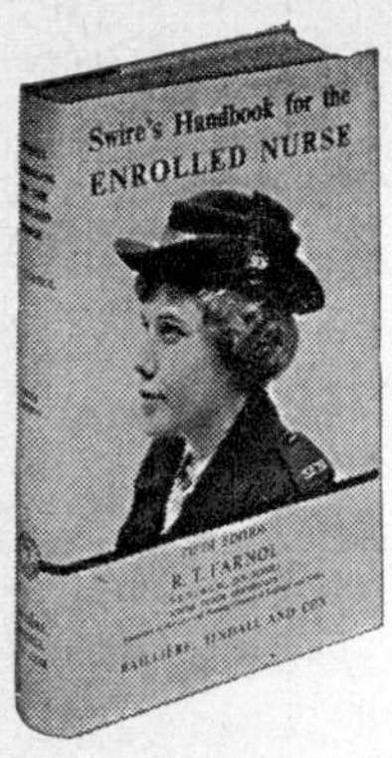

SWIRE'S HANDBOOK FOR THE ENROLLED NURSE

Revised by R. THORA FARNOL, S.R.N., S.C.M., D.N.

The only textbook of its kind written expressly for the enrolled nurse with a full appreciation of her needs derived from practical experience. Covers the syllabus of the G.N.C. and provides a basis of practical knowledge for both training and after-years.

Fifth Edition. 336 pages. 155 illustrations.
17s. 6d. *Postage and packing 2s. 6d.*

NURSING THE PSYCHIATRIC PATIENT

JOAN BURR, R.M.N., S.R.N.

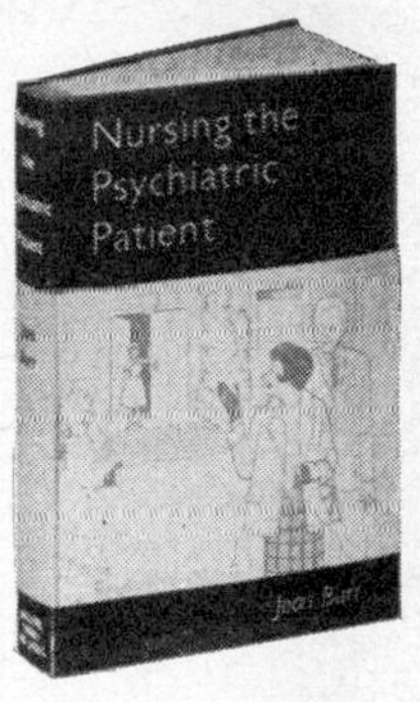

This book is written primarily for psychiatric pupil nurses, and psychiatric student nurses in the early part of their training. General student nurses seconded to a psychiatric hospital will also find it extremely valuable. Miss Burr displays a talent for describing difficult subject matter in a simple and readable way.

"I welcome this book as a very real contribution to the literature on psychiatric nursing. It deserves to be widely read and it has a place in any nurse training school library."—*Nursing Mirror.*

"This book has rapidly been acclaimed as an excellent addition to the psychiatric nursing textbooks already available, and it certainly provide a masterly account of what caring for the mentally ill is about."—*Nursing Times.*

First Edition. 308 pages. 10 drawings.
16s. limp covers, **25s.** hard covers.
Postage and packing 2s. 6d.

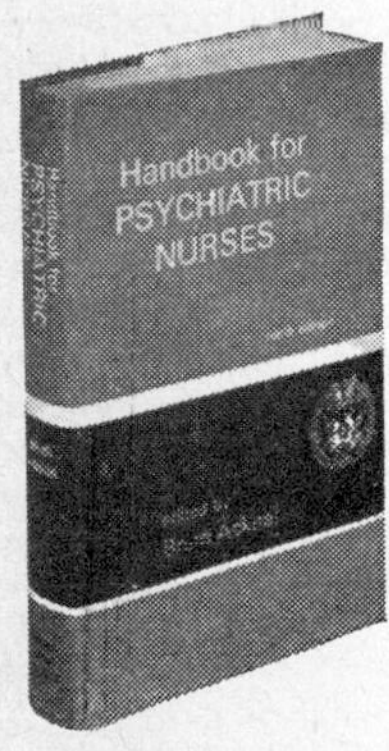

HANDBOOK FOR PSYCHIATRIC NURSES

Edited by BRIAN ACKNER, M.D., F.R.C.P., D.P.M.

Published in association with The Royal Medico-Psychological Association.

An entirely new edition of the "Red Handbook". A number of eminent contributors have assisted the Editor in the preparation of this standard textbook for the student psychiatric nurse.

Ninth Edition. 384 pages.
30s. *Postage and packing 2s. 6d.*

Baillière's

TO SEE IS TO LEARN! That is why Baillière's Atlases of the Male and Female Anatomy are so valuable for they enable you to see the relative size, shape, position and detail of every part and structure of the human body. Each atlas has a key naming

ATLAS OF FEMALE ANATOMY

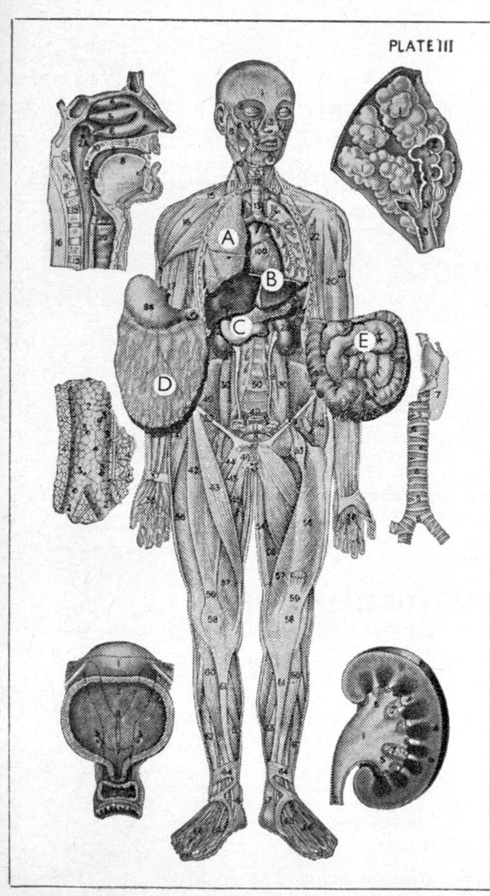

Five plates, printed in full colour.

Note in the illustration of Plate III on the left the letters A, B, C, D and E on certain organs. The organs so lettered are designed to lift up, thus enabling the organs beneath to be seen. By this means the relationship of the internal organs can be learnt *at a glance*. This unique feature makes learning by seeing easy, for not only is each internal organ fully visible, so that its shape and size may be memorised, but its exact position and relationship to other organs is made abundantly clear. The plates printed in full colour teach by seeing, and the text accompanying the plates explains how the parts of the body function. For studying the male anatomy see the description of Baillière's Atlas of the Male Anatomy.

Price 20s. each

"The best

Anatomical Atlases

every part and a clear and concise text explaining and teaching the anatomy and physiology of the body is also included. Printed in full colour. Size 17 in. × $8\frac{1}{2}$ in. each. By Miss Katharine Armstrong, S.R.N., S.C.M., D.N., and Douglas J. Kidd, M.M.A.A.

ATLAS OF MALE ANATOMY

Four coloured and three black and white plates.

To study human anatomy it is essential to consider both the male and the female body. That is why it is necessary to have two Atlases. The Male Atlas is just as important and essential as the Female Atlas. See how clearly (in spite of its reduced size) every detail stands out in the illustration of Plate IV on the right, which is printed in full colour in the atlas and shows the vascular system, the veins and arteries, the heart in various aspects, the pelvic contents etc. Plate IV is another example of "To see is to learn", and studied with the simple, clear explanatory text, learning becomes easy. To all who have to study anatomy Baillière's Atlases of the Male and Female body are indispensable.

Postage 2s. 6d. each

Atlases published"

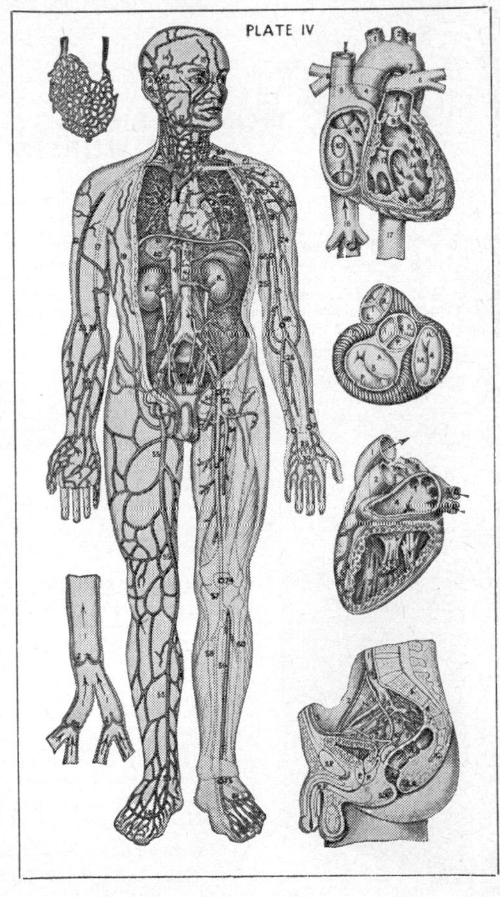

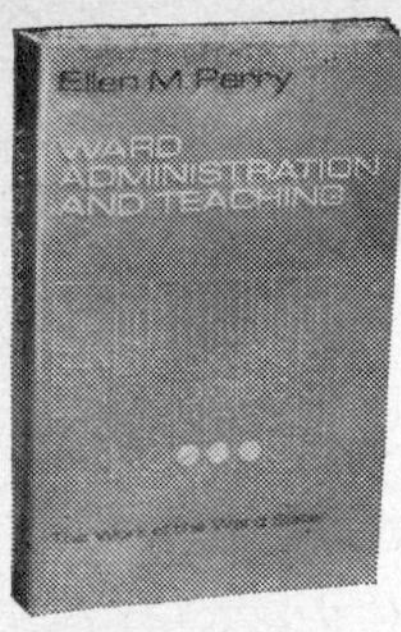

WARD ADMINISTRATION AND TEACHING

ELLEN L. PERRY, S.R.N., S.C.M., R.N.T.

This authoritative and valuable book is written primarily for nurses who are preparing for their first appointment as a ward sister or charge nurse. However, more experienced staff will also find it very useful since this new book fully reflects the present emphasis on management techniques in the profession. The author outlines the principles which should guide the nurse in charge of a ward in the planning, execution and evaluation of her work.

First Edition. 320 pages. 10 drawings.
30s. *Postage and packing 2s. 6d.*

APPLIED HUMAN BIOLOGY FOR NURSES

W. C. FREAM, S.R.N., B.T.A.Cert.(Hon.), S.T.D.

This is a vividly written, refreshing and informative textbook which integrates the basic biological sciences into the background of the nurse's training. The text covers the overall survey of the structure and functions of the human body as set out in Section II of the syllabus of the G.N.C. and the applied anatomy and physiology required in Section III.

"A truly fascinating book on human biology.... It will be an inspiration to any student, and tutors will find it an invaluable guide to teaching the subject."—*Nursing Mirror.*

First Edition. 408 pages. 258 illustrations.
28s. *Postage and packing 2s. 6d.*

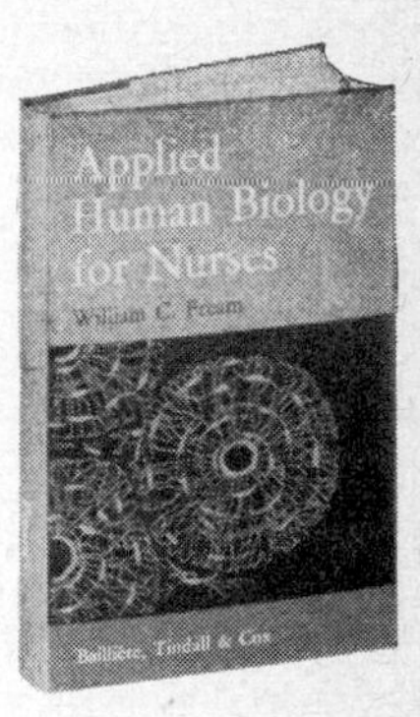

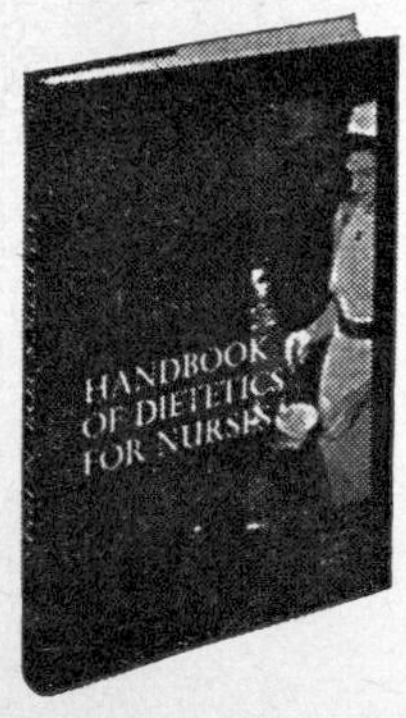

HANDBOOK OF DIETETICS FOR NURSES

CATHERINE F. HARRIS, S.R.N.

The second enlarged edition of a handbook written to cover the G.N.C. Syllabus, which will give the nurse a full understanding of the therapeutic value and use of food and diets. The principles of dietetic science and their practical application are fully covered, and specimen diet sheets are given for every condition known to benefit from dietetic treatments.

"A good reference book and a valuable addition to any library."—*District Nursing Review.*

Second Edition. 288 pages. 6 pages of plates.
25s. *Postage and packing 2s. 6d.*